GROWTH *and* DEVELOPMENT
Across the n

GROWTH *and* DEVELOPMENT
Across the Lifespan

A HEALTH PROMOTION FOCUS

GLORIA LEIFER, RN, MA

Associate Professor
Obstetric, Pediatric, and Trauma Nursing
Riverside Community College
Riverside, California

HEIDI HARTSTON, PhD

Clinical Psychologist
Stanford University Medical Center
Assistant Clinical Professor
University of California, San Francisco
San Francisco, California

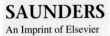

SAUNDERS
An Imprint of Elsevier

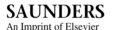

SAUNDERS
An Imprint of Elsevier

11830 Westline Industrial Drive
St. Louis, Missouri 63146

Growth and Development Across the Lifespan: A Health Promotion Focus   ISBN 0-7216-9879-4

NOTICE

Nursing is an ever-changing field. Standard safety precautions must be followed, but as new research and clinical experience broaden our knowledge, changes in treatment and drug therapy may become necessary or appropriate. Readers are advised to check the most current product information provided by the manufacturer of each drug to be administered to verify the recommended dose, the method and duration of administration, and contraindications. It is the responsibility of the licensed prescriber, relying on experience and knowledge of the patient, to determine dosages and the best treatment for each individual patient. Neither the publisher nor the author assumes any liability for any injury and/or damage to persons or property arising from this publication.

Library of Congress Cataloging-in-Publication Data
Leifer, Gloria.
Growth and development across the lifespan: a health promotion focus / Gloria Leifer,
Heidi Hartston.
    p.; cm.
Includes bibliographical references and index.
ISBN 0-7216-9879-4 1. Health promotion. 2. Health education. 3. Medicine, Preventive. 4. Nursing. I.
Hartston, Heidi. II. Title.
    [DNLM: 1. Human Development–Nurses' Instruction. 2. Health Education–methods–Nurses'
Instruction. 3. Health Promotion–methods–Nurses' Instruction. 4. Personality Development–Nurses'
Instruction. WS 103 L527g 2004]
RA427.8.L455 2004
613–dc22   2003058678

Vice President, Publishing Director: Sally Schrefer
Executive Publisher: Barbara Nelson Cullen
Senior Developmental Editor: Robin Levin Richman
Publishing Services Manager: Melissa Lastarria
Associate Project Manager: Bonnie Spinola
Book Designer: Teresa Breckwoldt

Cover art inset by David Nicholls/Corbis.

Printed in China.
Last digit is the print number: 9   8   7   6   5   4   3   2   1

Dedication

Dedicated to the memory of

Sarah Masseyaw Leifer
a nurse, humanitarian, and mother

and

Daniel Peretz Hartston, MD
a pediatrician, husband, and world traveler

and to the honor of

Heidi, Barnet, Amos, Eve, David, Zoe, and Elliot
who acquaint me with the beauty, joys, and challenges of my lifespan voyage

Gloria Leifer Hartston

To my mother,
with appreciation for your dedication,
your commitment to educating and healing, and
your talent in helping others develop their own healing abilities

Heidi Hartston

Special Contributor

Trena L. Rich, RN, MSN, ANP, CS
Infection Control Nurse Practitioner
Riverside County Regional Medical Center
Moreno Valley, California

Reviewers

Janis M. Browning, RN, BSN
Lamar State College—Port Arthur
Port Arthur, Texas

Linda Cox Curry, RN, BSN, MN, Phd, ACCE
Texas Christian University
Harris School of Nursing
Fort Worth, Texas

Karen Kathryn Haagensen, RNC
Howard College—San Angelo
San Angelo, Texas

Deborah T. Huntley, MS, RN, CS
Georgia Perimeter College
Atlanta, Georgia

Patricia Laing-Arie, RN, BSEd
Central Technology Center
Drumright, Oklahoma

Pamela Ann Mahmoudi, RN, MS, CCMA-AC
Sutter County Schools
Career Training and Education Center—Health Careers
Yuba City, California

Theresa Mendoza Mostasisa, RN, BSN, MS, PHN
Mills Peninsula Medical Center
Burlingame, California
City College of San Francisco
San Francisco, California

Anne W. Ryan, MSN, RN, C, MPH
Chesapeake College
MGW Nursing Program
Wye Mills, Maryland

Julie A. Slack, RN, MS, ICCE
Mohave Community College
Kingman, Arizona

Debra Gartman Spring, RN, BS, MS
Hinds Community College
Jackson, Mississippi

Judith L. Stauder, MSN, RN
Practical Nurse Program of Canton City Schools
Canton, Ohio

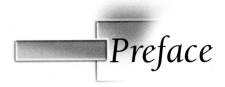

Preface

Understanding growth and development at each age and stage of the life cycle is a valuable tool for the nurse or health care worker that can be useful when assessing, planning, and implementing health care and education for patients. This text enables the student to study growth and development in a continuum or smooth transition across the entire lifespan and integrate concepts related to changes that normally occur in each stage of the life cycle.

The twenty-first century brings with it possibilities of increased population growth, intensified international conflict, and advanced scientific achievements, all of which can influence the world's social, economic, and health environments. Our abilities to improve health, enrich the quality of life, and lengthen the lifespan may become even more important as the future unfolds. Promoting healthy behaviors and healthy lifestyles is an integral part of improving quality of life.

Today, people want more control over their health care and want to be part of the decision-making process concerning their health care needs. The emergence of complementary and alternative medicine (CAM) reflects trends toward self-management and preventive care. The number of health-related publications, Internet resources, health spas, and self-help groups has increased rapidly over the past 10 years. This also reflects people's growing interest in, and concern with, health.

Healthy People 2010 provides a list of goals for health care workers and nurses related to providing care to a diverse population across the lifespan in a variety of settings. Focusing health care on illness prevention is less costly than focusing on the treatment or cure of an illness after it develops. Research validates the importance of a healthy lifestyle in preventing many types of illnesses.

This text explains concepts and theories about physical, cognitive, social, and personality development in each stage of the life cycle, from conception to death. It also provides an explanation of normal development, behavior, skills, and limitations at each life stage and a discussion of external influences such as culture and environment on normal development. Each chapter provides information that helps the student identify teaching strategies that incorporate personal priorities, skills, and limitations that characterize each stage of life. For example, teaching strategies or techniques that a health care worker would use for a young child would be different from the strategies used to teach an adolescent. Children learn as adults do, but because they are unencumbered by experiences, their processing and interpretation may be different. The approach to working with young adults would also differ from working with a family mourning the death of a relative, even though the shared goal of teaching may be to enhance the healing process.

Preventive health care is an important part of the objectives of *Healthy People 2010*. Understanding the influence of heredity, stage of life, and environment, on behaviors, can help the nurse or health care worker develop culturally competent education and care plans designed to meet the unique needs of individual patients. Teaching skills can help health care workers educate at-risk populations about healthy diets, exercise, mental health, and lifestyle choices. Utilizing every teaching opportunity in a culturally sensitive and developmentally appropriate manner will maximize learning and is the heartbeat of preventive care.

The course of growth and development has been charted by many researchers and theorists who formed a framework for understanding life-span development. This text reviews the theories and concepts to present typical physical and behavioral changes that occur at each stage in the life cycle. When a health care provider is familiar with normal developmental stages, alterations can be identified and typical patterns can be noted when designing approaches to patient care.

The theories of Dorothy Orem, a nursing theorist, include a supportive educative system of self-care in which the patient is educated and supported in his or her quest for sustaining optimal health. Assessing a patient's readiness and ability to learn is helpful in planning an effective teaching approach. Understanding normal growth and development, health challenges, and values at each stage of development is an integral part of providing effective support and patient education.

Predictable physical changes occur at each stage of development. Age-related changes in neurologic functioning also occur in predictable phases of the life cycle. Learning occurs in all phases of the life cycle, but different learning abilities and individual needs at each phase influence the effectiveness of teaching styles. Each stage of the life cycle involves specific developmental tasks or crises of the individual and the family that must be mastered during life's journey. An understanding of how physical changes and these developmental tasks affect each other is useful in assessing needs and designing a plan to help support family dynamics and empower both the individual and the family to participate in prevention and treatment of illness.

The Joint Commission on Accreditation of Health Care Organizations (JCAHO) has general standards for providing age-appropriate, in-hospital health care. Environmental, infection control, and safety standards of care are part of hospital policy in both the pediatric and adult units. For example, knowledge of age-related differences in drug administration, absorption, and excretion are expected staff competencies.

Most health outcomes measured in *Healthy People 2010* data are related to choices made by individuals during each stage of the life cycle. Health care workers and nurses are well qualified to focus on educating patients about health promotion and healthy life styles. Patients of all ages have the ability to make sound and healthy life style decisions empowered by information provided in a culturally sensitive, developmentally appropriate manner by informed health care workers and nurses. This text provides a comprehensive review of concepts of growth and development from conception to death, integrated with the goals of *Healthy People 2010* that can be utilized by nurses and health care workers in the achievement of their professional objectives.

INSTRUCTOR'S RESOURCE MANUAL AND TEST BANK

A printed Instructor's Resource Manual and Test Bank of approximately 375 NCLEX-PN® examination-style questions is provided.

ACKNOWLEDGMENTS

The birth of a book is a team effort. The authors wish to express sincere appreciation to those who contributed materially, as well as to those whose support and encouragement were vital to the outcome.

Terri Wood, former Senior Nursing Editor at Elsevier, seeded the vision and expressed confidence and support in the efforts of the authors to complete this text. Our sincere appreciation is extended to the many reviewers who shared their expertise and provided constructive comments. We would also like especially to thank Dr. Marjorie Hardy, Assistant Professor of Psychology at Eckerd College in St. Petersburg, Florida, for her detailed review of Chapter 4 and her helpful suggestions. Trena Rich, as research consultant, editor, and special contributor, kept the project moving with her incredible organizational skills and facilitated the meeting of deadlines in a painless fashion. The able assistance of the Elsevier nursing editorial staff, including Barbara Nelson Cullen, Executive Publisher; Robin Levin Richman, Senior Developmental Editor; and Catherine Ott, Senior Editorial Assistant, provided the necessary tools and helpful guidance through the publication process.

Professor Barnet Hartston deserves special thanks for his encouragement, support, and motivating ideas. Several of our photographic models, Eve, David, and Zoe Fleck, added sparkle to many of the illustrations that appear in this text; their patience was appreciated. Amos Hartston deserves special recognition for taking time out of his busy schedule to offer personal assistance and encouragement. The authors express appreciation to each other for the support and mutual respect generated by this collaboration.

Last, but not least, gratitude is extended to our students from Hunter College, California State University at Los Angeles, California State University at San Jose, and Riverside Community College for helping us understand their learning needs and inspiring us to continue the professionally challenging and personally rewarding careers of teaching and writing.

The utilization of information contained in this book is not dependent on scope of practice, so the text can be useful to those studying in multidisciplinary health-related fields such as nursing, psychology, counseling, early childhood education, or any field where the understanding of the needs, risks, and challenges of a specific age group influences a positive outcome of the interaction. We hope that the information contained in this text will provide the reader with the tools to enhance communication and develop effective plans of care for individual patients and their families.

Gloria Leifer Hartston, RN, MA
Heidi Hartston, PhD

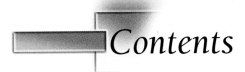

Contents

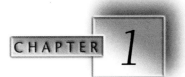

Healthy People 2010

OBJECTIVES

Upon completion of this chapter, the student will be able to:

1 Describe what Healthy People 2010 is meant to do.
2 List five public health issues related to Healthy People 2010.
3 Discuss how the health status of a population is measured.
4 State one health issue or goal for each stage of the life cycle.
5 Discuss the role of the nurse or health care worker in worldwide health improvement.
6 Discuss the role of the nurse or health care worker in achieving Healthy People 2010 objectives.

KEY TERMS

Determinants of health
Health indicators
Health status
Infant mortality rate
Life expectancy

WHAT IT IS

Healthy People 2010 is a 10-year report card describing health care accomplishments within the United States. It is also a prescription for what needs to be done in the next 10 years. The overall purpose of *Healthy People 2010* is to identify needs concerning health promotion and disease prevention, improve the quality of life for U.S. consumers, and eliminate unequal access to health care. Increasing access to quality health care and education for all social and ethnic groups is the core of the current plan. Published by the U.S. Department of Health and Human Services (USDHHS), *Healthy People 2010* is considered by many to be the most important document regarding health in the United States today. First written in 1979, *Healthy People* is the work of more than 350 governmental agencies, organizations, and experts in the health care field. By analyzing current statistics every 10 years, *Healthy People* provides a snapshot of progress, trends, and issues in the past 10 years and highlights future needs in health care by identifying specific goals for the following 10 years. Goals and objectives are being revised periodically based on what has been accomplished and what needs to be accomplished to improve the health of the people in the nation.

Healthy People 2010 lists 467 health objectives in 28 focus areas to be achieved by the year 2010 (Box 1-1). The publication is grouped within the four major stages of the life cycle: (1) infants, (2) children, (3) teens and young adults, (4) older adults and the geriatric population.

WHAT IT DOES

Healthy People 2010 identifies 10 leading **health indicators** that highlight current priorities for the nation. Each health indicator has objectives that will promote healthy

---

BOX 1-1   *Healthy People 2010* **Focus Areas**

1 Access to Quality Health Services
2 Arthritis, Osteoporosis, and Chronic Back Conditions
3 Cancer
4 Chronic Kidney Disease
5 Diabetes
6 Disability and Secondary Conditions
7 Educational and Community-Based Programs
8 Environmental Health
9 Family Planning
10 Food Safety
11 Health Communication
12 Heart Disease and Stroke
13 HIV
14 Immunization and Infectious Diseases

15 Injury and Violence Prevention
16 Maternal, Infant and Child Health
17 Medical Product safety
18 Mental Health and Mental Disorders
19 Nutrition and Overweight
20 Occupational Safety and Health
21 Oral Health
22 Physical Activity and Fitness
23 Public Health Infrastructure
24 Respiratory Diseases
25 Sexually Transmitted Diseases
26 Substance Abuse
27 Tobacco Use
28 Vision and Hearing

From U.S. Department of Health and Human Services (2000). *Healthy People 2010*. McLean, VA: International Publishing.

behaviors, protect the health and safety of communities, and improve efforts toward personal and public health issues that will prevent or reduce illness and disability.

Health Indicators

The following health indicators are U.S. public health issues and concerns linked to the 467 objectives of *Healthy People 2010*. The leading health indicators and some related objectives include the following:

- *Physical activity:* Encourage participation in regular physical activity that promotes cardiorespiratory fitness 3 or more days a week for 20 or more minutes per occasion for adolescents and 30 minutes per day of moderate activity for adults.
- *Overweight and obesity:* Reduce the proportion of children, adolescents, and adults who are obese. A healthy diet is included as an important part of this health indicator (Figure 1-1).
- *Tobacco use:* Reduce cigarette smoking by adolescents and adults.
- *Substance abuse:* Reduce the number of adolescents and adults using alcohol or illicit drugs.
- *Responsible sexual behavior:* Increase the number of adolescents who abstain from sexual intercourse, and increase the use of condoms in sexually active persons.
- *Mental health:* Increase the proportion of adults with recognized depression who receive treatment.
- *Injury and violence:* Reduce deaths caused by motor vehicle accidents, and reduce homicides.

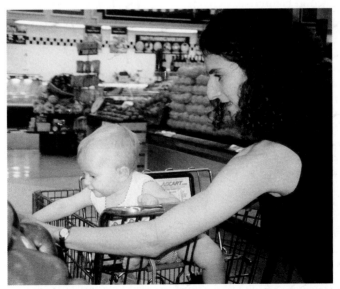

FIGURE 1–1 A child begins to learn about food and nutrition early in life during a food-shopping trip. This mother talks about the fruits and vegetables as she shops.

- *Environmental quality:* Reduce exposure to air that does not meet health-based standards for ozone, and reduce the number of nonsmokers exposed to environmental tobacco smoke.
- *Immunizations:* Increase the number of children who receive all vaccines recommended for universal administration for at least the first 5 years of life (Figure 1-2), and increase the number of adults vaccinated against pneumococcal disease and receiving annual immunizations against influenza (see Appendix A).
- *Access to health care:* Increase the number of persons with health insurance, and increase the number of persons who have access to ongoing health care; increase the number of pregnant women who begin prenatal care in the first trimester of pregnancy; provide immunizations and primary health care for all children.

Healthy People 2010 is "firmly dedicated to the principle that regardless of age, gender, race or ethnicity, income, education, geographic location, disability, or sexual orientation, every person in the nation deserves equal access to comprehensive, culturally competent, community-based health care systems that are committed to serving the needs of the individual and promoting community health."

Determinants of Health

Behavior and biology are interrelated. A disease affects biology, but behaviors can make a person susceptible or resistant to a disease. Social and physical environments impact behavior. For example, education can motivate healthy behaviors, but ozone in the environment can have a negative impact on biology (genetics). Therefore personal health behavior is closely related to the general environment in achieving the *Healthy People 2010* goals.

Both general policies and access to health care figure prominently into the entire cycle, illustrated in Figure 1-3.

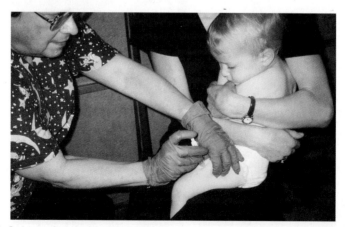

FIGURE 1–2 A mother holds her child in the "hug position" during immunization. Scheduled immunization programs for infants and children are listed in Appendix A.

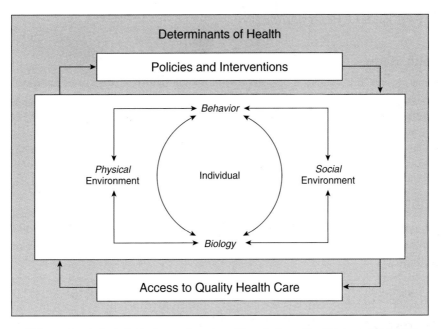

Biology refers to the individual's genetic makeup (those factors with which he or she is born), family history (which may suggest risk for disease), and the physical and mental health problems acquired during life. Aging, diet, physical activity, smoking, stress, alcohol or illicit drug abuse, injury or violence, or an infectious or toxic agent may result in illness or disability and can produce a "new" biology for the individual.

Behaviors are individual responses or reactions to internal stimuli and external conditions. Behaviors can have a reciprocal relationship to biology; in other words, each can react to the other. For example, smoking (behavior) can alter the cells in the lung and result in shortness of breath, emphysema, or cancer (biology) that then may lead an individual to stop smoking (behavior). Similarly, a family history that includes heart disease (biology) may motivate an individual to develop good eating habits, avoid tobacco, and maintain an active lifestyle (behaviors), which may prevent his or her own development of heart disease (biology).

Personal choices and the social and physical environments surrounding individuals can shape behaviors. The social and physical environments include all factors that affect the life of individuals, positively or negatively, many of which may not be under their immediate or direct control.

Social environment includes interactions with family, friends, coworkers, and others in the community. It also encompasses social institutions, such as law enforcement, the workplace, places of worship, and schools. Housing, public transportation, and the presence or absence of violence in the community are among other components of the social environment. The social environment has a profound effect on individual health as well as on the health of the larger community, and is unique because of cultural customs; language; and personal, religious, or spiritual beliefs. At the same time, individuals and their behaviors contribute to the quality of the social environment.

Physical environment can be thought of as that which can be seen, touched, heard, smelled, and tasted. However, the physical environment also contains less tangible elements, such as radiation and ozone. The physical environment can harm individual and community health, especially when individuals and communities are exposed to toxic substances; irritants; infectious agents; and physical hazards in homes, schools, and worksites. The physical environment also can promote good health, for example, by providing clean and safe places for people to work, exercise, and play.

Policies and interventions can have a powerful and positive effect on the health of individuals and the community. Examples include health promotion campaigns to prevent smoking; policies mandating child restraints and safety belt use in automobiles; disease prevention services such as immunization of children, adolescents, and adults; and clinical services, such as enhanced mental health care. Policies and interventions that promote individual and community health may be implemented by a variety of agencies, such as transportation, education, energy, housing, labor, justice, and other venues, or through places of worship, community-based organizations, civic groups, and businesses.

FIGURE 1–3 Determinants of health. (From U.S. Department of Health and Human Services (2000). *Healthy People 2010.* McLean, VA: International Publishing, Inc.)

Health Status

Evaluating specific details of the **determinants of health** enable us to develop an understanding of the **health status** of the population. The health status can be measured by birth and death rates, life expectancy, morbidity from specific disease, accessibility to health care, and health insurance coverage, as well as other factors. These factors are reported in publications such as *Healthy People Review* or *Health, United States*. The health status of the United States is a description of the health of the total population. The leading causes of death across the life span are depicted in Table 1-1.

PROGRESS ACHIEVED AND YET TO BE ACHIEVED

Each decade when the goals and objectives of *Healthy People* are identified, communities and health care professionals are expected to develop action plans to help achieve and maintain healthy behaviors and lifestyles, thus enabling access to and utilization of federal, state, and community programs and resources.

One example of the goals of *Healthy People 2010* is to increase quality and years of human life. **Life expectancy** is the average number of years a person born in a given year is expected to live. In 1900 the life expectancy was 47.3 years. In the year 2000 the life expectancy was 77 years. These statistics show definite improvement, but as of the year 2000 approximately 18 countries had a better life expectancy rate than the United States (Figure 1-4).

Life expectancy statistics can further be analyzed in terms of gender (women live an average of 6 years longer than men), race (white women have a greater life expectancy

TABLE 1-1

LEADING CAUSES OF DEATH BY AGE GROUP

Under 1 Year Birth defects Disorders related to premature birth Sudden infant death syndrome	*25-44 Years* Unintentional injuries Cancer Heart Disease
1-4 Years Unintentional injuries Birth defects Cancer	*45-64 Years* Cancer Heart disease Unintentional injuries
5-14 Years Unintentional injuries Cancer Homicide	*65 Years and Older* Heart disease Cancer Stroke
15-24 Years Unintentional injuries Homicide Suicide	

From U.S. Department of Health and Human Services (2000). *Healthy People 2010.* McLean, VA: USDHHS International Publisher.

Life Expectancy by Country

Female		Male	
Country	Years of Life Expectancy	Country	Years of Life Expectancy
Japan	82.9	Japan	76.4
France	82.6	Sweden	76.2
Switzerland	81.9	Israel	75.3
Sweden	81.6	Canada	75.2
Spain	81.5	Switzerland	75.1
Canada	81.2	Greece	75.1
Australia	80.9	Australia	75.0
Italy	80.8	Norway	74.9
Norway	80.7	Netherlands	74.6
Netherlands	80.4	Italy	74.4
Greece	80.3	England and Wales	74.3
Finland	80.3	France	74.2
Austria	80.1	Spain	74.2
Germany	79.8	Austria	73.5
Belgium	79.8	Singapore	73.4
England and Wales	79.6	Germany	73.3
Israel	79.3	New Zealand	73.3
Singapore	79.0	Northern Ireland	73.1
United States	**78.9**	Belgium	73.0
		Cuba	73.0
		Costa Rica	73.0
		Finland	72.8
		Denmark	72.8
		Ireland	72.5
		United States	**72.5**

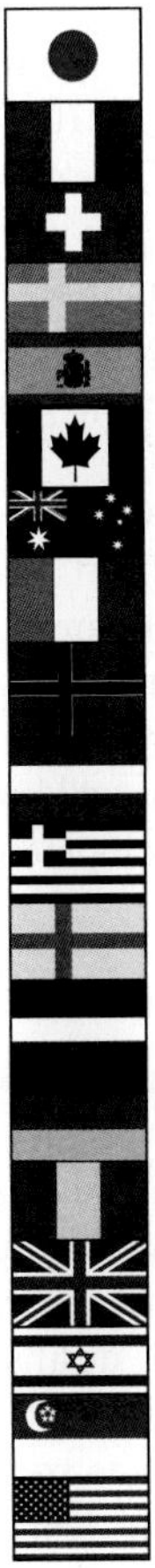

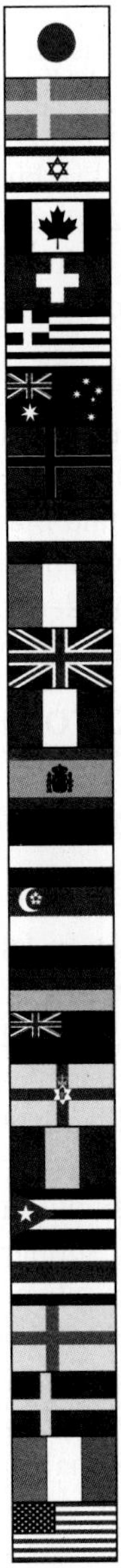

Sources: World Health Organization, United Nations; Centers for Disease Control and Prevention, National Center for Health Statistics, National Vital Statistics System, 1990–95 and unpublished data.

FIGURE 1–4 Life expectancy at birth. (From U.S. Department of Health and Human Services (2000). *Healthy People 2010*. McLean, VA: International Publishing, Inc.)

than other racial groups in the United States), and education status and income (a higher-income person may live 3 to 7 years longer than a lower-income person).

Progress toward stated goals has been seen in several areas since the inception of *Healthy People* in 1979, but much remains to be done. Another important indicator that measures the status of the nation's health is the infant death (mortality) rate. The **infant mortality rate** is the number of deaths that occur before 1 year of age per 1000 live births. In 1975 the infant mortality was 15 per 1000 live births. In 1997 the number decreased to 7.2 deaths per 1000 live births (USDHHS, 2000). However, according to the National Center for Health Statistics (NCHS), in 1999 the U.S. infant mortality rate is still ranked twenty-fifth among industrialized nations. There is obviously much work that still needs to be done to improve these statistics and achieve the specific goals as identified in *Healthy People 2010*.

The 1998–1999 review of the *Healthy People 2000* goals revealed that about 15% of the objectives were met in the areas of nutrition, maternal-child health, heart disease, and mental health. More than 40% of the objectives have been achieved in areas such as immunizations, breastfeeding, and breast cancer screening. Aspects of the goals and objectives of *Healthy People 2010* will be integrated throughout the chapters in this text. Specific tasks or risk factors will be identified, and health care interventions will be presented to promote a healthy lifestyle that leads to normal growth and development.

ISSUES AND GOALS RELATED TO PHASES OF THE LIFE CYCLE
Prenatal and Infant

Maternal and infant health is the core of the health status of the next generation. Some of the issues include:

- Reducing the infant death rate—the U.S. infant mortality rate has declined steadily since 1979, but as of 1999 the United States has remained twenty-fifth among industrialized nations (Center for Disease Control and Prevention, 2000), and the rate is higher in African Americans than Caucasians. Reduction from 8.4 deaths per 100,000 in 1997 to 3.3 in 2010 is the goal. The leading areas of progress in the last 10 years include reducing sudden infant death syndrome (SIDS) with the back-to-sleep educational program that urges parents to place their infants on their back rather than their abdomen when putting their infant down for a nap or for the night.
- Promoting the use of folic acid supplements early in pregnancy to reduce congenital malformations such as spina bifida.
- Increasing breastfeeding in the first year of life.

Little progress has yet been made in reducing the maternal mortality rate or reducing the occurrence of fetal alcohol syndrome (FAS). Continued effort is also needed in reducing the morbidity rate of asthma.

Childhood

The overall goal for this population is to increase health literacy and improve the quality, availability, and effectiveness of community-based programs designed to prevent disease and improve health. This goal can be achieved by the following:

- Health issues should be added to school curricula, teachers should be well informed, and school nurses should be available in all schools.

- High school completion should be encouraged, providing the education necessary for understanding the importance of healthy lifestyle choices. The target is that 90% of persons between 18 and 24 will complete high school by 2010. Encouraging school attendance, home schooling during prolonged illness, and school counseling services aids in achieving these goals.
- School nurses should provide health information regarding healthy life choices, including pregnancy prevention, sexually transmitted disease (STD) prevention, and drug use, as well as diet and exercise needs. In 1960 seven conceptual areas served as the basis for health education curricula. These areas included prevention of injuries, smoking, drug and alcohol use, sexual behavior, dietary patterns, and mental health. Environmental health (reduction of toxins in the air), consumer practices (education concerning food labels), and personal health (diet and exercise) have been added to the *Healthy People 2010* goals.

School health services started more than 100 years ago to reduce absenteeism caused by communicable diseases. Current school health programs reflect the concept that physical and mental health are related to academic and social success. School nurses assess development, screen for specific health problems, refer to community agencies, and provide immunization clinics.

Adolescent and Young Adult

Goals for adolescents and young adults include the following:

- Reducing the deaths of adolescents from 21.8 per 100,000 in 1998 to 16.8 per 100,000 by 2010 is a goal of *Healthy People 2010*. The leading cause of death in adolescents is motor vehicle accidents (MVAs). Other unintentional accidents are the second leading cause of death in this age group. Most of these deaths are preventable.
- Reducing the deaths of young adults from 93.8 per 100,000 in 1998 to 57.3 per 100,000 by 2010 is another important objective of *Healthy People 2010*. The leading cause of death in young adults is also MVA, with homicide and suicide running a close second. Most of these causes also are preventable. Only 24% of deaths in this age group were attributed to neoplasms (cancer) or other medical causes. Human immunodeficiency virus (HIV) in the adolescent is of growing concern, and alcohol consumption is a continuing problem. Sedentary lifestyles and the continuing problem of weight control in this age group add to health problems in later life.

Older Adult

Although the life expectancy has increased, the problems relating to maintaining an independent lifestyle remain a challenge. Goals for older adults include the following:

- Reducing the occurrence of periodontal disease in adults age 35 to 44 years will aid in their ability to keep their natural, permanent teeth and in maintaining nutrition. With the baseline occurrence rate for gingivitis at 48% for the years 1988 to 1994, a goal has been established for reduction to 41% by 2010.
- Increasing the number of adults who engage in some form of leisure time exercise from 60% in 1997 to 80% by 2010 will help improve the general function of the cardiovascular system. Reducing the number of deaths due to chronic obstructive

pulmonary disease (COPD) from 119.4 deaths per 100,000 in persons 45 years or older in 1998 to 60 deaths per 100,000 by 2010 is another goal of *Healthy People 2010*.

Geriatric Adult

Goals for the geriatric phase of life include the following:

- Reducing the number of illnesses and deaths related to vaccine-preventable illnesses is an important goal. A target is to increase the number of adults over age 65 who receive annual vaccines against influenza and pneumococcal pneumonia from 64% in 1998 to 90% by 2010.
- Because falls are the most common cause of injury and hospital admissions among the elderly population, another goal is to reduce the number of hip fractures from a baseline of 1055.8 per 100,000 in 1998 to 416 per 100,000 in 2010. More than 75% of all hip fractures occur in females. In 1994 a total direct cost of $20.2 billion was spent in the care and treatment of patients who sustained a hip fracture.

ROLE OF THE NURSE IN ACHIEVING *HEALTHY PEOPLE 2010* GOALS

Nurses play an important role in helping to achieve the goals of *Healthy People 2010* at all phases of the life cycle. For example, increasing the use of prenatal services reduces low-birth-weight newborns and prematurity. Promoting breastfeeding increases the health of the newborn and bonding between mother and infant. The school nurse is essential in setting the pace of health education by educating the school-age child concerning nutritional needs, diet and exercise, smoking and drug use, and healthy lifestyles. Employer-sponsored health promotion activities also contribute to the *Healthy People 2010* goals, and nurses have an integral role in that setting.

Providing health education services to patients in managed care organizations is a nursing responsibility. Approximately 70% of employees are covered by some form of health care insurance, which is an increase of 108% from 1993. Nurses also can encourage older adults to participate in at least one organized health promotion activity. Identifying health risks through screening programs can lead to early diagnosis and treatment of disease.

THE NURSE AND WORLD HEALTH

At the same time *Healthy People 2010* was being initiated and developed, efforts toward worldwide health improvement were also initiated by the World Health Organization (WHO). In 1978 the International Conference on Primary Health Care was held in Alma-Ata, Kazakhstan. The world community was urged to protect and promote the health of all people of the world, and a list of world health goals was developed. A charter for health promotion was adopted at an international conference in 1986 in Ottawa, Canada. This charter defined world health promotion as "those processes that enable people to increase control over and improve their health" (WHO 1986). The priorities included improving health policy, providing supportive environments, involving community, developing personal abilities, and working with public health services.

As a result of meetings held in various locations around the world in the 1990s, objectives were developed for improving the environment; eliminating poverty; and providing reproductive health services, adolescent health, women's empowerment, human rights, and tobacco control. According to Brundtland (2000), progress has been made in improving world health by decreasing infant mortality rates, increasing access to immunizations, and providing areas of safer environmental sanitation. However, much work is yet to be completed.

Global health efforts are necessary because health problems are no longer confined to local areas. Outbreaks of illness in one area of the world can quickly spread to other areas of the world due to increased utilization of airline travel. Improvement in technology is not the key to improvement in health—prevention is. Prevention of illness through education and access to early health care is essential. The cultural competence of health care workers and the willingness to be change-agents for the traditional health care delivery system is also essential.

Nurses and health care workers must work with the local community and form partnerships for health. Improving prenatal care, nutrition, and access to children's health care all over the world are important beginning efforts toward improving world health. The health care team can build a bridge of health that extends around the world. Providing culturally competent care in the local community is the starting point of that bridge. Working with organizations, political groups, and government agencies to help form legislation for policies and practices relating to health care is the responsibility of the individual as a nurse, as well as the individual as a citizen.

KEY POINTS

- *Healthy People 2010* is a 10-year report card issued by the USDHHS concerning what has been accomplished in the area of health care in the United States and what is yet to be accomplished in the next 10 years.
- *Healthy People 2010* identifies leading health indicators that are of concern in health maintenance.
- Leading *health indicators* include physical activity, obesity, tobacco use, substance abuse, mental health, violence, environmental quality, and access to health care.
- *Determinants of health* include genetics, biology, physical and social environment, social service, policies, and laws.
- The *health status* of a population is measured by statistics such as birth and death rates, life expectancy, and morbidity.
- Some goals of *Healthy People 2010* include increasing life expectancy, improving maternal-infant health, increasing access to health care, reducing periodontal disease, and reducing morbidity and mortality due to preventable diseases.
- Global efforts are necessary to improve health care because problems are no longer confined to local areas.
- Providing culturally competent care increases compliance with healthy lifestyles and can help in meeting the goals of *Healthy People 2010*.

CRITICAL THINKING

School nurses can contribute to the goals of *Healthy People 2010* by teaching relevant health topics to students. A school nurse is assigned to teach one class to a group of elementary school children and one class to a group of high school students. List two topics for each class that would be age appropriate and relevant to the goals of *Healthy People 2010*.

MULTIPLE-CHOICE REVIEW QUESTIONS

1 The health status of a population is measured by:
   1 The number of health facilities available
   2 The number of people in a country
   3 Statistics such as birth and death rates
   4 Membership in HMO organizations
2 Health care is best improved by:
   1 Increasing the number of doctors available
   2 Coordinated worldwide efforts
   3 Local health department programs
   4 Statewide programs
3 *Healthy People 2010* is a:
   1 Report card on the progress of health care and identification of priority future needs
   2 List of laws that concern health care requirements
   3 List of mandates related to medical practice
   4 List of health care facilities that will be available by the year 2010
4 Nurses play an important role in helping to achieve the goals of *Healthy People 2010* by:
   1 Treating the poor population who are ill
   2 Promoting breastfeeding and early prenatal care
   3 Working overtime to meet patient needs
   4 Working in a community-based clinic
5 Leading health indicators include:
   1 Physical activity, mental health, access to health care, and environmental quality
   2 Reduction in birth rates, death rates, and morbidity
   3 Health care conferences held locally and worldwide
   4 The number of new policies and laws related to health care

Government Influences on Health Care

OUTLINE

OBJECTIVES

Upon completion of this chapter, the student will be able to:

1 Trace the history of government involvement in health care.
2 Analyze health care legislation and its influence on health care delivery.
3 Discuss current health care policy issues, including health care reform.
4 List some factors that influence the cost of health care.
5 Describe two types of health care delivery systems.
6 Identify future trends in health care.
7 Discuss the nurse's role in political activity related to health care.

KEY TERMS

Informed consent
Federal register
Health maintenance organization (HMO)
Homeopathy

Managed care organizations
Medicare
Medicaid
Nurse practice acts
Occupational Health and Safety Act (OSHA)
Political action committees (PAC)
Preferred provider organization (PPO)
Scope of practice
Standards of practice

LAWS CONCERNING HEALTH CARE

In earlier times, people accepted the rights of leaders such as monarchs, the church, or specific people with knowledge or expertise to make health care decisions for them. These decisions evolved into judgments, and the judgments were based on individual case decisions. From repeated judgments, laws were developed that became part of a system of rules that governed the lives of people. In time, legislative groups or bodies were added to the lawmaking process, and eventually the U.S. congressional system was formed. Laws originally revolved around individual rights and property rights. In the nineteenth century, laws concerning health care were developed based on the fundamental principles of health care leaders such as Hippocrates, Dorothy Dix, Clara Barton, and Florence Nightingale.

The efforts of these and other leaders in the field of health care led to the development of **standards of practice.** Standards of health care practice are the foundation of laws that are passed for consumer protection. A system of courts and legislative bodies are organized around three levels of government: the federal, state, and local sectors. Most lawmakers are elected by the people to represent the needs of their community. The first legal health care issues concerned the definition of health related to the ability of slaves to work. Early court decisions influenced the methods of health care delivery systems and the providers within these delivery systems. Patient care problems included infected wounds, trauma care, and care for specific age-related diseases. Most of the caretakers were self-taught, and the health care needs of most patients were often provided for by family members. As health care needs increased and care became more complex, experts were called in for consultation. In 1750 the first hospital for the poor was established in Philadelphia.

HOSPITALS AND NURSING SCHOOLS

In 1873 the Bellevue Hospital School of Nursing was established in New York as a proponent of the Nightingale principles of nursing care. In 1887 the Mayo brothers in Minnesota established the concepts of private office healthcare practice and then group clinics. In 1881 Clara Barton founded the American Red Cross, which focused on community health needs. By the end of the nineteenth century, three schools of nursing existed in the United States. A group of nurse leaders formed the American Society of Superintendents of Nurse Training Schools. A code of ethics was adopted, based on the Nightingale pledge, and the structure was similar to the American Medical Association.

By 1903 licensure by a state government agency was required to practice nursing, and the original Society for Training Schools evolved into the National League for Nursing Education (NLN). In 1911 school alumnae formed the American Nurses Association. Gradually the belief that nurses needed higher education and increased theoretical knowledge led to the opening of a program at Columbia University in New York to train teachers of nursing. The founders of this program for nurse educators, Isabelle Hampton Robb and Mary Adelaide Nutting, advocated the professionalism of nursing.

Hospitals gradually became the centers for health care because they had more facilities than the private doctor's office. Health centers developed and specialization increased. Specialty service units appeared in hospitals, including medical, surgical, and obstetrical units. One of the earliest pieces of government legislation concerning hospitals was the Hill-Burton Hospital Construction Act of 1946, which provided grants to states for the purpose of building new hospitals. Nursing as a career flourished with the establishment of the Army Cadet Nursing Corps to care for military personnel. However, nursing in civilian life did not receive the respect it deserved and needed to flourish as a career choice. A standardized national competence examination was determined to be a requirement for nursing licensure. Most schools of nursing were managed in hospital settings, but in 1965 the American Nurses Association advocated that nursing education take place in a college setting and a respected profession of nursing was reborn.

The federal government provided funds to train vocational nurses who cared for patients in the community setting. The vocational nursing programs were about 18 months in length and focused on skills and theory correlated with clinical practice.

THE MULTIDISCIPLINARY HEALTH CARE TEAM

Health care soon grew into an industry that depended on multidisciplinary providers, such as doctors, nurses, laboratory technicians, X-ray technicians, social workers, and others. A team approach to health care developed with the nurse as an integral part of the team. The goal of the team is to ensure the optimum physical, social, and mental well-being of the patient. The team works together to provide this comprehensive care, and communication between team members and the patient is vital. The nursing care plan was developed as a tool for this communication. A care plan can be an individual patient care plan, a family care plan, or a hospital care path that outlines the needs of the patient and the planned approach to meet these needs. Standards of care were developed by professional organizations, and the state governments established **nurse practice acts** that define the **scope of practice** for each level of professional practice. The scope of practice is the identification of and legal limitations to the usual and customary skill practices of a professional. The usual and customary practices are determined by the educational preparation for that profession. Nurses are responsible for knowing the nurse practice acts of the state in which they practice. Their patient care activities are limited by the established scope of practice. Currently each state has their own nurse practice act, with some variations in scope of practice. However, a multistate licensing arrangement that may require a standardization of nurse practice acts is under consideration and may become a reality in the near future.

In 1973 Minnesota became the first state to establish the bill of patient's rights as law (Box 2-1). One of the most important patient rights is the right of **informed consent**.

BOX 2-1   **The Patient Care Partnership: Understanding Expectations, Rights, and Responsibilities**

When you need hospital care, your doctor and the nurses and other professionals at our hospital are committed to working with you and your family to meet your health care needs. Our dedicated doctors and staff serve the community in all its ethnic, religious, and economic diversity. Our goal is for you and your family to have the same care and attention we would want for our families and ourselves.

The sections below explain some of the basics about how you can expect to be treated during your hospital stay. They also cover what we will need from you to care for you better. If you have questions at any time, please ask them. Unasked or unanswered questions can add to the stress of being in the hospital. Your comfort and confidence in your care are very important to us.

What to Expect During Your Hospital Stay
- **High quality hospital care.** Our first priority is to provide you the care you need, when you need it, with skill, compassion, and respect. Tell your caregivers if you have concerns about your care or if you have pain. You have the right to know the identity of doctors, nurses, and others involved in your care, as well as when they are students, residents, or other trainees.
- **A clean and safe environment.** Our hospital works hard to keep you safe. We use special policies and procedures to avoid mistakes in your care and keep you free from abuse or neglect. If anything unexpected and significant happens during your hospital stay, you will be told what happened and any resulting changes in your care will be discussed with you.
- **Involvement in your care.** You and your doctor often make decisions about your care before you go to the hospital. Other times, especially in emergencies, those decisions are made during your hospital stay. When they take place, making decisions should include:
  - *Discussing your medical condition and information about medically appropriate treatment choices.* To make informed decisions with your doctor, you need to understand several things:
    – The benefits and risks of each treatment.
    – Whether it is experimental or part of a research study.
    – What you can reasonably expect from your treatment and any long-term effects it might have on your quality of life.
    – What you and your family will need to do after you leave the hospital.
    – The financial consequences of using uncovered services or out-of-network providers.

    Please tell your caregivers if you need more information about treatment choices.
  - *Discussing your treatment plan.* When you enter the hospital, you sign a general consent to treatment. In some cases, such as surgery or experimental treatment, you may be asked to confirm in writing that you understand what is planned and agree to it. This process protects your right to consent to or refuse a treatment. Your doctor will explain the medical consequences of refusing recommended treatment. It also protects your right to decide if you want to participate in a research study.

(Continued)

BOX 2-1	The Patient Care Partnership: Understanding Expectations, Rights, and Responsibilities—cont'd

- *Getting information from you.* Your caregivers need complete and correct information about your health and coverage so that they can make good decisions about your care. That includes:
  - Past illnesses, surgeries, or hospital stays.
  - Past allergic reactions.
  - Any medicines or diet supplements (such as vitamins and herbs) that you are taking.
  - Any network or admission requirements under your health plan.
- *Understanding your health care goals and values.* You may have health care goals and values or spiritual beliefs that are important to your well-being. They will be taken into account as much as possible throughout your hospital stay. Make sure your doctor, your family, and your care team know your wishes.
- *Understanding who should make decisions when you cannot.* If you have signed a health care power of attorney stating who should speak for you if you become unable to make health care decisions for yourself, or a "living will" or "advance directive" that states your wishes about end-of-life care, give copies to your doctor, your family and your care team. If you or your family need help making difficult decisions, counselors, chaplains and others are available to help.
- **Protection of your privacy.** We respect the confidentiality of your relationship with your doctor and other caregivers, and the sensitive information about your health and health care that are part of that relationship. State and federal laws and hospital operating policies protect the privacy of your medical information. You will receive a Notice of Privacy Practices that describes the ways that we use, disclose and safeguard patient information and that explains how you can obtain a copy of information from our records about your care.
- **Help preparing you and your family for when you leave the hospital.** Your doctor works with hospital staff and professionals in your community. You and your family also play an important role. The success of your treatment often depends on your efforts to follow medication, diet and therapy plans. Your family may need to help care for you at home.

  You can expect us to help you identify sources of follow-up care and to let you know if our hospital has a financial interest in any referrals. As long as you agree we can share information about your care with them, we will coordinate our activities with your caregivers outside the hospital. You can also expect to receive information and, where possible, training about the self-care you will need when you go home.
- **Help with your bill and filing insurance claims.** Our staff will file claims for you with health care insurers or other programs such as Medicare and Medicaid. They will also help your doctor with needed documentation. Hospital bills and insurance coverage are often confusing. If you have questions about your bill, contact our business office. If you need help under-standing your insurance coverage or health plan, start with your insurance company or

(Continued)

BOX 2-1 **The Patient Care Partnership: Understanding Expectations, Rights, and Responsibilities—cont'd**

health benefits manager. If you do not have health coverage, we will try to help you and your family find financial help or make other arrangements. We need your help with collecting needed information and other requirements to obtain coverage or assistance.

While you are here, you will receive more detailed notices about some of the rights you have as a hospital patient and how to exercise them. We are always interested in improving. If you have questions, comments, or concerns, please contact _____.

The nurse is responsible to sign as witness that a patient has received information regarding risks, advantages, and alternatives available to a procedure in a language that can be understood by the patient.

The U.S. government passed a rehabilitation act and various mandates that require the provision of health care services to physically handicapped persons, mentally handicapped persons, and pregnant women. These rights must be adhered to if the hospital is to remain accredited or approved, which means the hospital meets specific standards of care. Although the government does not accredit hospitals, a hospital that is not accredited may not be eligible to receive state or federal funding assistance.

GOVERNMENT'S ROLE IN HEALTH CARE

The right of the government to play a role in the health care of the people is established in the Constitution of the United States, Article 1, section 8, which states that the role of the government includes providing for the general welfare of the people and provides the spending power to achieve this role. Therefore the government can act to protect the health, welfare, and safety of the people. An example of this power is the requiring of specific immunizations for schoolchildren before they are allowed to enter school to protect the health of the community.

The role of the government in health care began gradually. President Roosevelt's New Deal, designed to revive the country from the Great Depression, provided government spending for health care. The National Insurance Plan proposed by Mayor Wagner of New York combined with the passage of the Social Security Act of 1935 were the sparks that ignited expanded government involvement in public health care. In 1937 the Unemployment Compensation and Old Age Benefit laws were passed.

Department of Health and Human Services

The Department of Health and Human Services (USDHHS) was named in 1980. It originally was established in 1939 under the title of the Federal Security Agency. Under the guidance of this department, the three levels of government (local, state, and federal) provide functions such as direct services, financing, information, and policy setting.

Direct services

Direct services include providing health care to American Indians, military personnel and their families, and prisoners. It is also concerned with managing screening clinics for diseases such as tuberculosis and immunization clinics for children.

Financing

The government pays for health education programs and finances health care through **Medicare, Medicaid,** and Social Security programs (Box 2-2). The government also provides grants for medical and nursing research and education.

Information

Government agencies such as the National Institute of Health (NIH) and the Centers for Disease Control and Prevention (CDC) write periodic reports concerning vital statistics, census data, and results of health surveys. Information is published in *Health, United States,* offering a snapshot of the health status of residents in the United States.

Policy setting

The Children's Bureau, established in 1912, studied the needs of children and established agencies to provide services, such as the Woman, Infants, and Children program (WIC), and defined essential community health and nursing responsibilities. Government policies influenced the survival of health care groups. The Sheppard-Towner Act of 1921 influenced social welfare policies. In 1945 the United Nations (UN) was formed by the joining of many nations for the promotion of common goals that included human rights, peace, and the economic and social advancement of all people. The UN is located in New York City and meets annually with the World Health Organization (WHO), which was created in 1946 to establish worldwide policies and services to promote health and health research. WHO endorses nurses and nursing education as essential to attaining the goal of health for all people (see Chapter 1).

Most health care legislation in the United States is delegated to the USDHHS, although specialties such as environmental health or occupational health may have a separate agency to focus on those specific problems. The public health sector of the USDHHS oversees the health care of U.S. citizens. The Public Health Service has a Bureau of Professions that is responsible for the Division of Nursing, Division of Dentistry, Division of Medicine, and so on.

Federal legislation concerning health care is recorded and published in the **Federal Register.** Local governments have similar publications. Revisions of various regulations are based on research findings and public input, and periodic hearings are held. When a law is passed, monitoring of the private sector for compliance occurs. See Table 2-1 for examples of federal legislation.

Although an individual U.S. citizen has the right to privacy and freedom, a federal law can mandate isolation if it is deemed necessary to protect the health or welfare of the individuals in a community, such as with tuberculosis or smallpox infections. In some states the state government mandates health insurance for all college students, which is paid for by student fees. Occupational health is regulated by the **Occupational**

BOX 2-2	**Medicare and Medicaid**

- **Medicare** is a type of insurance program in which benefits are received after contributions are made through payroll deductions
- **Medicaid** is more of a welfare program in which benefits are provided on a basis of need or poverty.
- These programs determine physicians' fees by a complicated formula. Many services may not be covered or may require a co-payment at the time services are rendered.

Safety and Health Act (OSHA), which requires standards of safety be maintained by employers to protect the health and safety of employees and mandates reporting of injuries sustained by workers. Workers have the right to know if they are working in a toxic environment. Workers injured on the job also have the right to receive health care and financial compensation for any life-altering injury that occurs while on the job. State laws also license and certify home care and hospice facilities.

State governments also regulate, to some extent, insurance companies and labor unions. Some federal laws can affect the social development of young adults. For example, 18- to 25-year-old males must register with Selective Service. In the event of a crisis requiring a military draft, they might be called into active service in a sequence based on random lottery number and date of birth, which may interrupt career or marital plans. Both federal and local laws regulate the age at which one can drink alcohol, drive a car, and work. The government also defines the age at which senior citizens are eligible for full Social Security benefits. This age has been designated at 65 years for a long time, but may be changed to 67 or 68 years of age by the year 2027.

There are also governmental influences on the family, including tough divorce laws in some states and lenient divorce laws in other states. Most states currently have lenient abortion laws and favor the concept of giving custody of children to the biological parent whenever possible in an effort to provide consistent caregivers who will meet the developmental needs of children.

DELIVERY OF HEALTH CARE

The cost of health care in the United States has increased over the past 20 years. Health insurance policies were introduced, but increasing costs threaten their survival. The National Committee for Quality Assurance was established to review and accredit **managed care organizations** (MCOs). Managed care organizations try to standardize and control costs of health care. Maintaining quality care while ensuring cost containment is today's challenge in health care. The **health maintenance organization (HMO)**, a group practice that cares for prepaid members, and the **preferred provider organization (PPO)**, which contracts with professionals to provide care to a specific group of patients at an agreed-upon fee-for-service rate, are types of managed care organizations (Knight, 1998).

TABLE 2-1

EXAMPLES OF FEDERAL LEGISLATION RELATED TO HEALTH CARE

1798	The Marine Hospital Service Act provided medical care to merchant marines (eventually became U.S. Public Health Service).
1878	The Port Quarantine Act prevented people with infectious diseases from entering the United States.
1879	A National Health Department was established.
1901	The Pure Food and Drug Act monitored the manufacture, labeling, and sale of food and drugs (later became the Food and Drug Administration [FDA]).
1912	The Children's Health Bureau established and implemented child labor laws. Meets every 10 years with focus on children's needs.
1921	The Sheppard-Towner Maternity-Infant Care Act provided funds for health and welfare of mothers and children.
1935	The Social Security Act passed Title VI to assist states in providing public health services. Enabled development of Medicare and Medicaid programs.
1939	The Federal Security Agency combined health, education, and welfare services.
1940	The Communicable Disease Center was established in Atlanta (now known as the Centers for Disease Control and Prevention [CDC]). The Nurse Training Act provided funds to encourage nursing education.
1944	The Public Health Act consolidated public health legislation into one law.
1945	The McCarran-Ferguson Act gave state governments the rights to regulate health insurance plans.
1946	The Hill-Burton Act provided for new hospital construction with provisions for care of the uninsured.
1947	The Army Nurse Corps was established.
1948	The National Institute of Health (NIH) was established.
1954	The Taft Sanitary Engineering Center was established to improve environmental health.
1955	The U.S. Medical Library was formed to provide access to medical literature.
1964	A health amendment provided increased funds for nursing education.
1965	The Title VIII Social Security Amendment created Medicare to care for older adults and the disabled. Title XIX provided access to health care for the poor via Medicaid.
1970	The Occupational Safety and Health Act (OSHA) focused on workplace and environmental health.
1971	The Environmental Protection Agency was formed to monitor all environmental programs.
1972	The National Security Act was amended to encourage health maintenance organizations (HMO) and preferred provider organizations (PPO) to manage health care. Provided grants for HMO development.
1973	The Health Maintenance Organization Act required employers to offer federally qualified HMO coverage for employees and mandated state supervision.
1980	Infant Formula Act required standards for the manufacture of infant formulas.
1981	The Omnibus Budget Reconciliation Act provided money for grants for various health promotion projects such as nursing homes, skilled nursing facilities, and home health agencies.

(Continued)

TABLE 2-1

EXAMPLES OF FEDERAL LEGISLATION RELATED TO HEALTH CARE—cont'd

1982	The Tax Equity Fiscal Responsibility Act (TEFRA) amended the Social Security Act establishing the diagnosis-related group (DRG) system, which changed health care radically by establishing strict rules for reimbursement.
1985	The Consolidated Omnibus Reconciliation Act (COBRA) ensured continuation of health insurance for a time after loss of coverage due to job termination.
1989	Reimbursement of nurse practitioners for care provided was approved.
1990	The Health Objectives Planning Act resulted from the 1979 *Healthy People* report, which identified and monitored the nation's health care goals. Established *Healthy People 2000* and *Healthy People 2010*.
1996	The Health Insurance Portability and Accountability Act (HIPAA) enabled portability of health insurance, privacy of medical information, and coverage for preexisting conditions.
1997	The Welfare Reform Act regulated restrictions for Aid to Families with Dependent Children (AFDC).
2002	Laws prohibit smoking in some public buildings. The use of mercury alloys in dental amalgam for certain patients and the use of mercury in medical devices such as blood pressure machines were prohibited. Asbestos abatement programs for school buildings were created. Lead and chemical poisoning prevention and screening programs were established. The Homeland Security Act addressed the public health and safety of the nation in the event of a terrorist attack.
2003	HIPAA regulations were enforced nationwide.

There is pending legislation to offer multistate licensing for nurses (Lasseter, 1999). This will involve standardizing the nurse practice acts of the various states who agree to the interstate practice. The mobility of nurses, the growth of traveling nurse programs, and the use of Internet services have led to the need for interstate licensing of nurses.

INCREASING COSTS OF HEALTH CARE

Increasing health care costs lead to higher premiums for membership in health care insurance plans. Part of the health insurance costs may be the responsibility of employers who then recoup their costs by increasing the cost of their consumer product, which in turn may raise the cost of living. Government-sponsored health care programs use resources that could be otherwise used to help reduce the federal budget deficit. Therefore the costs of health care are of interest to all people in the United States. Federal, state, and local governments also have a vested interest in controlling health care costs. Cost controls involve dealing with issues such as national health goals, entitlement, the right to health care, utilization of resources available, and identification of the changing health care needs of the people.

Prevention and early intervention seem to be the keys to reducing health care costs and are the core of *Healthy People 2010* (see Chapter 1). Examples of *Healthy People 2010* objectives related to proposed health care legislation are summarized in Box 2-3.

Efforts at health care reform have forced some states to develop subsidized health care plans that increase access to care, promote managed care plans designed to control costs, regulate physicians fees, and advocate insurance reforms.

HEALTH CARE REFORM

In 1994 President Clinton submitted a major health care reform plan to Congress for approval. The plan contained "sin taxes" to help pay for the increasing costs. (Taxes on cigarettes and alcohol were the focus of sin taxes because these products contributed to health problems.) However, the plan was opposed by the states that had close ties with the tobacco industry. Some small businesses also opposed the plan because they feared increased costs of paying employee benefits would force them out of business, whereas others felt that the implementation of specific aspects of the plan would be too expensive. Historically, people in the United States oppose big government getting involved in health care programs and generally resist socialized medicine. Any health care reform must involve managing costs, promoting access, and identifying who will pay for it. Many people believe that increased technology has added to the general increase in the cost of health care because high technology provides help only to a small proportion of the population and insurance companies may pay for only a small portion of the procedure. The focus on illness prevention and early detection and intervention will lead health care delivery systems into the ambulatory care setting rather than increased in-hospital care.

The Genome Project (see Chapter 5) enables health care providers to predict, detect, and treat illnesses before they become expensive, chronic problems. The cloud that looms over the health care of the future may be the issue of rationing care. Restricting

---

| BOX 2-3 | *Healthy People 2010* and Proposed Legislation |

Some of the objectives of *Healthy People 2010* will require the assistance of government legislation to achieve the target goals set by 2010. They include the following:

- Increase the number of K-12 schools with school nurse ratio of 1:750.
- Increase statewide surveillance systems to collect data concerning causes of injuries.
- Extend blood alcohol level requirements for drivers 21 years of age and older.
- Increase smoke-free environments.

access to health care or limiting coverage for specific problems may help to control costs but may be a difficult concept for U.S. citizens to accept. Many critics of the U.S. health care system believe that we now have a fragmented, uncoordinated program focused on acute care treatment of illness without universal access to preventative care.

GROWTH OF SELF-CARE

Self-care is a valuable adjunct to health care reform. The focus of health care has changed from treatment of illness to prevention of illness. That change in focus involves a movement from hospital-centered care to community-based ambulatory care. People are increasingly interested in actively participating in their own care, and as a result self-care strategies have become popular. The Internet provides a resource for education about illness prevention and self-help techniques. Self-care is not a new concept. Midwives and lay practitioners were popular in the eighteenth and nineteenth centuries. In the 1830s and 1840s the interest in self-care peaked and hydrotherapy (therapy using water) and homeopathy (the use of minute portions of chemicals for their healing power) flourished. The formation of the American Medical Association and philanthropic organizations such as the Rockefeller Foundation and the Carnegie Foundation advocated professional care, and self-care was devalued. In 1959 Dorothy Orem developed the self-care model related to nursing practice. In the 1960s Martha Rogers, a nursing theorist, proposed a holistic view of health care, and in 1989 another theorist, Jean Watson, focused on the value of the nurse-patient relationship in the promotion of health. Today the desire of the individual to have control over what is done to his or her body has resulted in a resurgence of self-care. Some health care organizations, such as Kaiser Permanente Foundation Health Plan, distribute self-care guides to all members. Internet and CD-ROM programs are available to offer advice and guidance for health promotion. Self-care and nutrition classes, as well as exercise facilities, are readily available and in popular use.

Complementary and alternative medicine (CAM) is practiced by individuals in the community, and many practices have been adopted into traditional care settings (Burcham, 1999). Outreach programs target local populations for screening and education based on needs assessments of the community. Providing safe environments in educational institutions and including self-care health concepts in school curricula are essential elements of modern health care reform. Nursing education programs are increasing students' experiences with healthy individuals in community-based settings. Culturally competent care of a diverse population is being integrated into medical and nursing school programs. Occupational health programs, in the form of supporting employee health, and Web sites for dissemination of health care information are also important to the future of health care.

FUTURE OF HEALTH CARE

Federal legislation and funding serve to increase the participation of government in health care. Throughout the twentieth century, the U.S. Congress enacted bills related to health care for U.S. citizens. Increasing health care costs, increasing need for health care, and growth of various health care delivery systems have resulted in the need for continued federal intervention. Public health programs have the potential of improving health and reducing the cost of health care. In the future, health care agencies may depend on self-care education to promote health and prevent disease, because it may be an effective cost-containment technique. Government agencies that provide vital statistics aid in identifying areas of need and developing intervention strategies.

Political influence is promoted by **political action committees** (PACs). PACs influence legislation by offering monetary contributions to legislators who support their needs and by providing lobbying efforts to create an awareness of needed legislation. The American Nurses Association and other medical organizations have PACs to represent the needs of nurses and patients. Many nurses serve as elected public officials, and nurse legislators help in interpreting health care issues.

Nurses will play a key role in the future of health care by supporting and educating patients; providing cost-effective, quality care; and becoming involved in the legislative decisions of local, state, and federal governments. Nurses realize that the role of government related to health care influences the delivery of health care. For that reason, nurses need to be active in the political arena to ensure that the needs of nurses and patients are considered when discussing, creating, and passing laws related to health care.

KEY POINTS

- The role of government in health care was established in article 1, section 8 of the U.S. Constitution, which provides spending power to promote the general health, welfare, and safety of the people.
- Standards of health care practice are the foundation of health care legislation.
- The Hill-Burton Hospital Construction Act of 1946 provided funding to build new hospitals.
- The Army Cadet Nurse Corps was established to care for military personnel, and nursing as a career began to flourish.
- The multidisciplinary health care team includes doctors, nurses, lab technicians, X-ray technicians, social workers, and others.
- Local governments established nurse practice acts that defined the scope of practice for each level of professional nursing practice.
- Minnesota was the first state to establish the Patient's Bill of Rights as law.
- A hospital that is not accredited may not be eligible to receive state or federal funding assistance.

- The Social Security Act of 1935 expanded government involvement in public health care.
- The Department of Health and Human Services of the federal government provides direct services, information, and health care legislation.
- The United Nations meets annually with the World Health Organization to establish worldwide health policies, services, and research.
- Federal legislation that is passed is published in the Federal Register.
- Occupational health is regulated by the Occupational Safety and Health Association (OSHA), which sets standards of health and safety in the workplace.
- The federal government provides legislation and funding to support the goals of *Healthy People 2010*.
- Political influence is promoted by political action committees (PACs), in which nurses can advocate for patient needs and interpret health care issues.

CRITICAL THINKING

Nurses or health care workers may have the opportunity to join political action committees to assist in increasing awareness of the need for health-related legislation. Discuss two topics relevant to health care reform that this committee might promote.

MULTIPLE-CHOICE REVIEW QUESTIONS

1 The purpose of the nurse practice act is to:
  1 Define the scope of practice for each level of professional nursing
  2 Define the length of nursing education programs
  3 Determine criteria to license nursing schools
  4 License nurses to practice
2 Most schools of nursing are currently located in:
  1 A hospital
  2 A high school
  3 An independent occupational setting
  4 A college
3 The right of the government to play a role in health care originates in:
  1 The U.S. Constitution
  2 Laws decided by local courts
  3 The Democratic Party
  4 An annual vote by the people

4 The functions of the U.S. Department of Health and Human Services (USDHHS) include:
   1 Writing licensing exams for health care professionals
   2 Prioritizing medical practices
   3 Operating clinics for the indigent population
   4 Setting policy, providing information, and financing health care programs
5 Political Action Committees (PACs) influence health care by:
   1 Writing health care laws
   2 Supporting legislators who vote on health care policies
   3 Studying the needs of local communities
   4 Promoting higher salaries for nurses

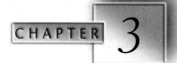

CHAPTER *3*

The Influence of Family on Developing a Lifestyle

OBJECTIVES

Upon completion of this chapter, the student will be able to:

1 Define the various types of family structures.
2 List the developmental stages of a family.
3 Define family systems theory.
4 Give examples of family system stressors.
5 Discuss the effect of the family lifestyle on child development.
6 State three childrearing styles.

7 List three developmental theories.
8 Define culture.
9 List the effects culture has on personal values, beliefs, and behaviors of family members.
10 Define what makes a family dysfunctional.
11 Discuss one positive and one negative influence of technology/electronic media on the family and child development.
12 State the effect of the community on the family and child development.

KEY TERMS

Blended family
Cultural assimilation
Cultural competence
Cultural relativism
Culture shock
Developmental stage
Developmental task
Dysfunctional family
Ethnocentrism
Family systems theory
Posttraumatic stress disorder (PTSD)
Sibling rivalry
Theory

DEFINITION

The family has been defined as a basic human social system that involves commitment and interaction between its members. This commitment includes a responsibility for the physical and emotional well-being and successful development of the children in that family. For most people, the family is the strongest and most influential group to which a person belongs. A healthy family is not necessarily a family where all members are at the optimum level of health. A healthy family is one that can successfully adapt to crises, challenges, and changes during the life cycle. The role of the nurse or health care worker is to help the family adapt to these challenges. Nurses must understand the many factors that influence family functioning and child development. Comprehensive care involves the patient and the family unit.

Family Structure

Family composition and cultural backgrounds have changed dramatically in the United States over the last 40 years. The traditional nuclear (two-parent) family, where the father works outside the home and the mother remains at home to care for the children, has given way to many other variations. Although one third of the children in the

United States are in a nuclear, traditional environment (Popenoe, 1989), the daily availability of the father to the children is often decreased due to the demands of the workplace. The father may leave the house to travel to work before the child awakens and returns after the child is asleep for the night. Flexibility is needed to maintain paternal role modeling, mutual respect, and equality of involvement in childrearing.

Dual-career families have become the norm in modern America. Both parents work outside the home, and design a lifestyle that helps support the need and rationale for that type of family structure. Conflicting demands among work responsibilities, continuing education for career advancement, and the demands of childrearing often create pressures that require careful scheduling, close communication, flexibility, and mutual support. Children of dual-career families are often expected to be more independent at an earlier age, and parents tend to overestimate the ability of the child to manage without direct supervision. Acute illness, chronic illness, or discipline and behavior problems can create additional stresses in this type of family structure (Box 3-1).

All family variations have some form of influence on childrearing and development. Table 3-1 lists the types of family structures found in the United States. An essential core of parenting within any family structure is commitment to the child. The parenting arrangement may be challenged by divorce, environmental poverty, or illness or death of a parent. Communication between parent and child helps the child adjust to a specific lifestyle, which may be different from his or her peers. Children need to have a sense of belonging, support, and consistency in their lives to achieve optimal development (Figure 3-1).

EFFECT OF FAMILY ON GROWTH AND DEVELOPMENT OF THE CHILD

There are many factors within the family structure, including interactions and lifestyles, that can affect the growth and development of a child. The more common aspects of family variations are discussed in this chapter.

Size of Family

The interpersonal relationship between siblings is unique. The presence of a brother or sister in a family group helps provide support and gives early experience in developing

---

BOX 3-1	Ten Potential Challenges in Dual-Career Families

1 Need for child care arrangements
2 Time to participate in child's activities
3 Time to support and encourage academic achievements
4 Time to support and encourage peer interaction
5 Time for child-focused family activities
6 Need for close scheduling and travel away from home
7 Lack of energy for home and child care activities
8 Difficulty with unexpected illness or injury management
9 Increased need for child to self-manage
10 Maintaining healthy nutrition options at mealtimes

TABLE **3-1**

VARIOUS TYPES OF FAMILY STRUCTURES

Type of Family*	Description
Nuclear	Traditional—husband, wife, and children (biological or adopted)
Extended	Grandparents, parents, children, and relatives
Single parent	Women or men establishing separate households through individual preferences, divorces, death, or desertion
Foster parent	Parents who care for children who are sent to them via the court system because of dysfunctional families, absent families, or individual family problems
Alternative	Communal family
Dual career	Both parents work because of desire or need
Blended	Mother or father, stepparent, and children
Polygamous	More than one spouse at the same time
Homosexual	A single gay person or two persons of the same sex who may have children from a previous relationship, who have adopted children, or have children via artificial insemination
Cohabitation	Heterosexual or homosexual couples who live together with their children but remain unmarried (a type of cohabitation may be experienced by college students who live in a dorm or off-campus school housing with men and women sharing facilities together)

Modified from Leifer, G. (2003). *Introduction to maternity and pediatric nursing* (4th ed.). Philadelphia: W.B. Saunders.
*Not all may be legally sanctioned.

skills necessary for social interaction. Older children can help younger siblings grasp language skills, but the firstborn or only child may have a longer, more intense verbal interaction with the parent. This one-to-one relationship may result in the development of a wider vocabulary and better conversational skills at an earlier age. Although social experiences may be limited for the single child, the popular use of day care and pre-school provides an opportunity to develop social skills and decreases the feeling of loneliness for an only child.

Spacing of Siblings

The age of the older child at the time of the birth of the sibling contributes to the response of the older child. When the new baby arrives, a 1-year-old child may whine and cling, whereas a two-year-old child may regress in toileting or feeding behaviors and a 4 year old may develop temper tantrums. A child older than 5 years of age may feel protective of the new arrival. Shared experience in siblings less than 4 years apart increases the occurrence of sibling rivalry. **Sibling rivalry** is a competition or struggle between two or more children in a family. It can contribute in a positive way to development by offering the opportunity for children to develop interpersonal skills and deal with conflict, but it can also cause stress and chaos in a family.

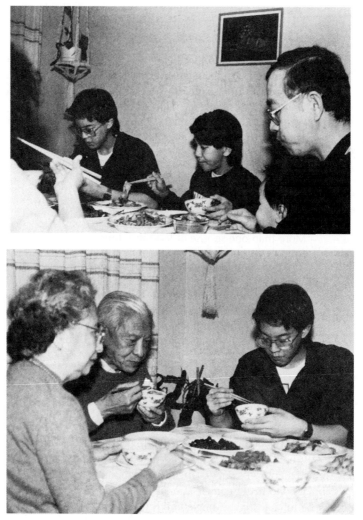

FIGURE 3–1 Several generations gather around the dinner table for holidays or other celebrations. Such activities strengthen the family structure. (From Betz, C.L., Hunsberger, M., & Wright, S. [1994]. *Family-centered nursing care of children* [2nd ed.]. Philadelphia: W.B. Saunders.)

Divorce

The psychological health and development of the child may be affected by the divorce of his or her parents. The child may be thrust into a single-family home or a newly blended family if remarriage occurs. Children of divorce often have a higher incidence of behavioral or learning difficulties later in life. The effect of joint custody on the child is partially determined by the motivation for such an arrangement. The best motivation would be to ensure continuing relationships with both parents, but other reasons often include convenience or lack of commitment by one or both parents. The presence or absence of hostility between the parents is an important factor that influences the psychological adjustment of the child regardless of the type of custody arrangements made.

The child should be prepared for the divorce and assured he or she had no role in the breakup of the marriage. However, self-blame is common despite assurances. Children should be told how the divorce will affect them and their needs, as well as what they can expect in terms of living arrangements and continued relationships with both parents. Children need permission to continue to love both parents and feel free to express these feelings. Table 3-2 reviews typical responses to divorce according to age group and developmental level and related guidance or interventions that can be offered by the nurse and the health care team.

Stepchildren and Foster Children

Nearly half of all children born in the United States experience life in a blended family (Levine, Carey, & Crocker, 1999). A **blended family** is one in which each parent brings children from a previous marriage into a new family unit. The children may have to adjust to a new home and school environment with new rules and new roommates (stepsiblings) who are strangers. This often accompanies a dilution of attention from the biological parent, who must divide attention among a larger family group. Resentment between stepsiblings may occur. A stepparent may be given a name other than mother or father if the children feel guilty that they are replacing their biological parent.

Children who enter foster care must face a strange environment without the support of even one biological parent. There is added uncertainty regarding the length of placement, which can result in insecurity and lack of trust in others. In the year 2000 there were more than 545,000 children in foster care in the United States (Table 3-3). Seventy-two percent were in foster homes, 8% were in group home settings, and 1% were in supervised independent living (USDHHS, 2000). Federal legislation in 1980 and 1995 promoted family reunification as the goal of foster care so that relatives are now first sought out to care for a child displaced from the biological family.

Chronic Illness

Having a child, parent, or dependent relative with a chronic illness can strain sibling relationships and place a toll on the emotional, psychological, and economic resources of the family. The well child may be expected to be more independent and carry more responsibilities or step into a caregiver role that may keep him or her away from normal activities with peers. Although some well children may react with anger at the ill family member, many children may develop a greater capacity for empathy because of their experiences with the person who is chronically ill (Table 3-4). Communicating the needs, limitations, and feelings of the ill relative and acknowledging the needs and feelings of caregivers and the impact on the family can make the crucial difference between resentment and attachment for each member of the family. Caregiver group support may be available in local communities.

TABLE 3-2

RESPONSES TO DIVORCE BY AGE GROUP

Age Group	Signs and Symptoms	Interventions Needed
Preschool	Regression Returns to thumb sucking Intensified fears Sleep disturbances Fear of abandonment	Maintain household routines Reassure love of child Spend added time with child Establish and maintain bedtime rituals
School age	Shows open grieving Feels rejected Fears being replaced by absent parent Difficulty in concentrating, resulting in poor grades Fears expressing emotions	Allow child to love both parents Help child move from parent to parent Diminish worry about present and future Attend school events Do not use child as confidant or as spouse substitute
Adolescent	Worry about fate of own future marriage Must rethink values and morality of the world May become depressed or suicidal May be expected to assume greater family responsibilities	Avoid delegating too much home responsibility Encourage discussion with neutral party Encourage to pursue own interests Help utilize support systems
Adult	Increased dependence on eldest child Open expression of fears, anxieties, and anger Inability to focus on needs of children	Counsel to join a single parent support group Encourage professional counseling Refer to social or financial aid resources
Geriatric	Depression, loneliness, helplessness, bitterness Increased dependence on children and grandchildren	Encourage joining groups Increase activities that are of personal interest

The death of a child in the family may cause a parent to be overprotective of the surviving children, thus depriving them of normal independence with their peers. The nurse can explain and discuss terminal illness and its developmental and behavioral consequences by identifying family strengths, coping styles, and strategies. A comprehensive plan for care, continuing education, and promotion of optimal growth and development can then be designed and implemented by the health care team.

The family that has a newborn child with a chronic illness or deformity goes through a grieving process. This process includes shock, disbelief/denial, anger, depression, withdrawal, adaptation, and adjustment. Any new crises can cause setbacks to previous stages and delay the coping and adjustment of family members. The health care worker must recognize these stages, determine the resiliency of the

TABLE 3-3

CHILDREN IN FOSTER CARE

State	Entering Foster Care This Year			Exiting Care During the Year			In Care on Last Day of Year		
	FY 1998	FY 1999	FY 2000	FY 1998	FY 1999	FY 2000	FY 1998	FY 1999	FY 2000
Alabama	2,803	2,734	2,661	2,851	2,062	2,334	5,198	5,511	5,621
Alaska	1,092	1,180	1,096	635	732	913	1,940	2,248	2,193
Arizona	4,300	4,372	4,644	2,190	4,853	5,056	5,608	7,034	6,475
Arkansas	2,737	2,489	3,542	2,094	2,160	3,679	3,138	2,919	3,045
California	52,997	43,587	45,685	50,049	39,156	50,112	112,767	117,937	112,807
Colorado	7,147	7,183	6,942	5,202	5,675	5,512	7,951	7,639	7,533
Connecticut	5,222	3,098	2,763	3,682	2,169	2,368	6,683	7,487	6,996
Delaware	1,023	1,002	950	333	811	886	1,480	1,193	1,098
District of Columbia	1,408	1,231	775	979	659	315	3,397	3,466	3,054
Florida	13,980	21,118	18,765	7,934	8,117	15,507	26,320	34,292	35,656
Georgia	3,724	7,218	7,028	3,632	6,267	4,657	9,937	11,991	11,204
Hawaii	1,774	1,718	2,002	1,410	1,700	1,768	2,441	2,203	2,379
Idaho	851	999	1,125	572	806	991	963	959	1,034
Illinois	9,229	7,856	6,643	12,627	14,112	11,505	48,737	40,270	33,125
Indiana	6,328	4,808	5,576	9,524	4,313	5,197	5,070	8,933	7,482
Iowa	5,331	5,343	5,620	5,257	5,443	5,414	4,920	4,854	5,068
Kansas	6,683	3,376	3,191	3,400	1,562	1,788	8,488	6,774	6,569
Kentucky	N/A	4,096	4,749	N/A	3,551	4,091	N/A	5,698	6,152
Louisiana	3,051	2,912	3,157	2,399	2,854	3,146	6,301	5,581	5,406
Maine	1,646	1,014	1,052	712	535	721	3,595	3,154	3,191
Maryland	4,467	3,936	3,928	3,296	2,933	3,110	12,890	13,455	13,113
Massachusetts	N/A	7,368	7,381	N/A	7,749	6,392	N/A	11,169	11,619
Michigan	10,220	10,929	10,707	5,207	6,740	7,802	18,583	20,300	20,034
Minnesota	9,574	10,724	10,803	8,171	9,743	9,939	8,521	8,996	8,530
Mississippi	1,821	1,750	2,005	1,325	1,676	1,726	3,359	3,196	3,292
Missouri	6,504	6,341	7,216	4,950	5,304	5,509	12,495	12,577	13,181
Montana	1,503	1,596	1,588	1,223	1,331	1,327	1,991	2,156	2,180

(Continued)

TABLE 3-3

CHILDREN IN FOSTER CARE—cont'd

State	Entering Foster Care This Year			Exiting Care During the Year			In Care on Last Day of Year		
	FY 1998	FY 1999	FY 2000	FY 1998	FY 1999	FY 2000	FY 1998	FY 1999	FY 2000
Nebraska	N/A	2,806	3,134	N/A	2,100	2,514	N/A	5,146	5,674
Nevada	N/A	N/A	673	N/A	N/A	387	N/A	N/A	1,615
New Hampshire	N/A	573	511	N/A	440	538	N/A	1,448	1,342
New Jersey	4,747	4,768	4,649	4,246	4,178	4,645	9,182	9,494	9,258
New Mexico	1,480	1,829	1,780	1,137	1,691	1,716	821	1,941	1,912
New York	19,749	18,172	16,601	20,324	20,497	20,243	53,555	51,159	47,208
North Carolina	5,464	5,391	5,458	3,993	4,317	4,481	11,314	11,339	10,847
North Dakota	1,056	965	1,006	671	827	851	1,170	1,143	1,129
Ohio	N/A	15,946	15,396	N/A	12,819	14,131	N/A	20,078	20,365
Oklahoma	6,346	6,484	6,558	5,337	4,746	5,364	7,233	8,173	8,406
Oregon	5,212	5,253	5,108	4,512	4,839	4,611	7,266	7,371	7,400
Pennsylvania	13,019	13,299	12,235	10,933	12,419	11,926	23,070	22,690	21,631
Puerto Rico	2,171	2,703	N/A	1,615	1,510	N/A	6,629	7,760	N/A
Rhode Island	1,623	1,403	1,409	915	1,018	1,348	2,844	2,621	2,302
South Carolina	3,191	3,036	3,190	3,689	3,022	3,140	4,644	4,645	4,566
South Dakota	N/A	1,308	1,441	N/A	1,106	1,042	N/A	1,101	1,215
Tennessee	N/A	5,968	5,480	N/A	3,481	4,370	N/A	10,796	10,144
Texas	7,025	8,938	9,939	7,665	8,200	8,283	15,182	16,326	18,236
Utah	2,196	2,383	2,148	1,956	2,332	2,264	2,468	2,273	1,805
Vermont	783	750	788	655	722	684	1,316	1,445	1,318
Virginia	2,639	2,776	2,768	1,354	2,200	2,139	7,213	7,264	7,391
Washington	7,541	7,369	7,590	7,123	7,376	7,129	8,872	8,688	8,945
West Virginia	2,011	2,151	2,392	1,767	1,973	2,256	3,082	3,169	3,388
Wisconsin	5,566	6,015	4,645	4,846	5,323	4,366	10,076	9,637	10,148
Wyoming	689	715	786	688	683	731	759	774	815
TOTAL	257,923	290,979	287,279	223,080	250,832	270,924	499,469	568,473	545,097

(From Children's Bureau, Department of Health and Human Services, 2002, Washington, DC: USDHHS.)

TABLE 3-4

UNDERSTANDING OF CHRONIC ILLNESS AT VARIOUS AGES

Age	Concept of Illness
Preschool	Magical thoughts
Early school age	Concrete, rigid ideas
	Little comprehension, although can list symptoms
Late school age	Child shows greater understanding of cause of illness
Adolescent	Understands abstract principles and concepts involved in the illness
Adult	Can understand cause and effect of illness and their role in coping

family to create a support network, and help them utilize resources within the family and the community.

Use of Child Care Services

Individual *child care* or group *day care* is a replacement for the direct care by a parent and is currently used more often than nannies, extended family members, sibling care, and private babysitters. Seventy-six percent of preschoolers with employed mothers received day care with someone other than a parent. Forty-five percent are in day care centers and 18% with nannies or relatives. More than 1 million families nationwide received federally funded day care services (Capizzano, Adams, & Sonenstein, 2000). Child care services are regulated for health and safety by the American Public Health Association but vary widely in ability to nurture growth and development. High-quality day care settings can contribute to cognitive development. The terms *day care* and *child care* do not indicate details about services provided. Some are babysitting-type services, and some provide early childhood education, based on known concepts of growth and development, by qualified staff. Day care is discussed further in Chapter 7.

UNDERSTANDING FAMILIES THROUGH THEORIES

A **theory** is a group of concepts that forms the basis for understanding observations. An accepted theory is logical, consistent, and integrates past and current research. Theories give us a way of studying family interaction or individual growth and development. The theories are useful because they help us understand why things happen the way they do and help us identify interventions needed for individuals or families that experience problems. Various theories of individual growth and development are discussed in detail in Chapter 4.

Family Systems Theories

Family systems theory is based on the understanding that family functions are interconnected. This means that what happens to one family member affects the entire family. No illness is seen as an isolated, individual event. Everything is viewed in the context of family interactions. For example, when a child has a problem such as anorexia, the entire family is affected. The problem of the child affects the family system, and the family system affects the general maintenance or recovery of the problem that the child is experiencing. Many problems of the individual, such as anorexia, can be manifestations of a dysfunctional family system. Therefore interventions, according to the family systems theory, must involve the whole family, not just the affected individual. Often, stabilizing the family group helps to stabilize the problem of the individual.

Murray Bowen, of Georgetown University, was one of the pioneers of the family systems theory, and Salvador Minuchin, of Argentina, first wrote about the values of family therapy in 1974. They stated that there are interactions among the biological, developmental, psychological, and social factors in the family that determine individual behaviors of each family member. There is a natural tendency in families to seek a stable state. For example, if one child is very aggressive and constantly breaks rules, another child in the family will assume the role of the good child to maintain family stability. This process is called *family dynamics*. Child guidance worker John Bowlby (1951) was a pioneer in describing how a child's distress was a reflection of a family in distress and treatment of both was essential to return to optimal health. It is therefore important for health care workers to understand the organization and communication within the family unit. Today, managed health care favors the treatment of the entire family rather than just the affected individual, because the results are quicker and last longer.

The Family Apgar

In 1978 George Smilkstein coined the term *Family Apgar* as a tool to assess family function. It was initially used by physicians and psychologists, and in 1982 an article in the *Journal of Family Practice* supported the reliability of the Family Apgar.

The Family Apgar is a way of looking at the family's ability to adapt, grow, develop, and resolve issues. Box 3-2 reviews the aspects of the family that are involved in determining family health and developing a family plan of care.

The role of the health care worker on the multidisciplinary health care team is to observe a family's function and ensure that the needs of each family member are being met. Referral to available community resources, which may include social agencies, school professionals, psychologists, or pediatricians, can help identify problems and

---

BOX 3-2 **Family Apgar**

- **A**daptation—sharing of resources and helping of family members
- **P**artnership—lines of communication and participation of family members
- **G**rowth—how responsibilities are shared among family members
- **A**ffection—visible and invisible emotional interactions among family members
- **R**esolve—how time, money, and space are used for solving or preventing problems among family members

Modified from Smilkstein, G. (1978). The family apgar: a proposal for a family function test and its use by physicians. *Journal of Family Practice*, 6(6), 1231-1238.

initiate the appropriate interventions early on. Accepting the nontraditional family and helping the adults care for their own physical and psychological needs are the first steps in helping the parents to care for their children and promote optimal growth and development of the entire family unit.

Developmental Theories

There are various theories of growth and development, and each theory emphasizes specific areas of development, such as motor, cognitive, social, and so on. Details of theories of development are presented in Chapter 4. Piaget offers a developmental theory of cognition, whereas Freud's theories involve behaviors that are motivated by unconscious wishes. Because the interaction of the individual with the world is a key element of development, psychosocial theories of development are also important to understand.

A **developmental stage** is defined as a period in life characterized by the mastery of specific skills or behaviors. Each stage incorporates achievements from the previous stage and contains skills, behaviors, or tasks necessary to enter and successfully master the tasks of the next stage.

Erik Erikson is one of the most well known psychosocial theorists, and his concepts are presented in Chapter 4 and throughout this text. Dealing with psychosocial conflicts using coping strategies and the use of support systems or significant relationships have an important effect on the developing personality.

Robert Havighurst was a theorist who described a sequence for the learning of developmental tasks at each stage of development, including tasks of late adulthood and for the aged. His view emphasized that society determines the skills that need to be acquired at each stage of development, but he pointed out that readiness to learn or teachable moments for acquisition of these skills need to be utilized or difficulties in later life can occur.

Betty Neuman, a nursing theorist, believed that nurses and the health care team members should care for the total patient and family needs, with special efforts to maintain interaction of the family within their environment. Specific interventions to reduce stress and achieve maximal wellness are the basis of the theory.

Evelyn Duvall, a family theorist, proposed specific stages of family development. Each stage of development is unique with new competencies to be mastered. Various stages of physical and psychosocial development occur at the same time, so all processes are *integrated*.

GROWTH AND DEVELOPMENT OF THE FAMILY
Developmental Tasks of the Family Life Cycle

The family has a life cycle of its own, which is described by events and influenced by the environment (Table 3-5). Deviation from the smooth flow of the family developmental cycle can result in dysfunctions.

A **developmental task** is a competency or skill that helps a person cope with the environment or advance personal development. Tasks occur in sequence, and mastery of developmental tasks of one stage are usually required to master developmental tasks of the next stage of development. There are physical, cognitive, psychological, motor,

TABLE 3-5

GROWTH AND DEVELOPMENT OF THE FAMILY

Stage of Development	Developmental Tasks
Marriage	Establish mutual goals and values. Define roles and responsibilities. Respect extended families.
Childbearing	Adjust to intrusion of child. Expand roles and responsibilities. Meet the needs of the child without losing sight of each other.
Childrearing	Meet own needs and continued achievements, as well as the needs of the children. Establish a child care philosophy.
Child launching	Maintain a supportive home base while letting go of the children to encourage their own fulfillment. Accept challenges to family values by children.
Contracting family	Experience empty nest syndrome as children leave home. Reintegrate and rediscover marriage relationship. Increase community involvement. Adjust to the grandparent role.
Aging family	Develop new roles and interests within limits of abilities. Fulfill lifelong dreams. Adjust to retirement. Cope with loss and loneliness. Adjust to declining income and energy. Maintain positive self-esteem. Maintain contact and relationship with children and grandchildren.

Modified from Duvall, E., & Miller, B. (1985). *Marriage and family development* (6th ed.). New York: Harper & Row.
NOTE: Each stage of family development has its own set of phases within that stage of development.

and psychosocial developmental tasks. Both the individual and the family have developmental tasks to be achieved at specific stages of development across the life span, such as the following:

- *Physical competencies*, which include functional abilities that result from motor and neurological development
- *Emotional competencies*, which include self-awareness, empathy for others, and utilizing strategies to cope with stress or frustrations
- *Social competencies*, which include the ability to form positive interpersonal relationships

The concepts of several theorists are presented in Chapter 4 and in each chapter covering the life cycle. Refer to psychology or anthropology texts for other details concerning individual theorists.

Role of the Nurse and Health Care Worker

Understanding the developmental stages and tasks of the family and the individual enables the health care team to provide individualized care based on that knowledge. Optimum growth and development results when the person or family masters each task in the various stages of the life cycle. When working with patients or families, health care team members must consider the developmental stage of the family and the individual, as well as cultural influences, before designing or carrying out a care plan that will meet comprehensive needs.

Childrearing Styles

Various family styles of functioning can be adopted by a couple in the beginning phases of family development and may be influenced by their cultural backgrounds. Some parents utilize an autocratic style, where decisions are made without the input of the children. Respect and obedience is expected without discussion. In the democratic family style, children are encouraged to participate in decision making, and all members of the family exhibit mutual respect. This is the ideal childrearing style because it nurtures positive self-esteem of all family members. The laissez-faire style offers complete freedom of all members with no rules, minimal if any discipline, and no effort at impulse control. Whichever style of childrearing and family development is selected, consistency of that style by both parents is essential for the development of stable family dynamics.

A functional family is a stable family unit (firmly established with constant members) with consistent rules whose members are able to deal with conflict, stress, and problems in a way that promotes the physical and psychological well-being of its members. A **dysfunctional family** is a family unit that does not offer consistency of members or rules, may exhibit poor interpersonal relationships among its members, deals poorly with conflicts and problems, and often cannot reach out to the community for help. Dysfunctional family styles often result in antisocial behaviors of family members, where behavior of individuals may violate the rights of others. Early referral by the health care team can help family members recapture self-esteem and break the cycle of family dysfunction in future generations.

When a family member has a problem, the nurse or health care worker must determine how the problem is perceived by the family, if coping skills exist, and if support systems are available. This is the core of a family care plan. The role of the nurse or health care worker is to help the family manage the problem. Referring the family to available community resources as appropriate and providing follow-up care are important in the plan of care.

Effect of Culture on the Family

Culture is defined as a set of learned values, beliefs, customs, and behaviors that is shared by interacting individuals, such as a family.

Cultural assimilation is a process by which members of a specific cultural group lose the characteristics of that group and adapt practices of another group. This is often referred to as "Westernization" of a culture when time spent in this country results in the adoption of an Americanized view of family function and behavior.

Cultural relativism is the concept that normalcy comes from the standard social practices of a specific culture. What is normal practice in one culture may not be considered normal practice in another culture.

Cultural shock is the effect of a sudden, drastic change in the cultural environment of an individual or family.

As people travel around the world with ease and frequency and families move from continent to continent, different cultural groups interact. Cultural backgrounds affect methods of communication and perceptions and response to health and illness. For example, in one culture, the response to a disability may be to hide it, whereas in another culture reentry into society is the treatment goal.

Ethnocentrism is the belief that one's own culture is the standard of behavior and is better than other cultures. Nurses and health care workers need to understand their own cultural beliefs and recognize how they may differ from their patients. It is unrealistic to expect the patient to change his or her cultural beliefs and practices. Health teaching plans must be designed to avoid conflict with the cultural beliefs and practices of the patient and family. Methods of communication are related to cultural practices. Understanding the culture and knowing who to communicate with in the family is essential in providing effective health care.

Cultural competence involves cultural awareness, acceptance, and respect toward behaviors and practices that are different from one's own. Achieving cultural competence is aided by knowledge, skills, and encounters with others of different cultures. Knowledge of various cultures and the ability to adapt the delivery of health care so that it does not violate the culture or religion of that group are the core of cultural competence. The nurse and health care worker must overcome cultural barriers to communication and behavior to provide effective health care to a culturally diverse society. Some cultural beliefs and practices related to stages within the life cycle are discussed in the following chapters. Cultural assessment includes values, socioeconomic status, communication patterns, nutrition, language, religious practices, health beliefs, and cultural aspects of the disease and illness.

ELECTRONIC MEDIA AND TECHNOLOGY: INFLUENCE ON FAMILY AND DEVELOPMENT

Media exposure includes newspapers, magazines, music compact discs (CDs), videotapes, movies, Internet sites, and television (TV). Electronic media has enabled families to be in immediate contact with the thoughts and actions of others around the world. The increased exposure of children to TV, computers, Internet sites, and video games may have some positive, as well as negative, influences on the development and behavior of children and adults, according to some recent studies.

The optimum style of TV viewing is family viewing, with adults selecting the programs and sharing thoughts with the child about what they are watching. However, studies have shown that many of the programs are not routinely viewed by the family together. Many programs typically selected by the child are developmentally inappropriate for the age of the child (Andreason, 1994). Thirty-two percent of children under 7 years of age and 53% of children between the ages of 12 and 18 have their own TV in their room (Shaefer, 2002). In a survey completed in 1999, most parents were not able to name their child's favorite TV program or video game.

In many homes the tragic attack on the World Trade Center in New York City on September 11, 2001, was viewed as it was happening and reviewed on TV for months afterward. This event brought terror into the private homes and lives as it was occurring.

Unlike reading a book, the use of electronic media such as TV does not require prior education to view. TV viewing is a passive experience. However, the developmental age of the child influences the child's ability to understand complex story plots that involve narration, cultural references, or interruptions in the continuity of the story. The character movement, sound effects, animation, and high-pitched voices in TV programs capture the attention of young children. Attention is maintained if the content of the program is understood by the child. Although some studies have shown that exposure to violent TV content can provoke aggressive acts in children who have a tendency for aggression, some authorities believe that desensitization may occur with repeated viewing of such content. There are many controversial opinions concerning the long-term effects of viewing TV violence on the behavior of children.

The Children's Television Act of 1990 has defined prime time or family-viewing time for programs and has placed some controls on programs aired during the hours young children may be watching. The American Medical Association (AMA) has offered guidance for health care workers in helping parents to monitor their children's TV viewing habits as part of healthy living counseling (Box 3-3).

Violent video games are of more concern than violent TV programs because interactive practice, repetition, reward, and reinforcement are elements within the video game, and these are the basic elements involved in learning a behavior. Learning and imitating aggressive behavior is a definite risk of interactive violent video games.

Some studies have shown that physiological changes occur during the interactive playing of video games. Release of a chemical called dopamine in the body increases, and dopamine is known to be related to learning, attention, and motor integration (Koepp et al, 1998). Another study (Funk, 1993) revealed that the powerful combination of demonstration, reward, and practice creates a learning environment, and the author related that finding to the fact that violence is a learned behavior. The lesson in

---

| BOX 3-3 | **Teaching Parents How to Manage the Media** |

- Monitor TV and video games that the child views.
- Do not use the TV or video games as a babysitter.
- Develop family guidelines for renting videos.
- Help the child interpret advertising.
- Provide opportunities for active play and socializing in balance with media viewing.
- Contact sponsors and TV stations and demand quality programming during hours when children are most likely to be watching TV.

some violent video games may be that violence is fun. Associating violent acts with a pleasant experience may provide the basis for learning violent behavior. This method of learning is the basis of training soldiers in how to shoot guns. Practicing shooting on video games increases hand-eye coordination that results in expert marksmanship in the real act of aiming and shooting a gun. A laboratory study (Emes, 1997) showed that children as young as 7 or 8 years of age acted out aggressively during free play after playing violent video games. Third- and fourth-grade students who played a violent video game provided more aggressive and hostile interpretations of stories with vague endings than children without violent video game exposure.

Because of the continued improvement in the realistic graphics of video games, further research concerning their effects is needed. The content of videogames, combined with daily, prolonged video game activity can also result in fatigue and sleep deprivation, which may lead to poor school performance. Most agree that video games should not replace other childhood activities such as athletics, chores, outside play, hobbies, reading, music, and homework. Often parents set limits on the time spent playing video games but do not restrict the type of game played and are often unaware of the violent nature of some video games. Parents need to be educated concerning the rating of video games and the amount of time the child should spend playing the games.

Video games can also have medical effects on players. The flicker frequency on the screen can trigger a seizure in a child who has photosensitive epilepsy. Also, an increase in blood pressure and oxygen consumption, breathing patterns, and adrenaline levels on a daily basis may contribute to heart disease later in life. Research is ongoing concerning effects of very low frequency (VLF) magnetic fields exposure during video games and TV viewing.

There are many positive outcomes of TV and Internet use by children. *Sesame Street* is an example of a TV program that provides positive messages and education for young children. A computer game and the Internet can provide interactive stimulation that captures the attention of the child and can offer help in developing processing skills and problem-solving abilities (Figure 3-2). Drills and repetition with periodic rewards can spark interest, maintain attention, and increase developmental abilities. Computer-assisted instruction is now offered in schools and community libraries and is also accessible at home at minimal cost. Distance learning enables an adolescent or adult to obtain college credit for courses without leaving home. Attitude and behavior remediation in the form of on-line driving schools are also available and popular. Video games can help increase hand-eye coordination, and many games are available without violent content.

The negative influences of the Internet on a child's behavior comes with the development of chat rooms and meeting places where sexual predators obtain private information and design personal meeting opportunities. The use of "cookies" to track interests and target the viewer for marketing ads requires parental supervision of the child's viewing choices to minimize negative effects.

The young adult can find sources of information on topics that formerly required hours spent in a library. Whether it is a hobby, a personal interest, or a specific need, further information is at the fingertips of the adult and is presented at all reading levels. Some critical thinking, in the form of evaluating the source of the information to determine validity, is important. Banking and other forms of financial activity can be

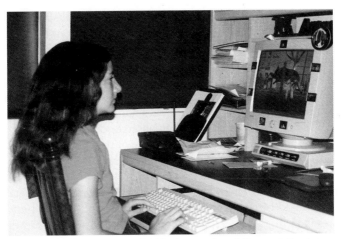

FIGURE 3–2 Computer games can provide interactive skills, and the Internet can offer a wealth of information to children and adults.

accomplished via the Internet. Older adults can find information about a health concern on the Internet, which can increase understanding of their own health problems and augment the teaching of the health care team. Print (font) size on the screen can be adjusted for the visually impaired. People for whom English is their second language (ESL) can have their Internet site information translated into their native language to enhance their pleasure and understanding. Digital video discs (DVDs) in the form of music, videos, or health information are available for use on the modern television and computer. Disabled persons confined to the home can enjoy personal contacts with the outside world. Often the E-mail abilities of the computer enable the elderly to maintain close communication with family and friends without the burden of writing a complete letter and finding a stamp to mail it.

EFFECTS OF A DISASTER ON FAMILY AND DEVELOPMENT

Disasters in the United States and around the world have been part of life in every generation. Disasters can occur in the form of a natural disaster, such as a hurricane, earthquake, or flood, or a human-made disaster, such as war. In the past, unless the family was personally involved in the location of the disaster, the event was recognized but soon forgotten and the impact on the individual family was thought to be minimal. Studies have revealed that children can suffer from **posttraumatic stress disorder (PTSD)** after witnessing parental violence within the family or any event that causes upheaval or disruption of their family life (Pfefferbaum et al, 2000). PTSD has been defined as the development of characteristic symptoms following an extreme traumatic stressor (APA, 2000). Some signs and symptoms of PTSD in children who have experienced a recent traumatic or abusive situation may be social withdrawal; appearing very serious (less playful) than other children their age; feelings of depression, anxiety, helplessness, or mistrust; giving up rather than displaying self-protective behavior; reacting quickly with fear; or having a dismal view of the future. Adults with PTSD, such as adult survivors of childhood trauma, may display similar emotions and behaviors. They may also develop an expectation of abuse or negative experiences and sometimes may unintentionally make choices and reactions that increase the risk of additional trauma. Symptoms of PTSD can be alleviated or prevented with psychotherapy. PTSD can affect the normal progress of growth and development. Today disasters are often viewed as they are occurring, in the privacy of the viewer's home via TV, and therefore can affect the family on a more personal level. Children observe adults on the TV screen struggle in the disaster area and then observe the response of their parents. Disasters near and far can be personalized by the family and therefore can influence family life and child development.

Studies have shown that boys born during wartime had developmental delays that may have been caused by an overattachment to the mother (Meijer, 1985). This overattachment resulted from an overprotective mother-child relationship directly influenced by the stresses of war. Emotional trauma from disasters can affect children emotionally and are influenced by parental reactions to the event.

Children respond to personal disaster by exhibiting anxiety, disorganization, confusion, inhibited activity, apathy, and withdrawal, as well as sleeping and eating dysfunctions. These responses can affect school performance and appetite, therefore impacting growth and development. In response to a disaster event, school-age children may regress to earlier developmental abilities and behavior patterns. Phobias, flashbacks, and reenactments during play are also common. Adolescents may respond with an increase in sexual promiscuity, vandalism, or substance abuse. These responses are the result of the child's perception of the disaster and the ability of the parents to cope as models of behavior. If a child is intimately involved in the disaster and strangers intrude in his or her life, these responses can intensify. Because children are dependent, they are more vulnerable to further trauma after a disaster occurs. If the community and the parents are personally affected, the child's functioning is disrupted. Symptoms of depression or stress that persist for more than a month after the disaster may warrant referral for a psychiatric evaluation.

Often parents are not aware of the child's responses or they tend to minimize the effect of the event on the child. The nurse and health care worker should be observant for signs of PTSD whenever in contact with a child in the aftermath of a disaster.

Children of rescue workers can develop anxiety concerning their parent's risky activities, and professional support may be indicated. The disaster of 9/11 demonstrated that the family does not need to be directly in the area of the disaster to have such aftereffects. Witnessing the disaster on TV in the privacy of their homes makes children almost as vulnerable as the on-scene victims. Nurses, health care providers, and teachers must advocate preparation and training for disasters and develop an awareness of risks in their own environment.

Role of the Health Care Team

Professionals who care for children have a responsibility to understand and respect the opportunities the fast-developing electronic media offer for learning and their role in revolutionizing education. There is also a need to help the child self-regulate choices of what to view and help parents utilize media in a positive way to promote a well-balanced lifestyle. Educating the public about quality programming and working with professional groups, industry, and regulating agencies to decrease the violence, pornography, and other negative aspects and promote quality programs are vital.

Nurses and health care workers must recognize that the response to disasters is influenced not only by a personal threat of injury or being close to the area of the disaster, but can be influenced by parental response to the event. Parents should be guided to provide extra emotional support to children, reassure them that their environment is safe, and try to maintain a familiar and consistent daily routine. Parents should be urged to discuss the disaster in honest terms at a level appropriate to the child's age. Drawings and play can be used to help children express their feelings. Parents can review how family members can help each other. Coping abilities of the children and the family should be monitored and referral for professional help offered as needed.

EFFECT OF COMMUNITY ON FAMILY AND DEVELOPMENT

Initially the family is the center of relationships that influence the development of the child. As the child grows, relationships expand and outside influences affect the family, as well as the child's growth and development. Teachers, coaches, clubs, teams, and peers each place demands on the family unit and have an increased effect on growth and development of its members. Most outside influences aid in learning social rules of behavior, help develop a sense of belonging, and contribute to the development of a positive self-image. The effects of outside influences during the stages of the life cycle are discussed in the following chapters.

FAMILY-CENTERED HEALTH CARE

In family-centered health care, the family is central to the plan of care for any individual family member. Identifying and valuing the strengths of the family network to cope, support, and assist in the care of a family member are essential. Today the family no longer hands over total responsibility of patients to health care personnel. Expanded visiting hours in the hospital setting allow family members to participate in care. Home care services have expanded to allow care of the patient in the home setting, with the family functioning as the experts and the nurse or health care team functioning as consultants in a true partnership experience that empowers the family. To achieve family-centered care, the nurse and health care worker must first listen to the family's perception of the problem and communicate the perception of the health care team, identifying similarities and differences. Armed with cultural competence and an understanding of the family as a unit, nurses and health care workers can provide meaningful, effective family-centered health care.

KEY POINTS

- The family is a social system that involves interaction with and commitment to its members.
- Family structures include the nuclear two-parent family, the dual-career family, the extended family, the single-parent family, the blended family, and others.
- Traditional family development includes marriage, childbearing, childrearing, child launching, the contracting family, and the aging family.
- A family systems theory is based on understanding that what happens to one member of the family affects the entire family.
- The family lifestyle; size, number, and spacing of siblings; and family health all have an effect on the growth and development of the child.
- Childrearing styles can be classified as *autocratic, democratic, or laissez-faire.*
- Culture is a set of learned values, beliefs, and customs that are shared by a family.
- Advances in technology and use of electronic media have enabled research of information and education to occur in the home setting.
- Interactive video games and television viewing involving violence can have a negative effect on the growth and development of children.
- Posttraumatic stress disorder can occur after viewing a live disaster scene on television and can affect growth and development.
- Community members such as teachers, coaches, clubs, and peers influence growth and development and place demands on the family unit.

CRITICAL THINKING

A newly divorced mother moves with her three children, ages 4, 7, and 15, into a new neighborhood. What interventions could a school nurse or health care worker use to help the family make a healthy adjustment to their new life?

MULTIPLE-CHOICE REVIEW QUESTIONS

1 A family is defined as:
   1 A structure consisting of two parents and at least one child
   2 A social system involving commitment and interaction
   3 Genetically related groups of people
   4 A group of people living together
2 A theory is:
   1 A logical, consistent concept based on research findings
   2 Concepts and thoughts accepted by most people
   3 An unproven concept based on an individual's observations
   4 A technique or intervention used to treat others

3 A family Apgar is:
   1 A tool to assess family function
   2 The financial status of a family
   3 A family systems theory
   4 A process of family therapy
4 A dysfunctional family includes:
   1 Stable family members
   2 Changing family membership
   3 Parents who manage the care of children
   4 Parents who utilize effective coping skills
5 The Children's Television Act of 1990 was designed to:
   1 Control programs aired when children may be watching
   2 Provide cartoons for young viewers
   3 Limit the number of hours children can watch TV
   4 Provide educational programs for preschool children

CHAPTER *4*

Theories of Development

OUTLINE

OBJECTIVES

Upon completion of this chapter, the student will be able to:

1 List theories of personality development.
2 Discuss one behavioral theory of development.
3 Discuss one psychosocial theory of development.
4 Discuss one environmental theory of development.
5 Discuss one cognitive theory of development.
6 Discuss the major forces that influence an adult learner.
7 Discuss how understanding developmental theories can enhance the ability to teach an individual who may be in a specific stage of development.
8 List some physiological, cognitive, personality, social, and emotional changes that occur over the lifespan.

9 Discuss the uniqueness of individual personality and behavior at each stage of the life cycle.

10 Practice a deeper understanding of self and family.

KEY TERMS

Behavioral theories
Behaviorist theory
Classical conditioning
Cognitive theories
Electra anxiety
Extrovert
Humanist theories
Information processing
Introvert
Looking-glass self
Moral reasoning
Oedipus complex
Operant conditioning
Psychodynamic theories
Social learning theory
Sociocultural theories

DEFINITION

A *theory* is a statement that explains principles that can predict behavioral development. It is designed to explain the development of a specific behavior and to suggest relationships of behavior to other developing social skills. A theory is based on research that helps to make observations and facts meaningful.

There is no single theory of development. **Psychodynamic theories** focus on personality trait development and psychological challenges at different ages; **cognitive theories** focus on advancement of the development of thinking; **behavioral theories** describe how behavior and behavioral learning changes; **humanist theories** describe the influence of human experiences such as love and attachment on behavior and personality development; and **sociocultural theories** describe how culture influences behavior. Each theory provides important insights into the different life stages. Human development is most accurately understood by integrating these theories.

IMPORTANCE OF UNDERSTANDING DEVELOPMENTAL THEORIES

Developmental theories focus on changes in physiology, psychology, and behavior that occur normally at different stages in the lifespan. Behaviors at different stages within the life cycle are influenced by culture, environment, past experiences, family, health status, and the reaction of the individual to all these events. The study of growth and development starts with conception and extends throughout the lifespan. Understanding what affects growth and development, in both a positive and negative way, helps nurses, health care workers, and educators predict behaviors, as well as responses, at each stage and therefore understand why adults may behave in certain ways. We now know that adults pass through predictable stages of development just as children do. Therefore studying growth and development in a continuum from birth to the geriatric adult provides a comprehensive understanding of how various life experiences affect growth and development at each stage of the life cycle. This understanding enables health care workers and educators to effectively intervene and foster positive physical and mental health care practices that will improve the lives of those they serve and teach.

Research concerning how babies decode speech has helped scientists develop computers that can decode speech. Understanding how behavior and personality are molded can help the nurse understand learning needs and teaching styles that will enable effective health education.

Specific changes occur in each phase of the life cycle (Figure 4-1). Therefore interventions at the appropriate time within each stage can effectively influence health practices and contribute to the achievement of the goals of *Healthy People 2010*. Anticipation of needs can help in the development of an effective health teaching plan.

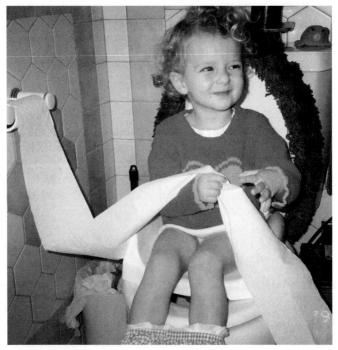

FIGURE 4–1 Toilet training. Learning self-control of bowel and bladder is a developmental task of the toddler. There are many child-size potties available, and eventually the child prefers adult facilities.

SELECTED THEORIES OF DEVELOPMENT
Psychoanalytic Theory (Freud)

Sigmund Freud was a psychoanalytic theorist who identified three interacting parts of a person's psychological functioning. They are as follows:

- *Id* (the unconscious) is present at birth and generates impulses that seek immediate pleasure and satisfaction.
- *Ego* is a view of the self or image a person wants to convey to others.
- *Superego* emerges between 3 and 5 years of age, delays immediate gratification for socially appropriate reasons, and represents recognition of good and bad. It is also known as a moral guide or a conscience.

Freud believed that conflict occurs when society gives mixed messages, causing the unconscious (id) to produce anxiety, which rises to the surface (conscious or ego) and become evident to the individual in his or her feelings and behavior. Freud described defense mechanisms that protect the ego by hiding unpleasant feelings from a person's conscious awareness and serves as a defense against anxiety (Box 4-1).

Freud believed that personality grows, develops, and changes during the lifespan but experiences in the early phases of development have a strong impact on the formation of the adult personality. Freud defined sexuality as any expressed bodily stimulation that is perceived to be pleasurable (Gormly et al, 1989). Freud described specific stages of psychosexual development (Table 4-1).

Psychodynamic Theory (Jung)

Carl Jung, a Swiss doctor, studied with Freud but did not believe sexuality was the basis of behavior development. He believed development extended into adulthood and that age 40 was the "noon of life." Jung believed the roots of personality are a reflection of the past culture of the family, which unconsciously molds the way a person perceives experiences as an adult. He was most recognized for describing personality traits, including the **introvert** (a quiet person who focuses inwardly on oneself) and the **extrovert** (an outgoing person who focuses on others in the environment). Jung believed that

---

| BOX 4-1 | Defense Mechanisms for Coping |

Rationalization: Developing a plausible excuse for unacceptable behavior.
Repression: "Forgetting" an unpleasant experience.
Projection: Attributing one's thoughts or feelings to another person.
Displacement: Expressing feelings (often anger) one has about one person toward another innocent person.
Reaction formation: Acting just the opposite of what one feels. For example, acting sure of oneself when one is really feeling insecure.
Regression: Reverting to immature behavior.
Identification: Joining a group so that its positive identity will be reflected on oneself.
Sublimation: Rechanneling unacceptable impulses into socially acceptable ones. For example, channeling aggression into playing football.

TABLE 4-1

FREUD'S STAGES OF PSYCHOSEXUAL DEVELOPMENT

Stage	Age	Description
Oral	First year of life	Focus is on mouth and the need to suck.
Anal	Toddler age	Focus is on learning self-control of bowels (see Figure 4-1).
Phallic	Preschool age	Attention is self-centered during this stage. Some type of masturbation often occurs at this stage. Child identifies with parent of opposite sex.* Superego develops at this time.
Latency	School age	Learns to suppress sexual urges and focuses on industry and achievement of skills.
Genital	Puberty	Deals with sexual urges involving the opposite sex (mature compared with phallic stage). Seeks mutual pleasure with a partner.

*Freud believed that the **Oedipus complex** arises during the phallic stage of development. Freud suggested that little boys compete with their father for the mother's love and attention. During this stage the boy prefers attention from the opposite-sex parent. As this stage ends, the boy decides to identify with his father and attention is desired from both parents again. The **Electra anxiety** occurs when little girls compete with their mother for the love and attention from their father. At the end of this stage, the little girl stops competing and identifies with the mother, again desiring attention from both parents. This occurs at about 5 years of age. Freud believed the experiences of the child played a role in forming adult personality but did not view the adult as a developing being. Thus Freud's theory has no identified stages beyond puberty.

the personality can be changed in the middle-adulthood phase, when repressed feelings are recognized and coping matures. Jung defined the process of recognizing one's own talent and abilities as *self-actualization*.

Stages of the Life Cycle: A Psychosocial Theory (Erikson)

Erik Erikson's theory describes the parts of personality development that are dependent on the social environment and social interactions. Each stage involves a social crisis or task that must be positively resolved to successfully pass to the next stage. For example, failure to establish trust with caregivers in the infant stage of development may affect the later life stage of intimacy, which is based on the ability to establish trust with another person. Successfully passing through each of these stages is thought to contribute to the overall development of the individual personality with unique strengths and weaknesses (Table 4-2).

The stage of adulthood proceeds through phases, which include occupation, marriage and family, friends, culture and religion, and leisure. Each phase has a period of stability, which could last several years, where values are pursued and choices are made. The phases are bridged by a transitional period of change, when reassessment occurs and modifications are made. For example, if a marriage occurred in one phase, divorce can occur in the transitional phase. Choices and changes are discussed in detail in the chapters concerning growth and development during the adult years.

TABLE 4-2

ERIKSON'S STAGES OF THE LIFE CYCLE

Stage	Age	Positive Achievement
• Trust vs. mistrust	Infant	Develops trust of others to meet one's own needs and as a result begins to trust oneself and others.
• Autonomy vs. shame and doubt	Toddler	Ability to act independently is equated with trusting oneself to be good.
• Initiative vs. guilt	Preschool	Imitates role models and follows rules. Experience self-control in social interactions.
• Industry vs. inferiority	School age	Develops ability to make friends and independently achieve school tasks.
• Identity vs. role confusion	Adolescent	Learns to know oneself and what one believes and develops a career goal.
• Intimacy vs. isolation	Young adult	Develops an ability to share all aspects of life with others.
• Generativity vs self-absorption	Middle adult	Can contribute to society in a meaningful way.
• Integrity vs. despair	Older adult (geriatric)	Maintains a sense of life achievement and absence of deep regret.

Erikson's theory involves generativity. Erikson believed that parents grow as their children develop and are influenced by parent-child interactions at each stage. He described specific stages of parenting (Table 4-3).

Psychosocial Theory (Levinson)

Daniel J. Levinson was a theorist who elaborated on Erik Erikson's theories. Levinson believed that an interaction among environment, culture, and the individual was the "fabric of life." Levinson believed that each person enters an orderly sequence of events

TABLE 4-3

STAGES OF PARENTING BEHAVIORS

Stage	Parenting Behavior
Stage 1: Parental image	Picturing oneself as a parent
Stage 2: Authority	Questioning parental skills as the child becomes autonomous
Stage 3: Integrative	Feeling responsible to motivate child as the child becomes more independent
Stage 4: Independent teen	Learning how to support teen while maintaining the authority role
Stage 5: Departure	Relating to the child as an adult as child prepares for the future and leaves home

or structures in life. The tasks of each structure are specific and identifiable. For example, Levinson defines the preadult as being between 17 and 22 years of age. The preadult first leaves the protection of the family, and that period serves as a bridge between adolescence and independent adulthood. The early adult (age 22 to 45 years) is at the height of vigor and vitality and makes important choices such as marriage, career, and lifestyle. The middle adult, age 45 to 65 years, is described as a transition phase with a gradual decrease of mental and physical functioning. The late adult, age 65 to 80 years, is the grandparent generation whose task is to define new goals and levels of involvement with family, friends, and community. The late-late adult (geriatric) stage begins at 80 years of age and involves the task of facing death, although the individual often continues to be socially interactive. Details of these stages are reviewed in later chapters.

Cognitive Theory (Piaget)

Jean Piaget was a Swiss psychologist who emphasized cognitive milestones in development. Piaget described four stages of development related to learning to understand and relate logically to the world (Table 4-4).

Piaget's theory involves sensory and motor interactions with the environment. An infant learns how to grasp a block and what relationship it has to the infant's body. The infant then learns that if he or she drops the block it will fall down and be out of reach. Gradually the infant learns that he or she can stack the blocks on top of each other, and eventually the infant can use the blocks to build something that represents a house or other objects in the environment.

TABLE 4-4

PIAGET'S FOUR STAGES OF DEVELOPMENT

Sensorimotor	Birth to 2 years	Gains developmental understanding of object permanence. Understands cause and effect. Understands differences in time of day.
Preoperational	2 to 7 years	Attributes life to inanimate objects. Child believes he or she is the center of world. Sees only the obvious. Understands only one bit of information at a time without seeing abstract relationships. Develops language skills. Uses pretend play. Begins to use logic to understand rules.
Concrete operations	7 to 11 years	Can understand more than one piece of information at a time. Has a realistic understanding of the world. Focus is on the present, not the future.
Formal operations	Adolescent	Can think abstractly and understand symbols. Can think in hypothetical terms. Is future oriented. Understands scientific basis of theories. Cultural practices play a role in helping adolescent understand "rules" and develop moral sense of what is right.

This interaction involves the thinking or processing of information of the child at different ages and stages of development. The **information processing** theory states that information is input, processed mentally, then followed by an output of judgment and decision making. This is believed to be the basis of problem-solving and critical thinking abilities. The basic technique of information processing does not change with age. Only the speed and efficiency of the processing improves with age to adulthood. Piaget's stages involve qualitative, not just quantitative, changes in thought.

Cognitive Theory (Loevinger)

Jane Loevinger stretched Piaget's model of development into the stages of adulthood. She believed that the ego adapts to demands and is an important basis for critical thinking. Loevinger believed ego development was progressive, with observable milestones throughout adult life.

Constructive Theory (Kegan)

Robert Kegan expressed a constructive developmental theory similar to Piaget's. Kegan believed there was a lifelong interaction with the environment, in which the individual moves through periods of changes in stability that provide a meaning to life. The core of Kegan's theory was the need to be included in reciprocal relationships with others and the need to maintain independence.

Theory of Language and Culture (Vygotsky)

Lev Vygotsky believed social and cultural experiences were necessary for optimum growth and development. Physiological maturation of the brain enables language development, which influences how a child thinks and behaves. His theory suggests that language is a major force in the growth and development of the personality (Table 4-5).

TABLE 4-5

VYGOTSKY'S LANGUAGE AND DEVELOPMENT THEORY

Age	Verbal Ability	Response of Parents
Infant	Cries and coos.	Parent responds to cry by cuddling, provides toys to stimulate responses.
Toddler	Points at objects.	Adult gives names and definitions to objects the child points at.
Preschool 3 years old	Speaks to self during play or movement.	Parents may or may not listen to all the words.
4 years old	Uses inner speech to guide behavior.	Parents praise the child for demonstrating delayed gratification or self-control
School age	Engages in speech and social interactions.	Parents who listen to their child understand the child's interpretation of events and experiences. Parents allow child to discover what they can do themselves and with the help of others.

Table 4-5 shows how language skills and social interaction affect each other and contribute to learning. People learn what they can achieve for themselves, and, through social interaction, what they can do with the help of others. This has implications for health education.

Social and Economic Influences (Bronfenbrenner)

Urie Bronfenbrenner presented a combination of social and economic factors that influence growth and development (Table 4-6). This theory offers insight into how children may be treated differently in different environments and the effect that may have on a child's understanding of himself or herself.

Hierarchy of Needs (Maslow)

Abraham Maslow described a hierarchy of needs. According to Maslow, if basic needs are met, then the individual can move to higher levels of thought and self-fulfillment. These needs are described by using a triangle. The base of the triangle represents the basic physiological needs of survival. As the sides of the triangle narrow, achievement of needs at each level allows movement toward a higher level (Figure 4-2). Once basic needs are met, a person can move toward self-actualization. Self-actualization is the realization of one's own talent and abilities and the achievement of satisfaction in life's goals and desires. It is reaching the peak of one's potential. For example, in severe poverty, basic physiological needs for food and shelter may be unmet. The person cannot think beyond meeting these basic needs of survival and so will not proceed to higher goals and ultimate self-actualization. Some characteristics of self-actualization

TABLE 4-6

BRONFENBRENNER'S SOCIAL THEORY OF GROWTH AND DEVELOPMENT

Social Contacts	Influence on Personality Development
Parents Siblings	Gender of child influences how others treat child and that influences child's behavior. Parental expectations of the child influence child's perception of self-worth.
Teachers Babysitters	Teacher's and babysitter's perceptions of the child influence child's sense of self. The active or aggressive child can be frustrating to teachers and babysitters and the quiet child is often more valued.
School Neighborhood Community	Coach may value an athletically talented child. The academically talented child may not achieve similar recognition.
Political community	Funding for school community centers and programs influence ability of child to experience these social opportunities. Some energy and behaviors, if not appropriately channeled, may become antisocial; poverty can result in poor nutrition that can decrease the ability to learn and develop.

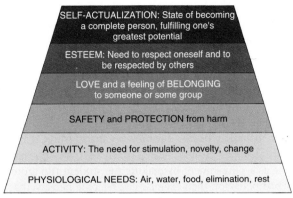

FIGURE 4–2 Modified version of Maslow's hierarchy of needs. (From Leifer, G. [2003]. *Introduction to maternity and pediatric nursing* [4th ed.]. Philadelphia: W.B. Saunders.)

include the accurate understanding of reality, judgments based on evidence, and the acceptance of self as independent and creative.

Environmental Theory (Rogers)

Carl Rogers believed people naturally form their own positive destiny, based on the concept of the self, if obstacles are removed. He theorized that mastery over the environment and positive relationships helped form the self-concept. A person has an idea of the type of person he or she would like to be. Sometimes there are differences between this idealized self and the actual self. If the ideal self shares a lot in common with the actual self, then that person discovers his or her full potential and achieves happiness. According to Rogers, self-actualization happens as a person realizes he or she can do many things to be like the ideal self.

Behaviorist Theory (Watson)

John Watson was known as the father of behaviorism. He believed the environment and experiences molded the personality. Inborn traits or drives are not the basis of his theory. Watson's theories are related to Pavlov's conditioning theory of personality development and Skinner's operant theory.

Behaviorist Theory of Personality (Pavlov and Skinner)

Ivan Pavlov and B.F. Skinner's theories describe learning and interaction with the environment as the center of development. This is known as the **behaviorist theory** of development. Behaviorists believe that personality and behavior are learned. Therefore they believe that there are no identifiable stages. Each experience helps to mold the adult personality.

These theorists believed that our environment and how we respond to the environment influence personality development. Pavlov developed the theory of **classical conditioning**. Conditioning has to do with associating (pairing) things in the environment. For example, when an individual eats a food that causes unpleasant symptoms of food poisoning, that individual may develop an aversion to that food. The food poisoning was paired with that food because they were experienced together. Because of this, that particular food is associated with negative feelings even without food poisoning occurring again.

Skinner attributed learning to **operant conditioning,** which involves behavioral consequences such as reward or punishment. For example, reinforcing positive behavior with a reward will eventually develop a regular practice of that behavior. Reward can be praise, special privileges, or material rewards such as toys, money, or candy.

These theories are useful in health education because positive reinforcement of information learned can result in positive health practices. The opposite is also true. If a coach uses exercise as a punishment by making the student run around a course or do 15 pushups after bad behavior, then exercise can become perceived as a negative activity and not considered to be a pleasurable experience. This can lead to a sedentary lifestyle and obesity later in life. Rewarding healthy behaviors such as exercise or medical compliance can increase the occurrence of these behaviors.

Social Learning Theories of Personality (Bandura and Mischel)

Albert Bandura and Walter Mischel were theorists who believed that social learning formed the basis for personality development (Bandura, 1977). **Social learning theory** involves exposure to and imitation of a behavior. Children often imitate what they see. If a father mows the lawn and receives praise for his work, the child witnesses the scenario and receives reinforcement of the positive aspects of that behavior. The child may copy that behavior out of curiosity or a desire to try out behavior of people they admire. In early childhood these models are the parents. In the school-age child, models may be peers. Therefore friends who belong to a gang and receive high praise from other gang members for their illegal or risky behavior can become the behavior models for the school-age child who is exposed to this type of social environment. The development of aggressive behavior and gender-specific stereotyped behavior may be intensified by the gangs or clubs the child is exposed to at this age.

Theory of Moral Development (Kohlberg)

Moral reasoning is the development of a set of social rules that enables a person to differentiate right from wrong. Moral behavior is based on perception and integration of these rules.

The Kohlberg theory consists of three levels that are closely related to Piaget's views (see Table 4-4). Kohlberg's stages of moral development (Table 4-7) remain a respected theory today, although modification of level three (the postconventional stage) has been suggested as a result of research findings. Carol Gilligan's work challenged the description of postconventional moral thought and also believed Kohlberg's research excluded women; therefore some findings may not be accurately applied to women. Moral behavior is generally considered to be learned, and therefore parents and schools provide rewards when the child demonstrates desired morally sound behaviors (Figure 4-3). Teaching a child right from wrong in a firm, loving way will result in the development of moral behavior. Helping a child understand how someone else feels in reaction to his or her behavior (empathy) is a preferred method of helping develop moral behavior.

TABLE **4-7**

KOHLBERG'S STAGES OF MORAL DEVELOPMENT

Stage	Age	Behavior
Preconventional	Toddler	Obeys rules to avoid punishments.
	Early childhood	Seeks to avoid punishment.
Conventional	School age	Conforms to rules to gain recognition or reward.
Postconventional	Adolescent and adult	Rules are followed that lead others to perceive one as "good." Develops a sense of responsibility.
	Older adult	Develops own set of principles that may overrule social laws or customs. Is independent.

Punishment often results in resistance and denial and turns the focus away from learning. Therefore it is not an effective tool for teaching moral behavior.

Development of Self-Image (Cooley and Mead)

Charles Horton Cooley had a theory called the **looking-glass self.** The theory states that the self-image is formed through three steps: (1) imagining how we portray ourselves to others; (2) imagining how others evaluate us; (3) combining these impressions

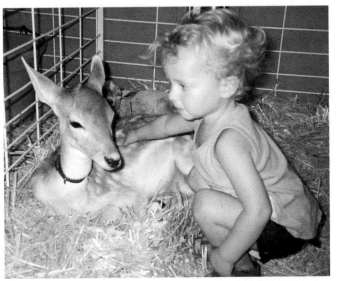

FIGURE 4–3 A young child understands the need to be gentle when touching animals. Critical thinking enables the child to be wary of this strange animal's responses.

to formulate a self-concept or idea of what we are like. For example, if a teacher criticizes a child, the child may think the teacher believes the child is stupid; therefore the child's self-image may incorporate appearing stupid.

George Herbert Mead furthered Cooley's theory by presenting three stages in the development of the self. In the first stage, children imitate those around them. The child uses a play broom to imitate the mother sweeping or a play lawn mower to imitate the father mowing the lawn. The child may vicariously feel proud of the clean floor or manicured lawn. When children are ready to experience the world of language, television (TV), and books, they are ready for stage two, which involves the use of language or other symbols during interaction with others, such as making a sad, pouting face; a happy face; and so on. In the third stage, the child pretends to be other people—for instance, a superhero such as Spider-man—and may play the role of the pretend person. In middle childhood the child understands his or her own role and the way it affects the role of others. A child learns what the expectations of others are and appreciates that each person assumes multiple roles in life, such as one person being a daughter, sister, mother, grandmother, and teacher.

Developmental Tasks of the Older Adult (Peck)

Robert Peck's theory is based on the developmental tasks of the older adult, which include dealing with retirement from work; adapting to the normal physiological decline due to aging; and facing the inevitability of death. Peck's theory involved the need to positively meet these challenges to maintain generativity (as described by Erikson) and avoid despair. Maintaining a positive self-image and feelings of self-worth, despite changing abilities and limitations, is essential to making a healthy transition in this stage.

Developmental Tasks of the Older Adult (Havighurst)

Robert Havighurst (1974) was a theorist who also described developmental tasks of late adulthood, which involve accepting oneself and maintaining meaning in life. The older adult's developmental tasks include adjusting to a decreasing health status, adjusting to decreased income, adjusting to the death of a spouse, adapting to changing social roles with peer groups, and adapting to a changing living arrangement.

Developmental Stages of Retirement (Atchley)

Robert Atchley described developmental stages in the older adult related to retirement. The five stages described by Atchley are listed in Table 4-8.

Many other factors influence growth and development. Cultural beliefs and practices have been discussed in Chapter 3. Gender differences also exist and affect development according to how the child is treated by others. At birth a girl is often dressed in pink frilly clothes and a boy in blue or brown. Toys selected by parents also enhance gender differences.

Poverty can decrease experiences available to the child, and it can also deprive the child of nutrition needed for brain and body development. The homeless child often does not have access to health care, and homeless adolescents may be exposed to drugs, sexual abuse, and other problems that affect growth and development.

TABLE **4-8**

DEVELOPMENTAL STAGES OF RETIREMENT

Stage	Focus
Preretirement	Dreams of retirement
Honeymoon	Enjoys freedom of retirement
Disenchantment	Designs new priorities as a result of boredom
Stability	Begins to feel needed and respected
Terminal	Changes because of need for reemployment or decline in health occur

There are developmental tasks to be achieved and challenges to be met in each phase of development through the lifespan. Psychological growth occurs through all stages of the life cycle and can modify a person's personality, behavior, and health.

KEY POINTS

- Personal development is influenced by many factors, including genetics, birth order, gender, and environment.
- A theory is designed to explain the development of specific behaviors and is based on research findings.
- Understanding developmental theories can help health care workers, nurses, and educators understand needs, learning styles, and behaviors at various stages of the life cycle.
- Understanding needs, learning styles, and behaviors at each stage of developmental enables the nurse, health care worker, or educator to plan teaching interventions that will contribute to the goals of *Healthy People 2010*.
- Understanding growth and development can help design teaching styles that will foster positive health care practices.
- Freud was a psychoanalyst who identified the id, ego, and superego and described stages of psychosexual development.
- Carl Jung believed development extended into adulthood, with age 40 as the "noon of life."
- Erik Erikson expressed a psychosocial theory that defined stages of the life from infancy through the older adult phase.
- Jean Piaget developed the cognitive theory of development that centered around understanding and relating to the world environment.
- June Loevinger stretched Piaget's theory of development into adulthood.
- Robert Kegan expressed a constructive developmental theory similar to Piaget's that involved lifelong periods of change and stability.
- Lev Vygotsky presented a theory of language and culture related to the developmental process.

- Urie Bronfenbrenner believed social and economic pressures influenced growth and development.
- Abraham Maslow described a hierarchy of needs theory leading to self-actualization.
- Carl Rogers believed people form their own destiny based on mastery of the environment.
- Ivan Pavlov and B.F. Skinner developed the behaviorist theory of personality development. They described how classical and operant conditioning influence behavior as it responds to the environment.
- John Watson was known as the father of behaviorism.
- K. Bandura and W. Mischel researched social learning theory as the basis of personality development.
- Lawrence Kohlberg described personality development based on moral reasoning. He believed moral behavior is a learned behavior.
- Charles Horton Cooley proposed the looking-glass self theory of personality development, and George Herbert Mead expanded the theory by presenting three stages in the development of the self.
- Robert Peck described developmental tasks of the older adult.
- Robert Havighurst described developmental tasks of late adulthood.
- Robert Atchley described developmental stages in the older adult related to the retirement phase of life.

CRITICAL THINKING

Using information from established theories of growth and development, explain why the diagnosis listed on the left might have the greatest impact on the development process of the age group listed on the right.

Diagnosis	Age Group
Fractured jaw	Infant
Fractured leg	Toddler
Fractured arm	School-age child

MULTIPLE-CHOICE REVIEW QUESTIONS

1 Which theorist described a hierarchy of needs that leads to self-actualization?
   1 Ivan Pavlov
   2 Abraham Maslow
   3 Lawrence Kohlberg
   4 Robert Peck

2 Health care workers need to understand developmental theories because it will
  help them:
  1 Pass the licensing examination
  2 Intervene effectively to promote positive healthy practices
  3 Design effective discipline for young children
  4 Analyze the goals of *Healthy People 2010*
3 Which psychoanalytic theorist first described defense mechanisms?
  1 Abraham Maslow
  2 Sigmund Freud
  3 Jean Piaget
  4 Lawrence Kohlberg
4 An understanding of object permanence is part of the stages of development
  described by:
  1 Jean Piaget
  2 Abraham Maslow
  3 Lawrence Kohlberg
  4 Sigmund Freud
5 Ivan Pavlov was a behaviorist who believed that personality and behavior develop
  under the influence of:
  1 Conditioning responses
  2 Genetic control
  3 Close parental guidance
  4 Chronological age

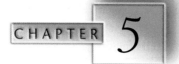

CHAPTER 5

Prenatal Influences on Healthy Development

OBJECTIVES

Upon completion of this chapter, the student will be able to:

1 State the goals of the Genome Project
2 Trace the steps of human fertilization and implantation.
3 Discuss the critical periods of fetal development.
4 Compare the similarities and differences in two types of twins.
5 Discuss the importance of prenatal health and nutrition to the health of the newborn and life expectancy.
6 Discuss the emotional changes that occur during transition to motherhood.
7 Discuss the importance of understanding culture as it affects the care of parents and newborns.
8 Discuss bonding and attachment between parents and newborns.
9 Describe the techniques of calming a newborn infant.
10 List the types of toys and activities that foster growth and development of the neonate.

66

KEY TERMS

Allele
Apgar score
Attachment
Bonding
Chromosome
Dizygotic
Dominant gene
Ectopic pregnancy
En face
Engrossment
Fetal alcohol syndrome
Fetus
Gene therapy

Genetic code
Genetic counseling
Genome
Gestation
Monozygotic
Multifetal
Mutated
Neonatal
Sibling rivalry
Syndrome
Viable
Virus vector

THE GENOME PROJECT: UNLOCKING THE SECRETS OF INHERITANCE

Growth and development are influenced by biology and by the environment. Research concerning the maternal-fetal origins of adult disease contributed to the development of the Human Genome Project. The National Institutes of Health (NIH) and the Department of Energy (DOE) assumed leadership of the many scientists who probed the secrets of human genetic makeup for this project. Various grants were awarded to finance the research. The project officially started in 1990, and a draft of the findings was published in 2001. The original goals of the project involved the following:

- Identifying the more than 30,000 genes contained in human DNA
- Determining the sequence of the billions of chemicals that are contained in DNA
- Developing tools for analysis of the findings
- Addressing the ethical, legal, and social implications (ELSI) involved
- Transferring the technology for use by the public in the private sector

A **genome** is a complete set of DNA that is contained in all human cells. (A *cell* is the basic working unit of all living systems.). The DNA in the genome is the genetic code of a cell that is carried on the chromosomes. A **chromosome** is a thread of protein and DNA contained in the nucleus of every cell. Each chromosome contains genes, and there are approximately 30,000 genes in a genome. The genes or **genetic code** within these cells carry information about all the proteins within the cell that will determine what characteristics will be inherited (Figure 5-1).

Heredity is controlled by pairs of genes from both the mother and father. This pairing of genes is called an **allele.** Genes can be dominant or recessive. A **dominant gene** will overpower a recessive gene most of the time, so that its characteristic will be inherited in about three out of four offspring. The fourth offspring may evidence characteristics of the recessive trait (Figure 5-2).

Inside the Cell

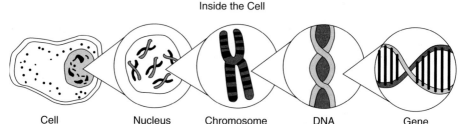

Cell   Nucleus   Chromosome   DNA   Gene

FIGURE 5–1 The cell contains the nucleus, chromosomes, DNA, and genes. (From Burroughs, A., & Leifer, G. [2001]. *Maternity nursing: An introductory text* [8th ed.]. Philadelphia: W.B. Saunders.)

The Genome Project involved gene mapping, which determined the makeup of human genes. The completion of the Genome Project in 2001 resulted in the identification of all human genes. Studying the characteristics and role of normal, as well as **mutated** (variations that may be abnormal), genes enables genetic therapy to be utilized to correct mutated genes and replace missing genes that cause specific syndromes. A **syndrome** is a group of symptoms or signs of an abnormal condition. It is known that specific genetic syndromes contribute to specific behavior patterns. Behavior patterns can result in a response from the environment, which can then affect a child's self-image, as well as growth and development. For example, a genetic abnormality that causes Down syndrome or an uncontrolled glucose (sugar) level in a diabetic mother or poor nutrition during pregnancy can each cause cognitive damage in the newborn infant that will impact the child's growth and development.

Genetic counseling is the communication between a geneticist (a specialist in inherited conditions) and the parents to discuss the risk of their infant inheriting genes that could result in an abnormality. It is known that behavior is molded by the influence of genes, as well as environmental factors. The success of the Genome Project will allow more detailed research concerning central nervous system problems and resulting behaviors that occur due to genetic problems. Because of the Genome Project, researchers have developed *therapeutic genes* that repair defective DNA, *suicide genes* that can be programmed to destroy defective genes, and *pure genes* that can replace a missing gene. **Gene therapy** involves placing a therapeutic gene on the back of a **virus vector** (a virus vector is a virus that has the ability to enter specific cells in the body). The virus vector carries the new gene into the cell that has a missing or defective gene. Gene therapy is in its infancy. Some problems and side effects must be controlled before gene therapy is available for widespread clinical use. However, gene therapy holds much promise. The ethical, social, and legal aspects of gene therapy will need to be clarified in the near future and standardized polices developed.

Screening Procedures and Therapies

In the past it has been possible to screen individual patients for the existence of some specific genetic problems without looking at DNA, such as using hemoglobin electrophoresis for types of anemia or the Guthrie test for phenylketonuria (PKU), a condition in which phenylalanine accumulates in the body and causes mental retardation. However, DNA-based genetic tests can detect carriers, identify susceptibility, and

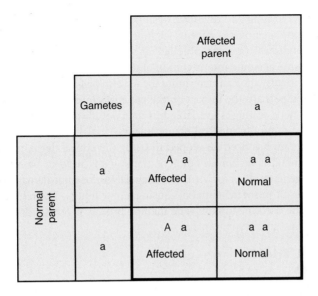

Characteristics of autosomal dominant inheritance

Males and females are affected with equal frequency.
Affected individuals will have an affected parent,
although expression may be variable (unless the
condition is caused by a new mutation
orgermline mosaicism).
Children of a heterozygous affected parent have a
50% probability of possessing the defective
gene, although it may be nonpenetrant.
Children of affected parents who did not receive the
affected gene will have unaffected children.
Traits can be traced vertically through previous
generations—a positive family history—unless
it is a new mutation, germline mosaicism, or
nonpenetrant.
Autosomal dominant disorders are more common than
recessive disorders and are usually less severe.

FIGURE 5–2 Transmission of dominant and recessive traits. One parent has a dominant gene (A) and one recessive gene (a) for a disease. The other parent has two recessive genes (a) for the disease. This chart shows the chances of their child being affected by the disease. (From Wong, D., Hockenberry-Eaton, M., et al. [1999]. Whaley & Wong's nursing care of infants and children [6th ed]. St. Louis: Mosby.)

enable diagnosis before symptoms occur. Carrier testing is possible and genetic counseling can be initiated for sickle-cell and thalassemia disease (where a genetic trait causes an abnormal shape or type of red blood cells), Tay-Sachs disease (which is a destruction of nerve cells that causes mental and motor deterioration and death during early childhood), and cystic fibrosis (which involves a malfunction of the exocrine glands that results in lung and digestive dysfunctions). Some adult-onset diseases can be diagnosed before symptoms appear, such as kidney disease, Huntington's chorea, and Lou Gehrig's disease (amyotrophic lateral sclerosis). However, genetic specialists are needed to ensure accurate interpretation of test results. This type of testing requires a team of professionals who can determine the psychological impact of this knowledge on the patient and perhaps the impact on the patient's employment eligibility, now and in the future. Genetic testing is available but may not always be affordable, appropriate, or relevant to optimum medical management.

The ELSI program has been developed to study the ethical, legal, and social implications of gene therapy. Techniques of gene therapy still need to be refined to ensure that inserting a gene on a vector virus to repair DNA does not damage the DNA in a way that could result in the potential of causing a new illness. The refinement of a suicide gene might be used to stop the gene therapy process if genetic damage is noticed. Research is ongoing and very promising.

THE PRENATAL PHASE
Critical Periods

Many of the critical periods during fetal growth occur during the first *trimester* of pregnancy (first 3 months), when basic structures are developing. Many of these factors can affect growth and development throughout fetal life, such as undernutrition, which can cause a reduction in the number of cells produced, resulting in health problems after birth.

Inadequate nutrition during fetal development can change the structure, physiology, and metabolism in the body and can predispose to the development of coronary artery disease or stroke in adult life (Barker, 1998). There are strong indications that coronary disease in adulthood originates in utero (Goldberg et al, 1994). A newborn who has a low birth weight with a small head circumference may be at risk for coronary disease. Low placental weight may be associated with predisposition for stroke in later life (Curhan, 1996). Every system in the body has a critical period in which nutrition, drugs, and other environmental factors influence its development and function. Illness, lack of nutrition, or exposure to toxins during this critical period can cause a maldevelopment or malfunction of a specific organ or system that may not manifest until adult life.

Lower respiratory tract infections in infancy may be an indicator of impaired lung growth that can increase the risk for chronic bronchitis in adulthood. Exposure to environmental factors such as smoking can increase vulnerability to serious bronchitis and respiratory problems in adulthood. The balance of maternal protein and cholesterol levels in late pregnancy and the amount of fat in the mother's diet can influence the development of later diseases in the child even though the infant may appear normal at birth.

The well-being of the mother and fetus can influence the life expectancy of the newborn. In accordance with the goals of *Healthy People 2010,* to prevent disease in the next generation we need to improve the nutrition of mothers and babies and reduce exposure to infection in early childhood (Barker, 1998).

Toxins

Teratogens (toxins) are harmful influences on fetal growth. Exposure to toxins during fetal development can cause abnormalities, illness, or miscarriage. Maternal ingestion of substances such as alcohol can interfere with cell growth in the developing fetus. For example, **fetal alcohol syndrome** is characterized by mental retardation and abnormal facial features. Recreational drug exposure during pregnancy can cause prematurity, seizure disorders, and learning disabilities in the newborn infant. Maternal cigarette smoking can cause decreased birth weight in the newborn. Mothers are alerted to avoid contact with litter boxes of cats during pregnancy because of the risk of developing a condition called toxoplasmosis, which can be devastating to the newborn. Radiation exposure during x-rays and lead contamination in the environment are examples of other environmental toxins that are harmful to a growing fetus.

Maternal illness must be prevented and certain immunizations avoided during pregnancy to prevent untoward effects in the fetus.

For example, the immunization for measles (rubella) involves use of a live virus that can cross the placenta and affect the growing fetus.

Maternal Adaptations During the Prenatal Phase

The changing patterns of childrearing, the increasing number of two-career households, and the increasing distance between extended family members influence the social support systems available to parents-to-be. Dependency on physicians is decreased because the large health maintenance organizations (HMOs) or health care facilities may not guarantee a regular personal physician to follow each pregnant woman throughout her pregnancy.

Parents need to be well informed to make healthy decisions about pregnancy, delivery, and child care. Parents need to be involved in developmental issues concerning their role as a parent and their impending change in lifestyle.

Attitudes are forming. If the pregnancy is planned and wanted, attitudes will most likely be positive. If the pregnancy is unplanned or unwanted, interventions and referrals may be necessary to help the parents develop a positive attitude or select alternatives such as adoption or abortion. The timing of the pregnancy in the life of the parents is also an important consideration. Adolescents may not have completed the transition to adulthood, may still be in the protective environment of their own parents' home, and so may need a more intensive adjustment period to establish their own independence.

The initial phase of establishing a family after marriage (see Chapters 3 and 10) involves adjusting to a marital adult affiliation with establishment of mutual goals, housing, financial responsibilities, educational pursuits, and lifestyle choices. Entering into the role of a parent who is responsible for a dependent child is, according to Erikson, the beginning of the stage of generativity. The mother is motivated to psychologically prepare for the arrival of the infant as she feels the fetus move in the womb (uterus); a state of attachment occurs, and rapport with the fetus develops. The partner attends parenting classes with the pregnant woman and is included in the attachment process as the fetus grows and develops (Figure 5-3).

The first stage in the development of a parent has three distinct phases, each with specific tasks (see Table 10-2). The first phase is response to finding out conception has occurred. The parents may be elated or disappointed. Lifestyle changes will be discussed. The second phase occurs in the second trimester (months 4 to 6 of the pregnancy), when fetal movement is felt, an ultrasound picture of the fetus is often seen, and the reality of the pregnancy becomes evident. Parents may worry about the health of the infant and plan for its place in the home (Figure 5-4). The third phase occurs in the third trimester (months 7 to 9), when plans for the actual birth of the baby become the focus. The father may worry about competing for attention and may feel left out. Old conflicts may surface. Parents may feel inadequately prepared for the responsibility of caring for the newborn. Parenting classes are available in most communities for referral as needed.

FIGURE 5–3 The father begins to bond with the fetus as the fetal heart and fetal movement can be felt.

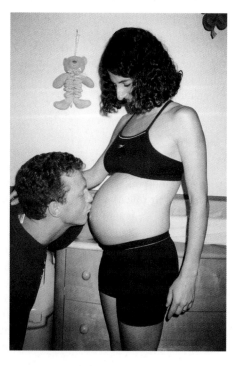

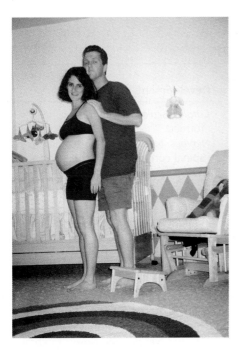

FIGURE 5–4 The parents-to-be proudly show the room prepared for the new baby, which includes a crib and a brightly colored mobile.

Fetal Development

Fertilization occurs when the sperm penetrates the ovum as it enters the upper portion of the woman's fallopian tube. The time in which fertilization can occur is brief because the sperm lives for up to 5 days, but the ovum lives for only 24 hours after ovulation (see Chapter 9 for discussion of puberty and the menstrual cycle). The ovum always contributes an X chromosome, and the sperm contributes either an X or Y chromosome. The combination of XX chromosomes produces a female fetus, whereas an XY combination results in a male fetus. Because it is only the sperm that carries the Y chromosome, the male partner determines the sex of the infant. However, the female has some influence on which sperm fertilizes the ovum, because estrogen levels and the pH of the reproductive tract affect the survival rate of the X- and Y-bearing sperm and the speed of their movement to the fallopian tube.

The *zygote* is the cell formed by the union of the sperm and ovum. The cell rapidly multiplies and develops. Within 1 week it enters the uterus and attaches to the upper posterior portion of the uterine wall. (If the zygote does not move freely through the fallopian tube, its increasing size will rupture the fallopian tube, and this condition is known as an **ectopic pregnancy.**) After implantation into the wall of the uterus, the cells differentiate into layers called the endoderm, mesoderm, and ectoderm. Each layer develops into different organs of the body. After 2 weeks of growth and development, the zygote is called an *embryo*. From the ninth week of life to birth, the developing baby is called a **fetus.** Fetal development is show in Table 5-1.

The third week after fertilization, the heart begins to beat and the neural tube (the beginning portion of the central nervous system) forms. For this reason, the mother

TABLE 5-1

EMBRYONIC AND FETAL DEVELOPMENT

Age	Length and Weight	Development
Week 3 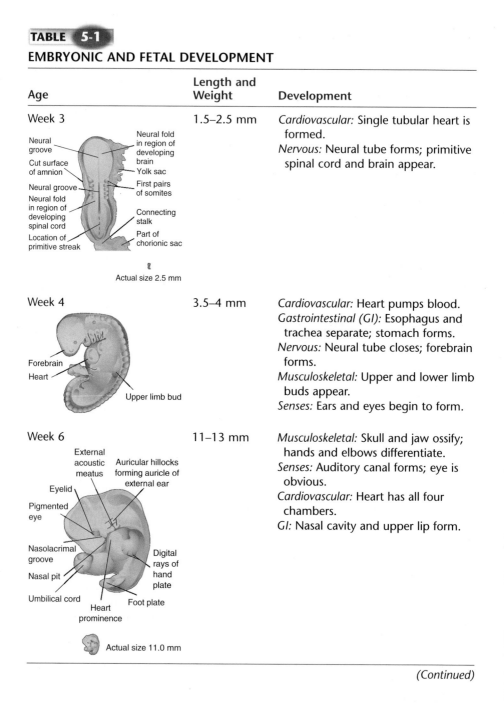 Neural groove / Neural fold in region of developing brain / Cut surface of amnion / Yolk sac / Neural groove / First pairs of somites / Neural fold in region of developing spinal cord / Connecting stalk / Location of primitive streak / Part of chorionic sac / Actual size 2.5 mm	1.5–2.5 mm	*Cardiovascular:* Single tubular heart is formed. *Nervous:* Neural tube forms; primitive spinal cord and brain appear.
Week 4 Forebrain / Heart / Upper limb bud	3.5–4 mm	*Cardiovascular:* Heart pumps blood. *Gastrointestinal (GI):* Esophagus and trachea separate; stomach forms. *Nervous:* Neural tube closes; forebrain forms. *Musculoskeletal:* Upper and lower limb buds appear. *Senses:* Ears and eyes begin to form.
Week 6 External acoustic meatus / Auricular hillocks forming auricle of external ear / Eyelid / Pigmented eye / Nasolacrimal groove / Digital rays of hand plate / Nasal pit / Umbilical cord / Heart prominence / Foot plate / Actual size 11.0 mm	11–13 mm	*Musculoskeletal:* Skull and jaw ossify; hands and elbows differentiate. *Senses:* Auditory canal forms; eye is obvious. *Cardiovascular:* Heart has all four chambers. *GI:* Nasal cavity and upper lip form.

(Continued)

TABLE 5-1

EMBRYONIC AND FETAL DEVELOPMENT—cont'd

Age	Length and Weight	Development
Week 8	30 mm crown-rump 6 g	Embryo has distinct human appearance. Purposeful movements occur. Tail has disappeared. Sex organs form. Beginnings of most external and internal structures are formed. Enters fetal period.
Week 17	150 mm crown-rump 260 g	Genitalia and leg movements are visible on ultrasound and may be felt by the mother. Bones are ossified. Eye movements occur. Fetus sucks and swallows amniotic fluid. Ovaries contain ovum. No subcutaneous fat is present. Thin skin allows blood vessels of scalp to be visible.
Week 25	28 cm (11.2 inches) crown-heel 780 g (1 lb 10 oz)	Wrinkled skin, lean body results from lack of subcutaneous fat. Eyes are open. Fetus is now viable. Mother feels stronger movement (quickening). Fetus has schedule of sleeping and moving. Vernix caseosa is present on skin. Lanugo covers body. Brown fat is formed. Lungs begin to secrete surfactant. Fingernails are present. Respiratory movements begin.

Week 8 illustration labels: Scalp vascular plexus, Eyelid, Eye, Nose, Mouth, Wrist, Umbilical cord, Toes separated, Sole of foot, Knee, Auricle of external ear, Shoulder, Lower jaw, Arm, Elbow. Actual size 30.0 mm.

(Continued)

TABLE 5-1

EMBRYONIC AND FETAL DEVELOPMENT—cont'd

Age	Length and Weight	Development
Week 29	38 cm (15 inches) crown-heel 1260 g (2 lb 10 oz)	Fetus assumes stable (cephalic) position in utero. Central nervous system is functioning. Skin is less wrinkled because of the presence of subcutaneous fat. Spleen stops forming blood cells, and bone marrow starts to form blood cells. Increased surfactant is present in lungs.
Week 36	48 cm (19 inches) crown-heel 2500 g (5 lb 12 oz)	Subcutaneous fat is present. Skin is pink and smooth. Grasp reflex is present. Circumferences of head and abdomen are equal. Surge of lung surfactant is produced.

Note: Full-term is considered 38-40 weeks. The crown-heel length is 48-52 cm (18-21 inches), and the weight is 3000-3600 g (6 lb 10 oz-7 lb 15 oz).

Table 5-1: Unn. figs. 5-1, 5-2, 5-3, 5-4, From Moore, K.L., & Persaud, T.V.N. (1998). *The developing human: Clinically oriented embryology* (6th ed.). Philadelphia: W.B. Saunders. Unn. figs. 5-5, 5-6, 5-7, 5-8, From Moore, K.L, Persaud, T.V.N., & Shiota, K. (1994). *Color atlas of clinical embryology*. Philadelphia: W.B. Saunders.

must take prenatal vitamins to ensure adequate intake of folic acid, which is essential for normal neural tube development. Conditions such as spina bifida can occur if there is a deficiency of folic acid when the neural tube is forming. The placenta takes control of fetal circulation at the end of the third month of pregnancy. The umbilical cord attaches the fetus to the placenta and a thin membrane separates maternal and fetal blood, because the two blood supplies do not normally mix. By 20 weeks of **gestation** (fetal life), the fetus is considered **viable** (able to survive outside of the uterus). However, the lack of a substance called surfactant in the lungs at this stage of fetal development would require that special neonatal intensive care be provided. Some surfactant is produced by 28 weeks' gestation, and another spurt of surfactant is deposited into the lungs of the fetus at 32 weeks' gestation. After 38 weeks of gestation, the fetus is considered to be full term and ready to be born. A woman should start prenatal care as early as possible. Adequate nutrition and exercise during pregnancy are beneficial, and monthly visits to the health care provider enable monitoring of the pregnancy to ensure a healthy outcome for both mother and baby.

Twins

Twins or other **multifetal** births (e.g., triplets, quadruplets, and so on) can occur. A fraternal twin is also called a **dizygotic** twin and occurs when two ova are released at ovulation and each ovum is fertilized by a separate sperm. The twins may or may not be of the same sex and are as alike as siblings. **Monozygotic** twins are called identical twins and occur when one single fertilized ovum separates into two separate embryos. These twins will be of the same sex and will be genetically identical (look alike). Many twins are born prematurely because the uterus becomes overdistended or the placenta is unable to supply the nourishment required to carry the pregnancy to term.

THE BIRTH PROCESS

Childbirth is a normal physiological process that affects the health of the mother and fetus. Labor and delivery are often a family affair with fathers or significant others participating and grandmothers closely involved. Attendance at preparation classes during pregnancy and the cultural background of the parents usually dictate the extent of the supportive role of the partner or grandmother in the labor and delivery unit. A woman can choose to deliver the baby in a traditional hospital setting, in a freestanding private birthing center, or at home. *Obstetricians* (doctors with special education in women's health), *nurse practitioners* (registered nurses with advanced practice education), or *nurse midwives* (registered nurses with advanced labor and delivery education) may be in attendance to monitor the process. A *doula* is a specially trained labor and delivery coach who may stay with the mother during labor and the birth of the baby. The birth process occurs in four stages. The first stage is the dilation (opening) and effacement (shortening) of the uterine cervix. The second stage is the descent and birth of the baby, and the third stage is the birth of the placenta (afterbirth). The fetal heart rate and the contractions of the uterus are monitored closely during the birth process. The fourth stage is the recovery stage, when bonding takes place and the family is united and monitored.

THE NEWBORN INFANT

As the infant is born and the umbilical cord it cut, many physiological changes occur in the infant's body to enable it to adjust to life outside of the uterus. The lungs expand and the circulation pattern that allowed bypass of the lungs during fetal life changes so that all blood will circulate to the lungs to receive oxygen. The cyanotic (blue) color of the skin quickly changes to pink as the infant cries and oxygenation is established. The infant is dried, placed in a pre-warmed bed and the head is covered to minimize heat loss until the infant can stabilize his own body temperature. The vital signs of the newborn are monitored and an Apgar score is assessed at one minute and five minutes after birth. The **Apgar score** is a rating of heart, respiration, muscle tone, color, and reflex irritability. A score from 1 to 10 gives an estimate of the condition of the infant and determines the need for further resuscitation efforts. The infant receives vitamin K to aid in blood clotting in the umbilical cord and an antibiotic ointment is placed in the infant's eyes to prevent ophthalmic neonatorum and *Chlamydia* infection, which if left untreated could lead to blindness in the neonate. An identification band with a special number is placed on the infant, mother and significant other and footprints of the newborn may be taken.

It is important for the nurse to promote bonding and attachment as soon as possible after birth (Figure 5-5). **Bonding** refers to a strong emotional tie between parents and the newborn. **Attachment** refers to an affectionate tie that occurs over time due to parent-infant interaction. Bonding begins during pregnancy, but it is most important that touch and visual interaction occur as soon as possible after birth. The newborn should be placed in the mother's arms, and put to breast if breastfeeding, as soon as possible after birth. The *en face* (face-to-face) position facilitates eye contact between infant and parent (Figure 5-6). The infant can see a short distance at birth and responds to close face-to-face encounters. The infant is most alert in the first hour after birth and then several hours of sleep and decreased motor activity will follow. Parent-infant bonding should be the focus of care during this first hour of life.

THE TRANSITION TO MOTHERHOOD

The transition to motherhood involves hormonal changes, changes in self-image, and reorganization of the tasks that face the new mother. Mood swings are common.

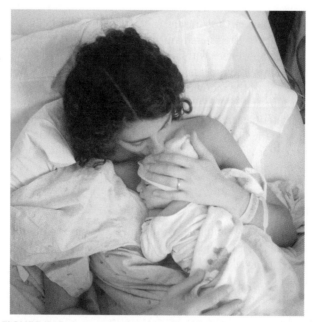

FIGURE 5–5 A new mother bonds with her newborn infant.

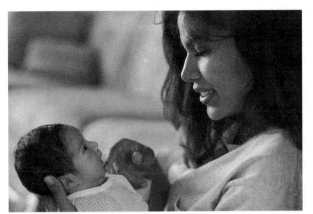

FIGURE 5–6 The "en face" position between mother and infant. The newborn gazes at the mother and responds to her voice and touch. (From Gorrie, T.M., McKinney, E.S., & Murray, S.S. [1998]. *Foundations of maternal-newborn nursing* [2nd ed.]. Philadelphia: W.B. Saunders.)

Irritability and fatigue may peak by the fifth day after delivery. Conflicting feelings of joy and depression are called the *postpartum blues*, and the symptoms are typically self-limiting. Discharge teaching concerning self-care and infant care, support, and reassurance should be offered. Rubin's descriptions of the psychological changes that occur after birth have been a framework for the care of new mothers for more than 35 years. The behavioral changes that occur help health care workers understand the new mother as she progresses through these stages (Table 5-2).

Fathers or Significant Others

Fathers or significant others develop an intense focus on the newborn, which is called **engrossment** (Figure 5-7). A realignment of relationships with his own parents, past experience with children, and relationship to his wife or partner are factors that will affect his bonding experience. When a new infant is added to the family, some of the

TABLE 5-2

RUBIN'S PSYCHOLOGICAL CHANGES AFTER BIRTH

Phase 1	"Taking in." The woman is passive, lets others care for her and infant, and talks about the delivery experience. The mother usually requests food and opportunity to sleep.
Phase 2	"Taking hold." The woman begins to initiate care of the infant and assumes responsibility for self-care. The woman is most receptive to teaching at this stage.
Phase 3	"Letting go." The parents recognize the reality of the new lifestyle and responsibilities they face and accept the gender and unique appearance of the new child.

Modified from Rubin, R.R. (1963). Maternal touch at first contact with the newborn infant. *Nursing Outlook, 11,* 828.

FIGURE 5–7 The "en face" position between father and infant. The intense fascination that fathers exhibit is called *engrossment*. (From Gorrie, T.M., McKinney, E.S., & Murray, S.S. [1998]. *Foundations of maternal-newborn nursing* [2nd ed.]. Philadelphia: W.B. Saunders.)

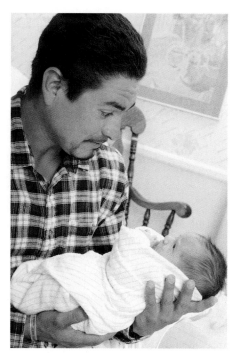

roles and responsibilities of the father or partner may also change. Fathers or partners may be expected to take more time and responsibility for the older sibling, who will need repeated reassurance and validation of continued love. A change in sleep patterns, new financial stresses, and changes in routines can be stressful for some fathers or partners. Plans for child care of other children while both parents are focused on the birth of the newborn need to be in place well before the occasion arises.

Siblings

The influence of the new child's birth on siblings depends on their age and developmental level. Toddlers may regress and be angry. Older children may enjoy helping with the newborn, and adolescents may feel embarrassed about their mother giving birth. A sibling relationship is a lifelong relationship that begins at birth and is characterized by both close friendship and intense rivalry. **Sibling rivalry** is the competition between siblings, usually for parental attention and love.

The initial relationship between a newborn and a sibling is established by the parent's interaction with each child (Figure 5-8). When the newborn is presented to the sibling as a person with feelings, the sibling is likely to develop positive attitudes and interactions. The birth of a baby is a positive and exciting event for the family, but often a sibling views the event as a loss. It is a loss of the sibling's place in the family. Relationships in the family change, expectations are different, and the parents may become somewhat less accessible when the parent must focus on the feeding and physical care of the new infant. A 2 year old may have a low tolerance to change in the relationship with parents, and a 4 year old may be still struggling to maintain impulse

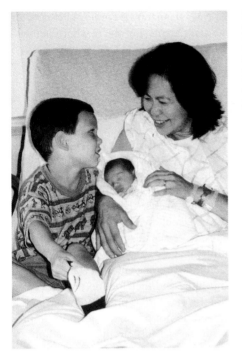

FIGURE 5–8 Reassuring her older child, this mother makes the initial introduction between a newborn and its sibling. (From Gorrie, T.M., McKinney, E.S., & Murray, S.S. [1998]. *Foundations of maternal-newborn nursing* [2nd ed.]. Philadelphia: W.B. Saunders.)

control. A sibling in the egocentric stage of development cannot be expected to clearly understand the needs of the new baby. Allowing the sibling to participate in the anticipation of the birth of the new baby may help in the adjustment and transition tasks. Providing an opportunity for the sibling to help with the care of the new baby, under the supervision of the parents, can help the sibling feel involved rather than displaced. Twins often have the opportunity to share experiences early, which can be positive, but when adults compare their achievements with each other, sibling rivalry can intensify. Sibling rivalry may also intensify when a new baby is born into a blended family, where a stepchild may foster resentment toward the new arrival. Major changes in child care arrangements, routines, or residential moves should be avoided in the first 6 months after a new baby arrives. Siblings are reliable and available playmates in the home and later may become role models and confidants for each other; therefore sibling relationships do have long-term benefits.

Grandparents

Culture and physical distance in living arrangements influence the role of grandparents in the lives of this new family. Some grandparents seek an interactive role, and some grandparents prefer minimal involvement. When parents and grandparents agree on their roles, conflict is avoided. Because the process of bonding and attachment between parents and newborn involves learning the cues of newborn behavior, it is essential that parents have the opportunity to spend time with the newborn in the first few weeks or months of life. Grandparents therefore can be most helpful if they assume the role of home manager, preparing meals, shopping, and helping with household tasks. When grandparents take on the care of the newborn, or when a nanny is employed to care for the newborn, the critical time for bonding between parents and the newborn is interrupted and may never be recaptured. This may affect the lifelong relationship between parent and child.

THE INFLUENCE OF CULTURE

The cultural background of the birth family may be different from the nurse or health care worker, but practices must be understood and respected. In some cultures the husband or partner is expected to be present during the birth process, and in others the presence of the husband or partner is discouraged. In some cases a male practitioner in attendance at birth may be forbidden. Some parents practice the hot-and-cold theory related to diet and any diet prescription needs to be carefully designed to ensure compliance. The postpartum phase may last 30 days or longer in some cultures, with the woman forbidden from leaving the home. Bathing may be delayed by cultural regulations; cold packs may be refused for perineal comfort. In some cultures women believe that the colostrum portion of breast milk is unhealthy and therefore do not breastfeed immediately after delivery. Ritual circumcision of the newborn is practiced in the Jewish religion and avoided in others. Some Asian women do not praise the newborn to protect the infant from evil influences. This behavior may be misinterpreted as a noncaring attitude or failure to bond.

Culture may also influence the accuracy of pain assessment. Nurses and health care workers often use a horizontal illustration of the score of 1 to 10 to assess the level of pain. Certain cultures read downward rather than left to right and may need a vertical chart for accuracy. In some cultures women suffer in silence, whereas in others women chant or moan loudly. Understanding pain and the influence of culture on the expression of pain is essential to providing comprehensive care. Interpreters should be used whenever possible for patients who speak little English. Family members should not serve as the interpreters when sensitive information is discussed, because a family member may interpret selectively (see Appendix B).

THE NEONATE: DEVELOPMENTAL TASKS AND RESPONSES

The main task after birth is the establishment of feeding patterns and habits. The infant learns how to latch on to the breast and suck to obtain nourishment that will last for 2 to 3 hours. If bottle-feeding, parents are taught techniques and types of formulas available. The mother must learn to recognize cues that indicate the infant is hungry *before* crying occurs. This is the first trust experience. The mother learns to recognize the different cries of the infant and knows if it means feeding, cuddling, or a diaper change is necessary. Various organized behavioral states of the newborn can be observed. They include (1) quiet sleep, (2) active sleep, (3) quiet alert, (4) active alert, and (5) cry.

The neonate sleeps 15 to 20 hours a day and is most responsive to interaction during the quiet-alert stage of responsiveness. Rocking an infant in a vertical fashion (upright) is likely to maintain alertness, whereas gentle rocking in a horizontal position (lying flat) while wrapped snugly will promote sleep. Each newborn infant has a unique temperament that will influence the intensity of responses to environmental stimuli. The **neonatal** period (first 30 days of life) serves to solidify parent-infant expectations and relationships. The newborn initiates environmental support by crying or turning away from excess stimulation and learns to self-console and eventually to interact socially by smiling. Nurses and health care workers can help cement a positive parent-infant relationship by observing parent-infant responses, educating parents concerning the abilities and behaviors of the newborn, and utilizing opportunities to promote bonding and attachment. Newborns who exhibit frequent startles or tremors, gaze away from the face of the caregiver, and appear irritable when stimulated require further professional assessment. Distressed parents who feel inadequate and believe their infant to be highly vulnerable need special guidance and support to assist their infant to achieve trust and grow toward autonomy.

> The alert neonate has predictable responses to environmental stimuli that parents learn to understand and anticipate. This interaction fosters effective parenting and infant growth and development.

During the neonatal period, the infant develops *conditioned responses*, which are unconscious responses to external stimuli. For example, the hungry infant who stops crying at the sound of a caregiver's presence, even though food is not yet offered, is exhibiting a conditioned response.

The neonate can hear clearly after the first sneeze clears the eustachian tubes. The newborn's sucking response is increased when stimuli are introduced, and sucking stops when attention is focused. The newborn is capable of feeling pain, and pain relief should be offered before any painful procedures. Swaddling, cuddling, wrapping, rocking, *nonnutritive sucking* (use of a pacifier), and a quiet environment provide comfort for the neonate. Oral sucrose (sugar) placed on a pacifier often serves as a mild pain reliever. The behavior and appearance of the newborn are influenced by reflexes that are present at birth and gradually disappear (Table 5-3). These reflexes help the neonate adapt to the environment and gradually disappear as voluntary motor ability develops. Assessment of the neurological system is achieved by testing for the presence of these reflexes.

Development of Intelligence

Intelligence is very difficult to define because it includes so many aspects and different types of abilities. Intelligence involves ability to learn from experience and adapt to the environment and its challenges. It includes the ability to reason, problem solve, and learn. Researchers have classified the study of intelligence to include *psychometric* variables such as reasoning, memory, perception, and abstract thinking; *computational* variables such as the ability to process information; *biological* variables such as neural (brain) functioning; and *complex system* variables that involve language intelligence,

TABLE 5-3

AGES OF APPEARANCE AND DISAPPEARANCE OF NEUROLOGICAL REFLEXES OF INFANCY

Response	Age at Time of Appearance	Age at Time of Disappearance
Reflexes of Position and Movement		
Moro reflex	Birth	1-3 months
Tonic neck reflex (unsustained)*	Birth	5-7 months
Palmar grasp reflex	Birth	4 months
Babinski reflex	Birth	Variable†
Responses to Sound		
Blinking response	Birth	
Turning response	Birth	
Reflexes of Vision‡		
Blinking to threat	6-7 months	
Horizontal following	4-6 weeks	
Vertical following	2-3 months	
Postrotational nystagmus	Birth	
Food Reflexes		
Rooting response (awake)	Birth	3-4 months
Rooting response (asleep)	Birth	7-8 months
Sucking response	Birth	12 months
Other Signs		
Handedness	2-3 years	
Spontaneous stepping	Birth	4-5 months
Straight line walking	5-6 years	

Figure of 1-3 months from Gorrie, T.M., McKinney, E.S., Murray, S.S. (1998). *Foundations of maternal-newborn nursing* (2nd ed.). Philadelphia, WB Saunders; figure of 5-7 months from Leifer, G. (2003). *Introduction to maternity and pediatric nursing* (4th ed). Philadelphia, WB Saunders.

*Arm and leg posturing can be broken by child despite continued neck stimulus.
†Usually of no diagnostic significance until after age 2 years.
‡Holding the newborn infant upright under the arms will induce eye opening.

spatial intelligence, musical intelligence, interpersonal intelligence, and so on. Each of these areas of intelligence may be studied separately, but they interact to form an individual's intelligence potential.

New molecular technology has enabled research into genetic influences on intelligence. Both genetics and environment influence the intelligence potential of a newborn infant. Poor nutrition, environmental toxins, or oxygen deprivation can inhibit optimum brain development. Family, schooling, and availability of preschool programs also will influence the infant's ability to reach the full potential of his or her intelligence. Bronfenbrenner (1993) proposed the theory that intelligence tests are imperfect measurements of intelligence. He believed that environmental influences affect the potential and rate of development (see Chapter 4). The environment can influence temperament and motivation that then influence the development of intelligence. Intelligence quotient (IQ) scores remain the valid measure of intelligence in research settings. IQ scores have been increasing about 3 points a decade, perhaps due to an increase in the complexity of our culture and an increase in the quality of our nutrition (Flynn, 1987). IQ tests are used to predict school success and identify children in need of professional intervention.

PLAY ACTIVITIES AND NEONATAL DEVELOPMENT

Because hearing and vision are present in the newborn, an appropriate toy would include a musical mobile that is placed above the crib within sight of the infant. Musical interludes can capture the attention of the newborn. A developmental task of the neonate is to learn how to focus on and follow objects as they move across the field of vision. An overhanging mobile in sharp contrasting colors will foster this development. The neonate can detect the smell of mother's milk by 6 days of age and prefers sweet tastes. The sense of touch is well developed, and stroking the cheek will cause the infant to turn toward the person stroking his or her face. An infant can be quieted and bonding promoted by placing the infant in skin-to-skin contact with the parent. A nude infant, placed on the nude chest of the parent, will quiet and snuggle. The neonate is in Piaget's sensorimotor stage of cognitive growth. Infants can learn and repeat behavioral responses. Looking, listening, and touching the environment help the infant master the tasks of this stage. Close contact with the infant will help parents recognize cues to specific needs so that cry time is minimized. The best time to interact with the neonate is during the quiet-alert state of responsiveness. The infant will quickly halt physical activity and become very still when approached and talked to. Eyes will focus on the parent's face and beginning communication will be evident.

KEY POINTS

- A genome is a complete set of DNA contained in all human cells.
- The goal of the Genome Project was to identify the more than 30,000 genes in the DNA; develop tools for analysis; and address the ethical, legal, and social implications of this knowledge and ability.
- The Genome Project may enable gene therapy to correct or replace abnormal genes.

- One of the critical periods during fetal growth occurs during the first 3 months of pregnancy, when basic structures are developing.
- The well-being of the mother and fetus can influence life expectancy of the newborn.
- The improvement in the nutrition and health of mothers and babies may prevent disease in the next generation.
- Exposure to toxins such as drugs and alcohol during fetal development can cause abnormalities in the newborn.
- According to Erikson, parenting a dependent child is the beginning of the stage of generativity.
- A combination of an XX chromosome from the mother and father will produce a girl and an XY combination will produce a boy fetus.
- Only the sperm carries the Y chromosome, and so the male partner determines the sex of the infant. However, the female has some influence on which sperm may survive to fertilize the ovum.
- An adequate intake of folic acid in the maternal diet is essential to prevent neural tube defects in the newborn infant.
- Fraternal twins are the result of two ova released at ovulation, each fertilized by a separate sperm. Identical twins are the result of one fertilized ovum separating into two embryos.
- *Bonding* refers to a strong emotional tie between the parents and newborn.
- *Attachment* refers to the affectionate tie that occurs over time due to parent-infant interaction.
- The influence of the new child's birth on siblings depends on their ages and developmental level.
- Breastfeeding, bonding, and attachment are developmental tasks of parents and the newborn.
- The neonatal period encompasses the first 30 days of life.
- Swaddling, cuddling, rocking, and use of a pacifier calm the newborn infant.
- Newborn reflexes help the neonate adjust to the environment and disappear as voluntary motor abilities develop.
- An overhanging mobile in sharp contrasting colors will foster the growth and development of the neonate.

CRITICAL THINKING

A woman has just confirmed that she is pregnant. List at least five ways she can reduce the risk of exposing her developing fetus to dangerous teratogens that may have a negative effect on fetal growth and development.

MULTIPLE-CHOICE REVIEW QUESTIONS

1 Neural tube defects such as spina bifida can be prevented by:
   1 Eating a well-balanced diet during pregnancy
   2 Intake of folic acid supplements during pregnancy
   3 Avoiding alcohol and smoking during pregnancy
   4 Early antibiotic therapy for infections during pregnancy

2 The *neonatal period* refers to:
   1 The first 30 days after birth
   2 The period between birth and 1 year of age
   3 The period immediately before birth
   4 The moment of birth

3 To promote growth and development in an infant, an overhead mobile should have:
   1 Contrasting colors
   2 Bright colors
   3 Animated characters
   4 Sound integrated with movement

4 Fraternal twins are the result of:
   1 Two ova fertilized by two separate sperm
   2 One ovum fertilized by one sperm
   3 Two ova fertilized by one sperm
   4 One ovum fertilized by two sperm

5 A complete set of DNA that is contained in all human cells is known as:
   1 A chromosome
   2 A nucleus
   3 A genome
   4 An allele

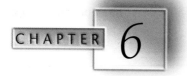

CHAPTER 6

The Infant

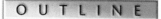

O B J E C T I V E S

Upon completion of this chapter, the student will be able to:

1 Define the term infant.
2 State the developmental tasks of infancy.
3 Describe the physical development of infants from 1 month to 1 year of age.
4 Discuss milestones of motor development.
5 Discuss the development of language.
6 Describe the theories of Piaget, Freud, and Erikson concerning infant development.
7 Define separation anxiety.
8 Discuss the development of attachment.
9 Describe the basic nutritional needs of infants from 1 month to 1 year of age.
10 List the immunization schedule for infants under 1 year of age.
11 State four safety precautions essential in infant care.

KEY TERMS

Autonomy	Norms
Cephalocaudal	Nursing caries
Coping skill	Object permanence
Defense mechanism	Ordinal position
Development	Personality
Expressive language	Pincer action
Growth	Preverbal
Infant	Receptive language
Length	Separation anxiety
Nonverbal language	SIDS

DEFINITION

The **infant** stage of development is the period between 4 weeks of age to 1 year of age. **Growth** indicates an increase in size, measured by inches (centimeters) and pounds (kilograms). **Development** indicates an increase in function and mastery of tasks for the specific phase in the lifespan.

The process of growth and development is orderly and proceeds from simple to complex in an expected pattern but at a variable pace. Growth spurts are common. The **norms** (average) presented are only guidelines concerning the age that specific abilities or skills are achieved. **Cephalocaudal** growth refers to the progression of the growth pattern that proceeds from head to toe. For example, infants are able to lift their head before they can sit and are able to sit before they can stand. *Proximodistal* growth refers to growth from the center of the body to the periphery. *Height* refers to a standing measurement, whereas **length** is measured while the infant is lying down. Height is generally a family trait, although nutrition and other factors may alter the attainment of adult height. A general estimation of potential adult height can be determined by the following formulas:

$$\text{Boys: } \frac{\textit{Father's height + mothers height in inches + 2.5 inches}}{2}$$

$$\text{Girls: } \frac{\textit{Father's height + mothers height in inches − 2.5 inches}}{2}$$

The length of the newborn is normally about 20 inches (50 cm), and by 1 year of age the birth length increases by almost 50%. A normal newborn weighs approximately $7\frac{1}{2}$ pounds (3.4 kg). The infant's birth weight doubles by 6 months of age and can be expected to triple by 1 year.

Many factors influence growth and development of the infant. Development is a process that continues throughout the life cycle, with mastery of specific tasks occurring in each phase of the cycle. Successful mastery of the tasks in one phase of the life cycle enables the person to easily proceed to the next phase of the life cycle. Development is an interaction among the child, the parent, and the environment. If there is a problem with the parents or environment, defense mechanisms or coping skills are activated or developed. A **defense mechanism** is a reaction that is protective to the individual or helps conceal conflicts or anxieties. Denial and projection of blame are examples of defense mechanisms. For example, if an infant is hurt, he or she may, by hitting or thrashing, blame the caregiver for causing the pain (an infant does not have the concept of an accident). A **coping skill** is a behavior that helps an individual adapt to or manage a stressful situation. If a goal is obstructed, the infant may find a way around the unachievable goal; modify the goal to an achievable level; or perhaps develop an alternative goal. For example, an infant may learn how to climb over a crib rail to reach a toy. Infants thrive with the support and praise of their parents. This interaction fosters an attachment between child and parent that provides a sense of security, enabling the infant to try to master developmental tasks. Mutual attachment involves not only a close feeling between the infant and parent but also a responsiveness to needs presented. If the needs of the infant are not responded to, the development of attachment will not be achieved as easily if at all.

Ethnic and cultural practices influence nutrition and behavior development.

The **ordinal position** in the family—that is, whether the infant is an only child, an older child, youngest child or middle child—may influence the age and rapidity of mastering developmental tasks.

Both the prenatal environment and the home environment influence growth and development of the infant. The development of the personality is the interaction between the biological and environmental factors. **Personality** is most often defined as a unique combination of characteristics that results in the individual's recurrent pattern of behavior. The influences of the family and family interactions on growth and development are discussed in Chapter 3. Theories of behavioral development abound, and a summary of popular theories is presented in Chapter 4. The role of heredity and prenatal influences are discussed in Chapter 5.

DEVELOPMENT AND TASKS OF INFANCY
Trust Versus Mistrust

The functioning of all humans is goal directed and involves the tasks of developing social competence and the mastery of skills necessary for functioning in their environment. Some tasks of infancy include weaning, self-feeding, walking, and acquiring language and communications skills.

Trust versus mistrust is the first psychosocial crisis in infancy that must be resolved (Erikson, 1994). In the first year of life, trust develops when infants learn their basic needs will be met. Infants who are left to cry it out cry more at 1 year than infants who are picked up and comforted or fed promptly when they evidence hunger. Infants who are fed on a rigid schedule rather than as a response to hunger signs generally show more spitting up and gastrointestinal (GI) disturbances and later behavioral problems (Behrman, 2004). By 2 months of age, parents react positively to the infants' responsive smile and a mutual bond (attachment) is secured.

Intelligence
Understanding Cause and Effect

Infants discover at an early age that there is a relationship between cause and effect, and experiences at each stage of the life cycle build on this discovery. Newborns suck their thumb to feel secure and will seek out the thumb or pacifier to achieve this feeling of comfort. A cry usually elicits a response from adults, and so the cry becomes a means of communication.

From 1 to 4 months of age the infant is focused on the parent and, when held, prefers the *en face* (face-to-face) position. After 4 months of age the infant begins to become more aware of surroundings and may prefer to be held outwardly or away from the parent, facing the activity in the room. By 4 months, infants discover their hands and feet. If a mobile gym is placed above them, infants discover there are predictable sounds and tactile responses that occur when reaching out to touch the mobile. The infant strives to recognize behavior patterns that elicit special responses from the environment. When infants feel secure, they will explore the world around them. Infants who have not developed an attachment to the parent figure do not explore readily. At 4 months the infant drops a spoon from the highchair and believes it is gone. By 7 months, the infant will continue to look for it. This is called **object permanence**, knowing the object is there even though you cannot see it. Playing peek-a-boo with the infant at this age helps to develop the concept of object permanence.

Memory

Studies have shown that infants in the first year of life can retain memory of a traumatic experience (Gaensbauer, 1995). General comforting may not be enough to achieve full emotional recovery for the infant. Newborns demonstrate a physiological response to pain, and so a stress response can develop and influence later behavior. For example, a choking episode (anoxia) early in breastfeeding may cause an infant to reject further attempts at breastfeeding. One study showed that a 10-week-old infant, repeatedly abused by the father and placed in a foster home, showed an aversion to male caretakers for many months afterward. This evidence has led psychologists to advise parents to talk about stressful events that may have occurred early in the lives of their children, so that the child does not have to deal with those memories by themselves (Gaensbauer, 1995).

Emotional Development

When placed face-to-face (*en face*) with an adult, an infant will mimic the facial expression of the adult. For example, if the adult's tongue is thrust out, the infant will eventually thrust his or her tongue out also. Smiling, eye widening, and puckering of the lips occur when the infant focuses on the adult or activity that the infant can see. When stimulation reaches a high level, the infant will turn away to rest and then return to the view when ready for further stimulation. If the adult turns away before the infant is ready, the infant will lean forward and attempt to get the parent's attention with sound and movement and will eventually cry with frustration if unsuccessful. When adult stimulation is not available, the infant will eventually lose energy and stop efforts at communication. Interaction between parent and infant is necessary in the first months of life and is important for later social development.

Separation anxiety begins at 6 months of age. The infant prefers the parent to a stranger. Leaving the room or leaving the infant with a babysitter or other caregiver can precipitate crying and distress in the infant.

Attachment

The process of attachment begins long before the infant is born, when the mother feels the fetus moving in the womb. The father feels the fetal movement by touching the mother's abdomen and feeling the fetus kick. Both parents can hear the heartbeat with the aid of a stethoscope or Doppler device. A relationship with an imagined child starts to develop. At birth the real child emerges, and if he or she is not too different from the imagined child, attachment easily intensifies. However, the infant must respond positively in this mutual interaction. An infant who is sleepy, does not focus on the face of the parent, has difficulty latching on to the breast for breastfeeding, or spits up or vomits feedings cannot contribute as much to the attachment process and the nurse or health care worker may need to help the process along.

Parents slowly develop an instinctive response to infants' cues. The way they cry, the pitch or its intensity, may indicate to the parent if it is a cry of pain, discomfort, hunger, or boredom. If the parent's response is prompt, attachment becomes secure. Providing time for *en face* interactions is important. The infant from birth to 3 months of age can respond with varied facial expressions. After age 2 or 3 months a responsive smile by the infant brings joy to the parent's efforts at interaction. By 5 or 6 months the infant clearly recognizes and prefers the parent to other casual caregivers. The infant also looks to the facial expression and body language of the parent in new situations and responds accordingly. For example, if a relative from out of town visits and the mother, while holding the infant, smiles and embraces the relative, the infant will likely smile and coo and respond calmly. However, if the person entering the room is a health care provider for a well child visit and the mother is concerned about the pain of the immunizations to be given, her facial expression and nonverbal behavior or body language (of a stiffened posture) will be communicated to the child, who may then cry as the health care provider approaches.

Separation anxiety emerges after 6 months of age. The infant cries or protests the parent leaving the room. *Stranger anxiety* peaks at 9 months of age when the infant is approached by a stranger in the absence of the parent. The mastery of object permanence indicates the infant understands that the parent is still available even though he or she is not visible at the moment. By 18 months, memory development helps the child remember the image of the parent and trust that the parent will return. Affectionate, responsive parents who respond to the needs of the child help develop a secure attachment and bonding. The process of attachment is a gradual one, but attachment abilities stretch across the life span. Mastery of this task is essential for the child to be successful in later attachments to school friends or partners in the adult phase of the life cycle. The temperament of the infant can influence the success of the attachment process. Parents usually have expectations concerning the temperament of their child. Parents may say, "He is a difficult child" or "She is an easy child." This usually means the expectations of the parents do not exactly fit the temperament of the infant, and the nurse or health care worker needs to guide the response of the parent to the temperament of the child (Table 6-1).

Parents who have psychiatric problems or marital stress or who both work long hours may not have the energy to respond to a demanding infant. Infants who receive

TABLE 6-1

TEMPERAMENT

Factors	Characteristics	Interventions
Activity level	Activity level of the infant can be high, medium, or low. It can be assessed by watching activity during feeding, bathing, or playing.	High activity: Provide opportunity for high activity. Low activity: Provide enough time for tasks.
Regularity	Regularity can be assessed by predictability of the infant's sleep-wake cycle, hunger, or elimination schedule.	Make provision for regularity by bringing food, diapers on trips.
Approach/ withdrawal	The infant may respond to a stimulus with gusto and exploration or with caution and avoidance. This applies to people, foods, and toys.	Use a time-limited trial and praise.
Adaptability	The ease at which an infant tolerates and responds to a new stimulus.	Provide multiple short exposures to events.
Threshold	The level of stimulation response. Can also indicate hyperreactivity to minor stimuli.	Limit stimuli before bedtime.
Intensity of response	Involves the energy.	Do not give in to buy peace.
Distractibility	Easily changes focus of interest.	Calmly redirect wandering attention.
Attention span	Loses interest rapidly.	Plan brief periods of activity; monitor completion of task. Warn if task must be interrupted for meal or sleep.

Modified from Levine, M., Carey, W., & Crocker, A. (1999). *Developmental-behavioral pediatrics* (3rd ed.). Philadelphia: W.B. Saunders.

inconsistent responses to their needs may withdraw from the risks of exploring the world around them, even when the parent is present. Some infants or toddlers may become clingy, angry, and rebellious or become nonresponsive to the soothing or care they do receive. Child abuse becomes a risk at this time. The nurse should be alert to signs and symptoms of child abuse (Figure 6-1).

This understanding of attachment behavior is one of the reasons for providing one consistent core teacher in elementary schools, whereas the high school has multiple teachers in one day because the typical adolescent has achieved independence, trust, and autonomy. It is also the basis of the rooming-in concept, where the parent is encouraged to stay in the room with the infant or child day and night when the child is hospitalized.

Observation of the parents' ability to comfort the infant, distract the infant, and respond to the emotional cues of the infant's behavior can be observed at each well child visit, and appropriate guidance should be offered as needed. For example, following a clinic immunization, the mother can be encouraged to hold, rock, or breastfeed her infant to calm the infant before leaving the room. Parents often need help with the separation experience. Sometimes it is not the child who cannot accept separation, but the parent who has the difficulty. Step 1 of separation starts with the placement of infants in their own bed, perhaps in their own room. Co-sleeping can prolong this first step in separation. Step 2 is leaving the infant with a relative or babysitter. Parents often do not realize that such separations help infants develop independence and enable them to

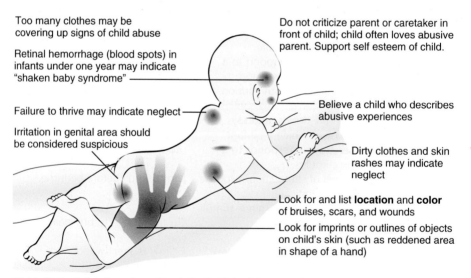

Too many clothes may be covering up signs of child abuse

Retinal hemorrhage (blood spots) in infants under one year may indicate "shaken baby syndrome"

Failure to thrive may indicate neglect

Irritation in genital area should be considered suspicious

Do not criticize parent or caretaker in front of child; child often loves abusive parent. Support self esteem of child.

Believe a child who describes abusive experiences

Dirty clothes and skin rashes may indicate neglect

Look for and list **location** and **color** of bruises, scars, and wounds

Look for imprints or outlines of objects on child's skin (such as reddened area in shape of a hand)

Divide the body into four planes Front, Back, Right side, and Left side.
Injuries occurring in more than one plane should be considered suspicious.

FIGURE 6–1 Assessing for child abuse. The nurse should be alert for inconsistent statements about injuries, bruises at various stages of healing, or delay in seeking care. (From Leifer, G. [2003] *Introduction to maternity and pediatric nursing* [4th ed.]. Philadelphia, W.B. Saunders.)

prepare for the next stage of autonomy. Coping skills are developed and trust is strengthened when the infant learns from many small experiences with short separations. Protest at the initial separation is to be expected but will diminish as the child learns to trust the caregiver and trust that the parents will return.

Hospitalization is a unique experience of separation that is filled with strangers, pain, and fear of the unknown. For this separation experience, it is strongly recommended that a parent room in with the child, and most hospitals have facilities to accommodate parents.

Parents who perceive their child as especially vulnerable and therefore avoid most separation experiences are exhibiting overprotective parenting, which can stifle the normal process of child development. Crises in separation experiences can recur later in life when the school-age child must leave the home environment to attend elementary school or when the teenage child leaves home to enter college. Leaving home may precipitate a recurrence of the separation anxiety.

Language Development

Language development consists of verbal language that is both **expressive** (can say it) and **receptive** (can understand it) and body language that follows a predictable course of development. *Body language*, also known as **nonverbal language,** is the language of the motions, postures, and gestures of the body and is learned as part of communication. There appears to be an innate ability to develop language skills. The first year of life, before the infant can express understandable speech, is called the **preverbal** stage of language development. In the early months of life the infant initially communicates needs by crying or smiling. The infant will stop all random motor activity when listening to a voice. At this time, the infant is learning the rhythms of the speech pattern of what will be his or her native or primary language. At 3 or 4 months of age, the infant will utter repetitive sounds, which develops into babbling, using combinations of vowels with some consonants. By 7 to 8 months of age, syllables using the *D, P,* and *B* sounds appear and parents are gleeful when they hear "ma" or "da." By 9 or 10 months of age, specific sounds are used consistently to refer to objects or events. At this age, infants shares their emotions by showing a favorite toy to an adult because they are sure it will bring the adult joy also.

The first words may occur between 10 and 13 months of age. Body language, such as pointing, leaning, or staring, assists the infant to make desires or needs understood. The first single words used often have multiple meanings. For example, "ball" can mean "that is a ball" or "give me the ball." Nonverbal behavior often assists the parent to understand what the infant means.

By the time infants are 1 year old, their brain is committed to the language that is used regularly in the environment around them. Initially, at birth, the infant was able to tune in to the covert sounds that often separate language with different sounds, such as English and Japanese. By the time the infant is a year old, the rhythm and pattern of the language is set and the ability to distinguish sounds from other languages wanes. Infants soon learn combinations of syllables that separate words by hearing them often and separating them according to the frequency heard. For example, in the phrase "pretty girl," babies learn that "ty" goes with "pret," not "girl." It is not "pret-tygirl," it is "pretty-girl." This is a learned skill and is an important reason parents should talk to their infants in a natural language and not use slang or baby talk (Figure 6-2).

Motor Development

The development of motor skills is closely related to the development of perception, emotion, and cognition. Reaching out and touching what they see enables infants to establish visual-motor skills. Many motor skills are dependent on the disappearance of newborn reflexes (which are discussed in Chapter 5). With the disappearance of the tonic neck reflex, where the extension of the arm occurs when the head turns to the side, the infant is able to bring both hands to the midline of the body into prayer position. At 3 months, the infant grasps whatever he or she touches. At 6 months, the infant shapes the hand to prepare to touch an observed object. By 9 months, the **pincer action** enables the infant to grasp with the thumb and forefinger. By 2 years, wrist action enables the use of spoons during feeding.

As posture and balance develop, infants first learn to lift their head, then to sit and stand, and then take their first steps around 1 year of age. Infants start to walk about 4 to 5 months after they are able to pull themselves up to a standing position (Table 6-2).

Autonomy

Autonomy refers to independence. Striving for independence starts early in infancy. Self-consoling behavior is an early form of independence. Infants learns to bring their hand to their mouth and suck their fingers to bring comfort or relieve boredom. Studies have shown that sucking on a sucrose (sugar)–coated pacifier offers pain relief to newborns undergoing circumcision. At 6 to 10 months of age, body rocking is used to

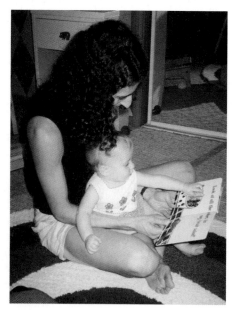

FIGURE 6–2 Reading to an infant promotes language development. Infants enjoy books that provide colorful pictures and varied textures.

TABLE 6-2

THE DEVELOPMENT OF LOCOMOTION, PREHENSION, AND PERCEPTION

	Locomotion	Prehension	Perception
1 Month	Chin-up.	Hand held closed. Fingers move without coordination from mind.	Able to focus on sharply contrasted angled mobile above.
2 Months	Chest up. Elevates self with arms.	Hand held open most of the time.	Selectively responds to patterns, colors. Imitates expressions. Is self-centered. Prefers to look at familiar sights.
4 Months	Rolls over at will.	Reaches for overhead objects with fingers, with hit-and-miss action.	Perceives differences in facial expressions.
5 Months	Sits alone momentarily.	Picks up toy with squeeze action.	
6 Months	Sits alone steadily with hands forward for support.	Grasps with thumb on one side and 3 fingers on other.	Can distinguish between familiar and unfamiliar sight. Separation anxiety begins. Sees self and parent as one.
8 Months	Sits with support. Pulls to standing position.	Thumb and index finger can hold object without pressing it into palm. Can transfer from one hand to the other.	Can distinguish happy from fearful face.

(Continued)

TABLE 6-2

THE DEVELOPMENT OF LOCOMOTION, PREHENSION, AND PERCEPTION—cont'd

	Locomotion	Prehension	Perception
9 Months	Creeps.	Uses finger to explore what eye sees. Has hand-mouth coordination.	Fears strangers. Recognizes self as separate from parent.
10 Months	Walks when led.	Can let 1 toy go at a time.	Separation anxiety peaks.
11 Months	Stands alone and can sit from standing position.	Pincer action enables infant to pick up small objects.	
12 Months	Walks 3 steps.	Hand obeys direction from mind. Aim is poor but can place toy in pan. Can attempt to feed self.	"Goal corrected partnership" enables infant to grasp onto parent because he or she anticipates being left with stranger.
15 Months	Can walk up stairs with support.	Mind is 100% in control of hands. Places round peg in round hole. Builds tower of 2 cubes.	

From Leifer, G. (2003). *Introduction to Maternity & Pediatric Nursing* (4th ed.). Philadelphia: WB Saunders, pp. 387–388.

achieve self-comforting. Nine month olds with newly developed pincer ability will insist on self–finger feeding and resist the attempts of parents feeding them at mealtime.

Sleep Patterns

A maturing central nervous system combined with parental responses aids in the development of a sleep pattern. By 3 months, most infants develop a pattern of sustained sleep between midnight and 5 A.M. A few do not develop this pattern before 1 year of age. In the first year, waking at night is considered normal. The goal is to help the infant develop self-regulatory skills so that the infant may return to sleep without prompting. This can occur faster if parents wait until there is evidence that the infant is fully awake before picking up the infant. In a semi-awake state, gentle body patting or use of a pacifier should be enough consoling assistance to help the infant return to sleep. Picking the infant up too quickly may delay the development of a sustained sleep pattern. The establishment of a prebedtime routine of a quiet activity such as rocking or reading to the infant helps with the acceptance of bedtime in the first years of life.

> The establishment of an appropriate sleep pattern is important because adequate sleep is related to memory, attention, learning, and general behavior.

Role of Play in Fostering Growth and Development

Piaget's sensorimotor theory of development of the infant is evident in the infant's play activities, which are activated by sensations and relate to the infant directly. Play is the work of a child. Age-appropriate play activities can effectively foster growth and development. For example, a newborn must learn to focus and follow with the eyes. Hanging a bright mobile with contrasting colors (such as black and white) above the crib within the sight of the infant can promote the development of this skill. At 3 months, an interactive mobile that is activated by kicking helps develop the cause-effect understanding. At 6 to 7 months of age, playing peek-a-boo helps solidify the object permanence concept. Dropping food from the highchair and having someone there to pick it up is also part of the learning process, although the messiness involved often tries the patience of parents. In the young infant, all toys are explored for taste and touch, but by 1 year the infant typically understands the function of the toy. A car will be pushed; a telephone will be put to the ear. All toys and activities are related to the child's body. Egocentric behavior is evidenced by 1 year olds who drink from a toy cup or place a toy telephone to their ear, but a toddler at 18 months of age will offer the drink to a doll. The 1 year old enjoys push toys that foster the newly mastered walking abilities.

According to Freud's theory of development, the infant is in an oral phase, which involves exploring with the mouth. Oral sucking, biting, and chewing toys are appropriate for this stage of development.

By applying learned skills to environmental experiences, children learn about the world around them. Often the nurse or health care worker needs to reassure the parents that picking up everything from the floor and placing it into his or her mouth or intentionally dropping food from the highchair tray onto the floor are developmentally normal behaviors and definitely not signs of a badly behaved child.

HEALTH MAINTENANCE
Nutrition

In the first year of life, the brain and the body grow and develop rapidly. Proper nutritional intake is essential to support optimum development. The newborn has a rooting reflex that seeks out the nipple and a sucking reflex that is elicited when the nipple touches the lips. A tongue extrusion reflex prevents ingestion of solid foods.

The best nutrition for the newborn is breast milk, which contains antibodies and easy-to-digest fats. For mothers who cannot breastfeed, most commercial formulas provide adequate nutrition, although the extra benefits of the antibodies and other protective ingredients are not provided.

Cultural factors influence breastfeeding choices. Some mothers from North American or European backgrounds are uncomfortable with the body contact and exposure required for breastfeeding. In American cultures, mothers' return to the workplace soon after delivery influences the choice to bottle-feed their newborns. In many cultures, breast pumping is not accepted as a relief for engorgement or a convenience for working mothers. In cultures such as Cambodian, Mexican-American, and Filipino, colostrum is discarded, and in some Asian cultures, sterile water may be given to the newborn until maternal milk flow is well established. In African-American cultures, solid food is added to the formula bottle in the early months of life. Breastfeeding may be medically contraindicated in most women with human immunodeficiency virus/acquired immunodeficiency syndrome (HIV/AIDS) and in women receiving medications that may pass into the breast milk and cause adverse effects in the newborn.

Newborns are usually fed on demand at 2- to 3-hour intervals and by 4 to 6 months of age may skip a nighttime feeding. If the newborn is lethargic, efforts to maintain a state of alertness will aid nutritional intake. Infants should be fed formula or breast milk for 1 full year. At 1 year of age the infant can be placed on whole milk. Low-fat milk should not be given to children under age 2, because the fats are necessary for development of the nervous system. At 6 months of age the tongue extrusion reflex has disappeared; the infant will no longer spit out solid foods and is therefore ready for strained rice cereal. Gradually, fruits and vegetables are added, but only one at a time to help the parent determine what foods may upset the infant's stomach and to identify a food allergy response. By 11 months of age, meat and eggs are added to the diet. By 1 year the infant typically eats table food three times a day and can join the family meal schedule.

Introduction of foods before 6 months of age is not for nutritional value, because the infant may not have the digestive enzymes necessary for complete digestion and utilization of the nutrients. Foods such as nuts, jellied candy, and large pieces of solid foods should not be offered to the infant because they present a choking hazard. Honey should not be given to children under 2 years of age because of the risk of botulism poisoning. Commercially prepared foods such as beets, turnips, spinach, celery, and collard greens are high in nitrates and should be used sparingly for infants under 1 year of age. Commercially prepared baby food in jars are vacuum packed, and parents should check the safety seals and expiration dates before purchase. When a jar is first opened, a pop is heard as the vacuum is broken. Foods should not be fed directly from the jar, and leftovers should not be returned to the jar because saliva contamination can alter the foods. Parents should avoid tasting the food from the same spoon used to feed the infant because organisms from their mouth will be passed to the baby.

The development of autonomy dictates the need for finger foods by 9 or 10 months, when the infant can be expected to prefer self-feeding. The temperament of the infant will influence the development of mealtime challenges. For example, infants with a high activity level should not be expected to sit for a long period at the family meal table. Infants who are highly distractible may not even finish a meal. Infants who are slow to adapt may not easily try new foods.

The nurse or health care worker can help the parent develop strategies to deal with temperament as it relates to feeding, so that conflicts will not arise. The prevention of obesity is a *Healthy People 2010* goal, and overfeeding during infancy is thought to be a contributing factor. The nurse or health care worker can provide parents with information regarding feeding concerns during the first years.

Teeth

The eruption of the first 20 *deciduous* teeth, which are also known as primary or baby teeth, usually begins at 5 to 7 months of age (Box 6-1).

The upper and lower central incisors are usually the first to erupt. At this time the infant enjoys toys that can be chewed. The primary teeth serve the purpose of helping the intake of nutrition by allowing the chewing of foods, and they also help in the formation of the jaw. If an infant or child loses a primary tooth due to an accident, a spacer is usually inserted by the dentist to preserve the space for the later eruption of the permanent tooth, thus avoiding expensive orthodontic care. The most common type of dental caries seen in infants is **nursing caries.** Nursing caries occur when the infant is put to bed while sucking on a bottle of milk or juice. The sugars in the milk or juice coat the teeth and promote tooth decay. If the infant insists on a bottle at bedtime, it should be a bottle of water to prevent the development of nursing caries.

BOX 6-1   ### Estimating the Number of Erupted Primary Teeth in the Mouth

The number of primary teeth that should be present in the mouth of an infant or toddler can be anticipated by use of the following formula:

Age in months – 6

Immunizations

Well child visits should be scheduled before the newborn is discharged. Community resources should be assessed and the parents informed about available help for breast-feeding problems, such as the La Leche League or Healthy Starts programs offered by some health insurance companies. Home visits are often available from the Visiting Nurse Association or the local health department or through the home health services of a hospital for new mothers or high-risk newborns. The growth, development, health, and nutrition of the infant should be checked every 2 months and appropriate immunizations scheduled (see Appendix A).

Well child checkups are the best time to answer questions the parents may have and provide anticipatory guidance concerning developmental stages and needs of the growing infant.

Accident Prevention

Accidents are a major cause of *morbidity* (illness) and *mortality* (death). The first injury prevention activity for the newborn, now required by law in most states, is the use of car seats for infants and children. When an infant is held in the lap of a parent, the infant becomes a high-speed missile in the event of a motor vehicle accident. The advent of front airbags in cars can be lifesaving for adults but can be lethal to an infant or child sitting in the front seat of a car that is in an accident. See Chapter 7 for car seat guidelines.

Falls are a common cause of injury to infants under 1 year. Keeping the crib side rails up prevents the infant from rolling out of the crib. The use of safety straps when infants are placed in highchairs or strollers also prevent falls (Figure 6-3). Gates are needed at the top and bottom of stairs to prevent the infant from falling. Placing the infant supine on the back to sleep and not using pillows in the crib can aid in preventing accidental suffocation and sudden infant death syndrome (SIDS). When the infant masters the pincer action of the thumb and forefinger, choking becomes a high risk because small objects picked up from the floor are typically placed in the mouth. Infants can drown in a shallow tub bath if left unattended even for a minute. Burns can be a risk for infants who pull on the cord of a hot iron, reach for the handle of a pot on the stove, or stick their finger into an exposed and inviting electrical outlet.

A childproof home is essential for the prevention of accidents. There are private agencies in many communities that will come to the home to evaluate safety and offer childproofing suggestions for parents. Local police stations or highway patrol stations may offer assistance assessing car seat installations.

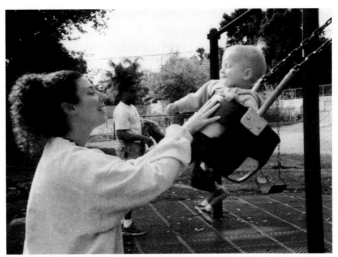

FIGURE 6–3 Using age-appropriate swings is important to prevent accidents. This child is secure in the swing and establishes eye-to-eye contact with the caregiver during play.

KEY POINTS

- Infancy includes the period between 1 month and 1 year of age.
- Developmental tasks involve the goals of developing social competence and mastery of skills necessary for functioning in an environment.
- Some developmental tasks of infancy include weaning, locomotion, self-feeding, and acquiring language.
- The development of a sense of trust begins in infancy.
- The infant's birth weight doubles by 6 months and triples by 1 year of age.
- The infant is in Piaget's sensorimotor stage of development.
- Object permanence involves knowing an object is there even though it is not within sight.
- The infant is in Freud's oral stage of development. Sucking and exploring textures with the mouth are normal behaviors.
- Separation anxiety starts at 6 months of age, when the infant protests if the parent leaves the room.
- Language development involves both verbal language and body language.
- Verbal language involves expression and reception (understanding).
- Egocentric behavior is evidenced by the 1 year old, who relates all toys to his or her own body.
- Breast milk is the best food for infants under 6 months of age.
- The infant should be placed on the back to sleep to prevent SIDS.
- By 1 year of age the infant eats table food three times a day.
- The most common type of dental caries in infants is nursing caries, which is preventable.

- By 9 months of age the pincer action enables the infant to grasp small objects with the thumb and forefinger.
- A childproof home is essential to prevent accidents.

CRITICAL THINKING

Accidents are the major cause of illness and death in children. List three types of accidents that commonly occur in the first year of life and discuss how they can be prevented.

MULTIPLE-CHOICE REVIEW QUESTIONS

1 The period of infancy includes the following ages:
   1 Birth to 1 month
   2 1 month to 1 year
   3 1 to 3 years
   4 1 to 12 years
2 A 1 year old who relates all toys to his or her own body is exhibiting which of the following types of behavior:
   1 Dysfunctional
   2 Selfish
   3 Sexual
   4 Egocentric
3 Separation anxiety typically begins at what age:
   1 3 months
   2 6 months
   3 1 year
   4 2 years
4 By 9 months of age a pincer action is well developed, enabling the infant to:
   1 Increase locomotion
   2 Grasp small objects with thumb and forefinger
   3 Scoop up toys within reach
   4 Achieve increased depth perception
5 By 1 year of age the normal infant should weigh approximately:
   1 Twice the birth weight
   2 Quadruple the birth weight
   3 Three times the birth weight
   4 30 pounds

Early Childhood

OBJECTIVES

Upon completion of this chapter, the student will be able to:

1 Define early childhood.
2 Describe the characteristics common to toddlers.
3 Describe characteristics common to the preschool child.
4 Discuss the developmental tasks of early childhood.
5 List three factors that help develop language skills.
6 List at least three guidelines in selecting a preschool or day care center.
7 Describe the characteristic play and appropriate toys for a toddler and preschool child.
8 List three safety risks common to the early childhood years.
9 Discuss the principles of guidance and discipline for children during the early childhood years.

KEY TERMS

Age-appropriate toys
Cooperative play
Corporal punishment
Dental caries

Discipline
Immunity
Oropharynx
Parallel play
Preschool phase
Toddler phase

DEFINITION

The early childhood period includes children from 1 to 6 years of age. Early childhood is typically separated into two phases; 1 to 2 years of age is the **toddler phase**, and 2 to 6 years is the **preschool phase**. During early childhood, physical growth slows and stabilizes.

DEVELOPMENTAL TASKS OF EARLY CHILDHOOD

Tasks to be mastered include acquiring **receptive language** and **expressive language** (understanding and speaking words); developing social interaction skills; mastery of self-control (such as toilet training); and beginning to develop a self-image and sense of autonomy. The toddler, between 1 and 4 years of age, is in Erikson's stage of autonomy versus shame or doubt. The preschooler, between 4 and 6 years of age, is in Erikson's stage of initiative versus guilt.

Increased motor ability allows expanded exploration in the family and within the community. The willingness to separate from the mother and explore enhances the development of autonomy and communication skills.

PHYSIOLOGICAL CHANGES

Most children learn to walk steadily between 12 and 15 months of age. By age 2 an exaggerated lumbar curve of the spine causes the abdomen to protrude. By age 3 the posture is more erect. The legs appear bowed between 12 and 18 months of age, and the feet strike the floor flat when walking. A knock-knee appearance develops between 18 months and 2 years. The gait gradually becomes steadier, and by age 2 the knees and toes appear more in alignment. At age 2, the child can run. By age 2½ the child can climb stairs gracefully; by age 3 the child can alternate feet when climbing stairs and can ride a tricycle. By age 4 the child can hop and by age 5 can skip.

Twenty primary teeth erupt by age 2, and the anterior fontanel of the skull closes at 18 months. Continued myelinization of neurons within the brain increases brain function. Although complete myelinization of the brain does not occur before 6 to 7 years of age, the rate of brain and body development during the preschool years influences behavior and motor coordination. The neocortex of the brain is responsible for thought, emotion, and higher-level brain functions. The frontal lobes are responsible for memory, attention, behavior, and emotions. For example, the skill of bike riding involves vision, hearing, sensation, balance, and using the thalamus and neocortex brain functions (Figure 7-1). A school-age child can ride a two-wheel bicycle, whereas a toddler struggles to learn skills involved in controlling a tricycle. The left hemisphere of the brain has been

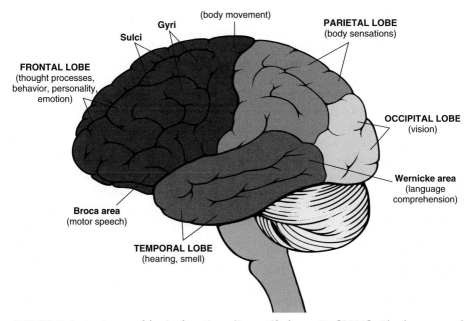

FIGURE 7-1 Anatomy of brain function. (From Chabner, D. [2001]. *The language of medicine* [6th ed.]. Philadelphia: W.B. Saunders.)

implicated in language disorders, cerebral palsy, and deafness (Olsen et al, 2002). Language-rich interactive play helps to enhance language development. Children who have difficulty in one area of brain development may be predisposed to other areas of developmental delay. Developmental screening should be part of every well child visit.

The preschooler gains about 5 to 7 pounds (2.7 to 3.2 kg) and grows about 2½ to 3 inches (6.25-7.5 cm) per year. Half of the adult height is achieved by age 2 (Levine, 1999), and the birth weight is quadrupled.

The toddler has a well-developed **pincer grasp** (the ability to pick up small objects with the thumb and forefinger) by age 1 and can touch the thumb to each finger sequentially by age 5. A 2 year old can copy a straight line; a 3 year old can copy a circle and use scissors. A 4 year old can draw a person with three body parts, and most 5 year olds can print their name. Between 18 months and 5 years the child shows a preference for using one hand or the other and so becomes left-handed or right-handed. Attempts to change hand preference are often met with frustration and are rarely successful. The eye muscles strengthen, depth perception increases during the preschool period, and 20/20 vision is usually achieved by age 4. When asked to find a specific picture on a page while reading a book, the toddler will examine the page in a random pattern to find the specific picture. However, in the same situation with a preschool-age child, the child will examine the page in an organized fashion (up and down or side to side), indicating reading readiness has occurred. Successful reading requires examining the page in an organized pattern.

Hearing is fully developed in the toddler and is necessary for speech development to occur. The eustachian tube connects the middle ear to the **oropharynx** (back of the throat). The eustachian tube is short and straight; therefore bacteria can easily travel from the throat to the middle ear and cause an ear infection. A child who is put to bed while drinking milk or juice from a bottle may have a pooling of the sugary fluid in the back of the throat that enables bacteria to grow. These bacteria then have easy access through the eustachian tube and can cause a middle ear infection. If a child must be put to bed with a bottle, only water should be in the bottle to prevent development of frequent ear infections, as well as **dental caries** (cavities).

During early childhood, fine motor skills develop, which include self-feeding, undressing, and then dressing themselves. Toddlers are able to eat with a fork and spoon but often prefer finger foods. At age 2 the appetite decreases.

Toilet training occurs as sphincter control develops and the child masters some form of communication to indicate the need to use the toilet. Modeling behavior with specially equipped dolls and celebrating successes aid in achieving toilet training, but the process cannot be hurried and may not be complete before 3½ years of age. Bowel control occurs before full bladder control, and nighttime or stress time accidents are common. Accidents should not be scolded or punished, because mastering sphincter control is related to the development of the self-concept.

NUTRITION

Good nutrition starts before conception. During the early childhood years the dependent child is fed by adults whose eating habits may be based on ethnic, cultural, folklore, or fad concepts. Some families are poor, some need guidance on how to select nutritious foods, some need guidance on how to cook foods to preserve the nutritious qualities, and many families do not consider food a priority in the home. However, adequate nutrition is essential for optimum physical and mental development of young children. The U.S. Department of Agriculture (USDA) and The U.S. Department of Health and Human Services (USDHHS) offer guidelines for good eating, as seen in the Food Pyramid for children 2 to 6 years old (Figure 7-2).

The Food Pyramid includes suggestions for portion servings appropriate for young children. High-fiber diets are not adequate for children because the foods are filling but do not provide the essential nutrients for growth and development. Children 1 to 6 years old are susceptible to nutritional deficiencies because growth is rapid and energy output is high. There are no known advantages of consuming excess nutrients or vitamins. Obesity should be prevented and support for growth and development provided through a varied and nutritious diet. Eating habits are developed during the early childhood years, and children may carry these healthy (or unhealthy) habits with them to adulthood. The effect of childhood nutrition on adult health and illness has been well established.

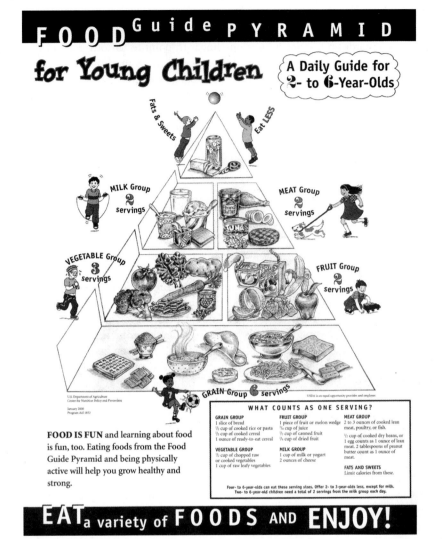

FIGURE 7–2 Food Pyramid for children 2 to 6 years old. (From U.S. Department of Agriculture, March 1999.)

PSYCHOSOCIAL DEVELOPMENT
Language Development and Communication Skills
The Toddler

Children develop receptive language before expressive language. That is, they are able to understand words before they can express them. Communication is evidenced in the neonatal period by the cry, coo, or smile. The initial purpose is to communicate needs, regulate another's behavior, attract attention, and socially interact.

By 1 year of age the toddler usually says the first clear word and responds to simple, single demands or statements such as "bye-bye" or "no!" By 15 months the toddler may speak 4 to 6 words and typically uses one finger to point to various parts of the body. By 18 months the toddler speaks about 15 words and by 19 months may speak in two-word sentences. By age 2 the child has a vocabulary exceeding 100 words and can follow two-step commands such as "Pick up the toy and put it away." The toddler can learn more than one language when learning to speak if both languages are used at home. It is when one language is used at home and a different language is used in school that difficulties tend to arise. By age 5 parents have usually assisted their child to achieve competence in their native language.

The Preschooler

Language development occurs rapidly during the preschool years. A typical 2 year old has a vocabulary of just over 100 words, whereas a typical 5 year old has a vocabulary exceeding 2000 words. In a preschool child the number of words in a typical sentence is equal to the child's age (Behrman, 2004). By age 2½ the child expresses possession, as in "My doll." By age 4 the past tense is expressed, and by age 5 the child can express the future tense. Although speech development is directly influenced by the experiences of others talking to the child and encouraging the child to verbalize, speech development follows a predictable sequence and occurs even without the benefit of encouragement or imitating the words of others, albeit at a much slower pace. Speech development is a reflection of mental and emotional development, and often mental retardation can be detected by age 2, when speech delay is obvious. However, speech can also be delayed under conditions of abuse and neglect.

By age 2 a child can be heard to repeat the commands of others. When tempted to touch a forbidden object, the child can be heard stating "Don't touch." From this observation it is apparent that the child's own internal language plays a part in the child's behavior. When the child's skill at language allows him or her to express basic fears, the need for acting out the fears or frustrations decreases. For this reason, language-delayed children are apt to have more frequent behavioral outbursts or temper tantrums.

The language skills acquired during the preschool years sets the stage for success for the school-age child in the task of achieving literacy at school. A school-age child is expected to enter the classroom with competency in his or her native language. Language milestones can be used to aid in the assessment of the child's development (Table 7-1).

If speech ability is delayed, such as the inability to use single words by 18 months, or few vocabulary words by age 2, or words not clearly understood by age 3, then a referral for speech and hearing evaluations should be offered (Table 7-2).

Cognitive Development

The sensorimotor stage of cognition ends when the toddler begins to use words to express ideas and solve problems. This marks the beginning of symbolic thought. By age 1 the toddler can push away an obstacle in front of him or her to gain access to a toy. By 18 months the toddler learns that dropping a ball, a block, or a stuffed toy down a stairway results in different rates of descent and heights of bounce. By age 2 the tod-

TABLE 7-1

LITERACY MILESTONES

Age	Motor	Cognitive/Language	Interaction
6-12 months	Reaches for book. Puts book to mouth.	Looks at pictures. Vocalizes, pats picture.	Face-to-face gaze. Parents follow baby's cues for "more" and "stop."
12-18 months	Holds book with help. Turns several pages at a time.	Points at pictures with one finger. Labels pictures with same sound.	May bring book to read. Child becomes upset if parent does not let child "control" reading.
18-36 months	Turns one page at a time. Carries book around house.	Names familiar pictures. Attention highly variable Demands story over and over.	Parent asks "what's happening?" questions. Parent shows pleasure when child supplies word.

From Levine, M., Carey, W., & Crocker, A. (1999). *Developmental-behavioral pediatrics* (3rd ed.). Philadelphia: W.B. Saunders.

dler remembers past experiences and adjusts behavior accordingly. A 1 year old may exhibit stranger anxiety when the parent leaves the room. By age 2 the child can anticipate a temporary absence (e.g., a parent going to work) in an accepting manner. Preschool thinking involves Piaget's preoperational or prelogical characteristics, such as magical thinking and egocentrism. Two year olds attribute life qualities to inanimate dolls or toys and typically feel their wishes caused things to happen. They feel their point of view must be the same as everyone else's point of view. Although preschoolers are empathetic, they believe what comforts them will also serve to comfort others. Through experience, preschoolers gradually learn about cause and effect and how to problem solve. Having one object represent another, such as a box representing a train, evidences symbolism and fantasy play. Pretend play is common at age 2. By age 3 children can understand the motivations of others that may differ from their own, and by age 5 they can role play scenarios with elaborate plots and characters. During the preschool years, while the child is trying to understand the differing opinions of others, the fears and forces may be represented by monsters, bad people, or invisible friends.

One of the major tasks of the preschool years is to develop impulse control of behaviors such as biting, kicking, and throwing toys. Impulse control is typically achieved by age 4, with minor relapses in times of stress. By 18 months the toddler develops a sense of self (Greenspan, 1996) and by age 3 is able to express complex feelings and ideas through pretend play (Figure 7-3). At age 4 the child can understand the wishes and emotions of others and how they differ from the child's own. Whatever the preschooler

TABLE 7-2

WHEN A CHILD WITH A COMMUNICATION DISORDER NEEDS HELP

Age	Behavior Indicating Help is Needed
0-11 months	Before 6 months the child does not startle, blink, or change immediate activity in response to sudden loud sounds.
	Before 6 months the child does not attend to the human voice and is not soothed by the mother's voice.
	By 6 months the child does not babble strings of consonant + vowel syllables or imitate gurgling or cooing sounds.
	By 10 months the child does not respond to his or her name.
	At 10 months the child's sound making is limited to shrieks, grunts, or sustained vowel production.
12-23 months	At 12 months the child's babbling or speech is limited to vowel sounds.
	By 15 months the child does not respond to "no", "bye-bye", or "bottle".
	By 15 months the child will not imitate sounds or words.
	By 18 months the child is not consistently using at least six words with appropriate meaning.
	By 21 months the child does not respond correctly to "Give me...", "sit down", or "come here" when spoken without gestural cues.
	By 23 months two-word phrases have not emerged that are spoken as single units (e.g., "Whatzit", "Thank you", "All gone)".
24-36 months	By 24 months at least 50% of the child's speech is not understood by familiar listeners.
	By 24 months the child does not point to body parts without gestural cues.
	By 24 months the child is not combining words into phrases ("Go bye-bye," "Go car," "Want cookie.")
	By 30 months the child does not demonstrate understanding of on, in, under, front, back.
	By 30 months the child is not using short sentences ("Daddy went bye-bye").
	By 30 months the child has not begun to ask questions, using where, what, why.
	By 36 months the child's speech is not understood by unfamiliar listeners.
All Ages	At any age, the child is consistently dysfluent with repetitions, hesitations; blocks or struggles to say words. Struggle may be accompanied by grimaces, eye blinks, or hand gestures.

From Behrman, R.E. and Kliegman, R.M. (2002). *Nelson's Essentials of Pediatrics* (4th ed.). Philadelphia: W.B. Saunders. Originally adapted from Weiss, C.E., & Lillywhite, H.E. (1976) *Communication disorders: a handbook for prevention and early detection.* St Louis: Mosby.

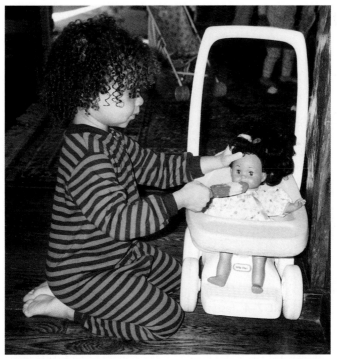

FIGURE 7–3 This child engages in pretend play as she feeds her doll.

cannot understand or express is often acted out in the form of negativism or tantrums as a vehicle of expression. The natural temperament of the child influences the intensity of responses to emotions such as joy, anger, or frustration. Many parents need guidance in helping their toddler manage these challenges in a positive way.

Moral Development

According to Kohlberg, learning self-control and learning to share with others are moral tasks of early childhood. Preschoolers look carefully at parents as models of moral behavior, and this is often acted out in their play. Preschoolers must organize and synthesize what they view at home, in the community, and on television. They constantly test limits either to confirm that a behavior is unacceptable or just to gain attention (Figure 7-4). A child of 3 becomes ritualistic and aware of rules that he or she feels must be obeyed and will feel guilty if scolded. A 2 year old cannot differentiate between intentional acts and accidents and readily assigns blame. A 3 year old can understand the difference between intentional acts and accidents but still may extend blame to another. By age 5 the child extends blame for only the intentional act and easily excuses the accident.

Some parents complain that their preschool child lies. Preschoolers do not have the abstract reasoning to lie for the purpose of deceiving anyone. They tell the truth as they interpret it or wish it to be true. Stealing is a behavior that a preschooler does not feel

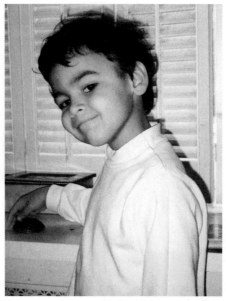

FIGURE 7–4 Testing the limits of acceptable behavior.

is wrong because ownership is not completely understood. Respecting the property of others is a learned behavior. A child will learn socially acceptable behavior through consistent, positive reinforcement and discipline.

Discipline

Discipline must have as its basic purpose, the guiding, teaching, or correcting of behavior, not punishment. Preschoolers are naturally egocentric and may not understand the rights and needs of others. The preschooler may hit the mother in anger yet expect to be loved, hugged, and comforted by the mother in his or her frustration.

The purpose of discipline for toddlers should be to help them develop self-control while maintaining a positive self-esteem. Limit setting should include praise for good behavior. A time-out response to unacceptable behavior is effective for children between the ages of 1 and 6 years. It places the child in a safe place with time for self-regulation. Timing for time out is usually 1 minute per year of age. The child is removed from the situation, placed in time out with just a very brief explanation of why it is happening, and reminded of the cause at the end of time out. With consistent use, the child will learn to anticipate that response to certain behaviors and learn to control those behaviors. **Corporal punishment** (spanking) focuses on the pain of the punishment, role models aggression, and rarely accomplishes the true goal of discipline. Young children may model the behavior of the parent and hit the parent. Children can also get used to the spanking, so that the parent has to hit harder and child abuse becomes a risk. Severe physical punishment may affect the psychological health of the child. Rewarding good behavior is the positive and most effective technique of discipline. A hug, smile, praise, or material reward for good behavior is effective. Consistency in parent response is the key to successful discipline. It is best to ignore the behavior of a child who whines or nags or has a tantrum and give frequent praise when the behavior is good. If a behavior gets attention, it will be used again and more intensely to get attention. *Operant conditioning,* as described by Skinner, occurs when the learner repeats behaviors that result in a positive outcome of his or her goals and stops behaviors that have negative outcomes. The operant theory of discipline is described in Table 7-3. An example of the operant theory during play is the use of an interactive mobile that is activated when the infant kicks and touches a footpad. The infant's kicking will increase if the infant enjoys the resulting sound and movement of the mobile.

When discussing discipline techniques with parents, the nurse or health care worker should be nonjudgmental and help parents develop a mutually acceptable plan that will be consistent and safe. Support groups, parenting classes, and counseling should be available for referral as needed.

Sexuality in Early Childhood

In the past, toddlers and preschool-age children were thought to be free of sexuality or in a period of sexual dormancy. Today it is recognized that children in early childhood do have the capacity for sexual pleasure and response, which includes penile erection, pelvic thrusting, rhythmic movements, and masturbation. Kinsey (1948) and other researchers have shown that children between the ages of 4 and 7 years experience play activities that involve viewing or touching the genitals. This behavior is normal curiosity (Table 7-4).

Parents have an impact on the molding of sexuality in their infants and children. The parents' response to the child's urinary and fecal elimination is an early influence related to sexuality. A negative response to a dirty diaper, the label of "stinky" to the soiled underpants of a toddler, or forced toilet training all influence the development of sexuality. Treating the natural process of bodily functions as secret or dirty promotes embarrassment or discomfort related to the genital area. Modesty appears gradually between 5 and 6 years of age. The acceptance or rejection of hugging and kissing as an expression of emotion by parents can influence sexuality and the ability of the child to

---

TABLE 7-3

THE OPERANT THEORY OF EFFECTIVE DISCIPLINE TECHNIQUES

Type of Discipline	Example	Effect
Positive reinforcement	Child gets a lollipop for helping mommy.	Increases the "helping mommy" behavior.
Negative reinforcement	Restrict privileges for bad behavior. Remove restrictions for good behavior.	Increases likelihood of desired behavior occurring again (useful in older children as well).
Negative punishment	Take away fun and interaction with others. Ignore behavior.	Decreases or stops unwanted behavior.

TABLE 7-4

SEXUALITY BEHAVIOR IN EARLY CHILDHOOD

Normal	Requires Referral
When diapers are changed, child may touch own genitals	Prefers touching genitals instead of playing with toys
Plays with feces	Repeatedly uses feces as a toy
Touches genitals, breasts of family and peers	Asks to be touched in genital area
Removes clothes, likes to play nude	Removes clothes in public repeatedly even after correction
Shows interest in watching bathroom functions	Often insists on watching bathroom functions of others
Plays "doctor" to inspect body of others	Forces peers to remove clothes
Places objects against genital area	Insists on placing objects against genital area of self or peers
Plays house, with mommy and daddy roles assigned to peers	Simulates sexual intercourse activities; draws genitals on figures

establish intimate relationships in later life. Preschool day care centers typically do not separate boys and girls bathrooms, and viewing the body is treated as normal and natural. Masturbation or sexual curiosity that interferes with normal play activities or acting out sexual intercourse with dolls or playmates may be an indication of sexual abuse, and the child should be referred for counseling.

Play

In the toddler period, play is a reflection of the child's experiences. The toddler may play putting baby to bed or shopping in the store. The 2 year old exhibits **parallel play,** in which he or she plays next to a friend but does not interact with the friend. The 3 to 4 year old exhibits **cooperative play,** in which a group of children can cooperate by playing out a scene together or building blocks together. By age 5 there is organized group play with assigned roles, such as playing house with one child assigned the mother role, one the father role, and so on. Play allows the child to imitate adult roles, play the aggressor, or assume superpowers and solve problems. The child's drawings often reflect their inner emotional issues or conflicts. Rules of play are absolute and fairness means equal treatment regardless of circumstances, according to the preschool child. Group songs and music are enjoyed by both the toddler and the preschool child, who respond with unique dancing and random movements (Figure 7-5). Many 2 year olds enjoy singing along with a tape, CD, or music video.

Age-appropriate toys are toys that are safe and promote the cognitive and motor development of the specific age group.

Day Care

The experience of spending time in day care or preschool is a big step toward developing independence. The child must accept that the parent will leave and trust that the

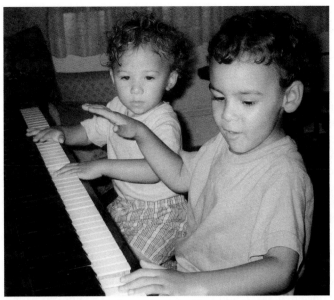

FIGURE 7–5 Preschoolers share a love of music. These brothers sing along while experimenting with a musical instrument. Note how the younger child (on the left) mimics his older brother.

parent will return. There are several types of day care settings in the community that may be available to parents who work outside the home.

The parents may choose a private *babysitter* to come into their home and offer personal attention to their child. Family day care centers provide child care for small groups of children, and often parents take turns providing the child care in this type of setting. Some employers offer day care within the workplace as a service to their employees. *Day care centers* offer structured play and rest activities for groups of children supervised by professional staff. *Preschool centers* offer structured activities that foster growth and development and teach coping skills. A good preschool program can help a child gain self-confidence and positive self-esteem.

Parents may be offered the following suggestions to help select a facility that will best meet the needs of their child:

- State licensing agencies offer lists of local day care centers and preschools.
- The school should meet accreditation standards set by the National Association for Education of Young Children.
- Staff should have school preparation in early childhood education.
- Student-to-staff ratios should be established with clear limits.
- Techniques of discipline, philosophy of care or education, safety, and sanitary conditions of the environment should be reviewed.
- Facilities for snacks and rest should be reviewed.
- Health history requirements for children should be reviewed.
- Toys and facilities for indoor and outdoor play should be reviewed.

- Parents should visit the school and observe staff-child interaction.
- Parents can speak to parents of other children in the school to get input.

TEACHING TECHNIQUES

When parents respond to the words of a toddler appropriately, they stimulate the development of communication. The use of picture books at regular interactive reading sessions with the toddler also aids in language development. Parents should not demand correct speech of a 2 year old, and pronunciation should not be a focus. If speech difficulties are associated with other oral problems, such as inability to blow a kiss or eat, medical evaluation should be sought.

Parents can be taught how to help the preschooler express feelings through words such as "You feel angry now and I understand." Teaching the preschooler how to express feelings verbally rather than acting out is a key to positive social development. Preschool children learning to be autonomous often rapidly shift between dependence and independence, joy and rage, and this changing behavior can cause parents to feel frustrated and inadequate. Parents need to be counseled concerning the normal development and behavior of the toddler and preschool child. The parent can often model the behavior that they wish their child to imitate. For example, introduction of toothbrushing can begin at age 2, and professional dental checkups can be initiated by age 3 (Figure 7-6). The behaviors of the child and responses of the parent should be discussed at well child visits. When a parent does not offer any positive statements about his or her child and the child misbehaves in preschool and at home, more detailed assessment may be necessary.

Safety and Accident Prevention

Accidents are a major threat during the early childhood years. Young children play hard and have little understanding of the potential dangers around them.

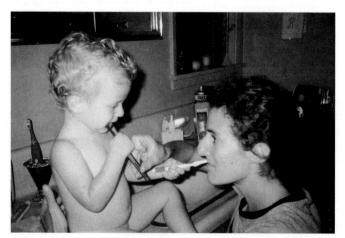

FIGURE 7–6 This mother guides the child's hand as the child brushes her own teeth. The child also "helps" brush the mother's teeth in this nightly ritual.

Parents need guidance concerning the need to childproof the house, keep stairways safe, and avoid clutter. Toys should be sturdy, age appropriate, and not have sharp edges. Preschoolers should not be allowed to carry breakable items or sharp objects. The appropriate use of car seats is essential. Children should not be left inside a car to play alone (Figure 7-7).

Pot handles should not overhang the stove because accidental burns are a common danger in the home. Medicines should have childproof bottle caps and should not be left within the sight or reach of a young child. Preschool children can be taught the dangers of talking with strangers and should know where to go if a parent or sitter is not in sight. Accident prevention techniques should be discussed at every well child visit (Table 7-5).

Immunizations

Immunity is defined as the body's resistance to disease-causing organisms. Newborns have immunity protection transferred via the placenta from the mother, but it lasts only for a few months. In infants and young children the immune system is immature and

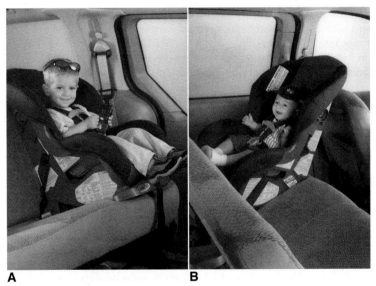

A   **B**

FIGURE 7–7 Car seats. **A,** The infant under 20 pounds is secured in a rear-facing car seat in the back seat of the car to prevent the large and heavy head from falling forward when the car stops suddenly or in case of an accident. The driver can look through the rearview mirror of the car toward a mirror mounted on the rear window to see the face of the infant. **B,** A child over 20 pounds is secured in a front-facing car seat in the back seat of the car. Note that the car seat belt clip rests firmly on the chest of the child, not under the chin. (Comfort Sport-Convertible Car Seat. Courtesy Graco Children's Products, Inc., Exton, Penn.)

HOW TO PREVENT HAZARDS CAUSED BY THE BEHAVIORAL CHARACTERISTICS OF TODDLERS

Behavioral Characteristics	Hazard and Prevention Strategies
Automobile	
Impulsive, unable to delay gratification, increased mobility, egocentric	Teach child street safety rules.
	Teach child the meaning of red, yellow, and green traffic lights.
	Caution child not to run from behind parked cars or snow banks.
	Use car seat restraints appropriately.
	Hold toddler's hand when crossing the street.
	Supervise tricycle riding.
	Do not allow child to play in the car alone.
	Driver must look carefully in front and behind vehicles before accelerating.
	Teach child what areas are safe in and around the house.
	Supervise child under 3 years at all times.
Burns	
Fascination with fire Toddler can reach articles by climbing, pokes fingers in holes and openings; can open doors and drawers; is unaware of cause and effect	Teach child the meaning of "hot." (One mother taught this by allowing child to touch beach sand warmed by the sun.)
	Put matches, cigarettes, candles, and incense out of reach and sight.
	Turn handles of cooking utensils toward the back of the stove.
	Beware of hot coffee; avoid tablecloths with overhang.
	Keep appliances such as coffee pots, electric frying pans, and food processors and their cords out of reach
	Test food and fluids heated in microwave ovens to ensure that center is not too hot.
	Beware of hot charcoal grills.
	Use snug fireplace screens.
	Mark children's rooms to alert firefighters in emergency.
	Keep a pressure-type fire extinguisher available, and teach all family members who are old enough how to use it.
	Practice what to do in case of fire in your home.
	Install smoke detectors.
	Cover electrical outlets with protective caps.
	Check bath water temperature before placing child in water.
	Do not allow child to handle water faucets.
	Protect child from sun with sunscreen and clothing.
Falls	
Exploring different parts of house; can open doors and lean out open windows;	Teach children how to go up and come down stairs when they show a readiness for this task.
	Fasten crib sides securely and leave them up when child is in crib.
	Use side rails on a large bed when child graduates from crib.
	Lock basement doors or use gates at top and bottom of stairs.

TABLE 7-5

HOW TO PREVENT HAZARDS CAUSED BY THE BEHAVIORAL CHARACTERISTICS OF TODDLERS—cont'd

Behavioral Characteristics	Hazard and Prevention Strategies
Falls—cont'd	
toddlers' depth	Mop spilled water from floor immediately.
perception	Use window guards.
immature	Use car seat restraints appropriately.
Capabilities	Keep scissors and other pointed objects away from the toddler's
change quickly;	reach.
may seem	Use childproof doorknobs and drawer closures.
quite grown	Secure child in shopping cart at store.
up at times,	Supervise climbing child in playground.
but still require	Clothing and shoelaces should be appropriate to prevent tripping.
constant	
supervision at	
home and on	
playground	
Suffocation and Choking	
Explores with	Do not allow small children to play with deflated balloons, as
senses, likes to	these can be sucked into windpipe.
bite on and	Inspect toys for small or loose parts.
taste things	Remove small objects such as coins, buttons, and pins from reach.
Eats on the run	Avoid popcorn, nuts, small hard candies, chewing gum, or large
	chunks of meat, such as hot dogs.
	Debone fish, chicken.
	Learn Heimlich maneuver.
	Inspect width of crib and playpen slats.
	Keep plastic bags away from small children; do not use as
	mattress cover.
	If child is vomiting, turn him or her on side.
	Avoid nightclothes with drawstring necks.
	Discard old refrigerators and appliances or remove doors.
Poisoning	
Ingenuity increases,	Store household detergents and cleaning supplies out of reach
can open most	and in a locked cabinet.
containers	
Increased mobility	Do not put chemicals or other potentially harmful substances into
provides access	food or beverage containers.
to cupboards,	Keep medicines in a locked cabinet; put them away immediately
medicine	after using them.
cabinets,	Use child-resistant caps and packaging.
bedside stands,	Flush old medicine down toilet.
interior of	Follow physician's directions when administering medication.
closets	Do not refer to pills as "candy."

(Continued)

TABLE 7-5

HOW TO PREVENT HAZARDS CAUSED BY THE BEHAVIORAL CHARACTERISTICS OF TODDLERS—cont'd

Behavioral Characteristics	Hazard and Prevention Strategies
Poisoning—cont'd	
Looks at and touches everything	Educate parents as to when and how to use ipecac syrup.
	Explain poison symbols to child and to parents not fluent in English.
	Keep telephone number of poison control center available.
Learns by trial and error	When painting, use paint marked "for indoor use" or one that conforms to standards for use on surfaces that may be chewed
Puts objects in mouth	by children.
	Wash fruits and vegetables before eating.
	Obtain and record name of any new plant purchased.
	Alert family of location and appearance of poisonous plants on or around property or commonly encountered when camping.
	Use childproof locks on cabinets.
	Use dishes that do not have high lead content.
Drowning	
Lacks depth perception	Watch child continuously while at beach or near a pool.
	Empty wading pools when child has finished playing.
Does not realize danger	Cover wells securely. Wear recommended life jackets in boats.
	Begin teaching water safety and swimming skills early.
Loves water play	Lock fences surrounding swimming pools.
	Supervise tub baths; be aware that a young child can drown in a very small amount of water.
Electric Shock	
Pokes and probes with fingers	Cover electrical outlets.
	Cap unused sockets with safety plugs.
	Water conducts electricity; teach child not to touch electrical appliances when wet; keep appliances out of reach.
	Keep electrical appliances away from tub and sink area.
Animal Bites	
Immature judgment	Teach child to avoid stray animals.
	Do not allow toddler to abuse household pets.
	Supervise closely.
Safety	
Easily distracted	Teach toddler stranger safety.
Trusting of others	Do not personalize clothes.
Falls frequently	Do not allow toddler to eat or suck lollipops while running or playing.
	Keep sharp-edged objects out of reach.
	Keep sharp-edged furniture out of play area.

Keep first aid chart and emergency numbers handy. Know location of and how to get to nearest emergency facility.
Modified from Leifer, G. (2003). *Introduction to maternity and pediatric nursing* (4th ed.) Philadelphia: W.B. Saunders.

the child is vulnerable to life-threatening infections. An active immunization program starts at 2 months, when the child is capable of producing his or her own antibodies.

The American Academy of Pediatrics (AAP) recommended immunization schedule for infants and children is listed in Appendix A.

Sometimes teaching a preschooler about health issues requires the child's' participation, interaction, or cooperation. A preschool child knows that when a pin or needle is stuck into a balloon, the balloon will pop. Therefore it is no surprise that in children's minds, when a pin (or needle) is stuck into their arm or leg, they fear that their body will pop or explode too. One possible approach is to allow the child to handle the syringe (without the needle) and give pretend injections to a doll. The immediate presence of a calm, reassuring parent who is holding the child in a firm hug will assuage fear and anxiety better than any verbal explanation or reassurance.

During toilet training (potty training), a child's refusal to sit on a toilet may stem from the fear of being flushed away. The child's fear is real and the parents cannot dismiss the fear and expect to gain cooperation.

When teaching parents, it is important to develop a partnership with them and understand their values so that anticipatory guidance can be provided. The nurse can offer the parents tools to help manage their child's behavior, including an understanding of the ongoing developmental process.

KEY POINTS

- The early childhood period is between 1 and 6 years of age and is separated into the toddler phase and the preschool phase.
- Tasks to be mastered during early childhood include understanding and speaking words, social interaction, mastery of self-control in feeding and toileting, and beginning to develop a self-concept and a sense of autonomy.
- Toilet training occurs as sphincter control develops and the child masters basic communication skills to indicate the need to use the toilet. Complete bowel and bladder control is typically complete by age 2½ to 3 years.
- Adequate nutrition is essential for optimum physical and mental development.
- A 2-year-old child exhibits negativistic behavior and tantrums due to frustrations and struggles for independence.
- Preschool thinking involves Piaget's preoperational or prelogical characteristics.
- A 2 year old cannot distinguish between intentional acts and mistakes.
- Impulse control is typically achieved by age 4.
- A 3 year old is ritualistic and feels all rules must be obeyed.
- According to Kohlberg, the preconventional stage of moral development begins in the preschool age.
- Discipline should have as its purpose the guiding, teaching, or correcting of behavior, not punishment.

- Toddlers and preschoolers do not completely understand the rights of others.
- According to Freud, a conscience begins to develop in the preschool phase and children begin to understand how their behavior affects others.
- Play is an important part of a child's life. Appropriate toys can promote growth and development.
- Twenty primary teeth erupt by age 2. One half the adult height is reached by age 2½, and the birth weight quadruples as well.
- The preschool child can learn more than one language when both languages are used at home.
- Language milestones can be used to assess the child's development.
- In a preschool child the number or words in a typical sentence is equal to the child's age in years.
- A preschool child learns socially acceptable behavior by positive reinforcement.
- Time outs should last 1 minute per year of age.
- A 2 year old exhibits parallel play, whereas a 3 year old engages in cooperative play with groups using a high level of imagination.
- Parents who hold, hug, and rock their children can influence the ability of the child to establish intimate relationships later in life.
- Accident prevention techniques should be discussed with parents.
- An active immunization program schedule starts at 2 months and continues through the preschool years. Many communicable diseases in childhood can be prevented through immunization.

CRITICAL THINKING

When discussing discipline techniques for children, the nurse or health care worker can help parents develop a plan that is mutually agreeable. Discuss three types of discipline techniques that can be used consistently and safely and are appropriate for the early childhood years. List examples of how these techniques can be implemented.

MULTIPLE-CHOICE REVIEW QUESTIONS

1 Tasks to be mastered during early childhood include:
   1 Walking
   2 Bowel control
   3 Abstract thinking
   4 Visual maturity
2 The toddler-age child is in Erikson's stage of:
   1 Trust versus mistrust
   2 Initiative versus guilt
   3 Autonomy versus shame and doubt
   4 Identity versus role confusion

3 The preschool-age child, between 4 and 6 years of age, is in Erikson's stage of:
   1 Trust versus mistrust
   2 Initiative versus guilt
   3 Autonomy versus shame and doubt
   4 Identity versus role confusion
4 Between 12 and 24 months of age, the child's speech normally includes:
   1 Only vowel sounds
   2 Both vowels and consonants
   3 Frequent babbling
   4 Three- to four-word sentences
5 In early childhood the best discipline technique includes:
   1 Rewarding good behavior
   2 Punishing bad behavior
   3 Setting rigid, structured rules
   4 Posting rules on the refrigerator door

Middle Childhood

OBJECTIVES

Upon completion of this chapter, the student will be able to:

1 Define *middle childhood.*
2 Describe the physiological changes that occur in middle childhood.
3 Describe the cognitive development that occurs in middle childhood and its effect on the development of learning styles.
4 Discuss the psychosocial development that occurs in middle childhood.
5 List at least three ways in which Erikson's task of industry can be fostered in middle childhood.
6 Trace the development of moral behavior in the school-age child.
7 Discuss the discipline techniques that are effective in middle childhood.
8 Describe the typical play activities of the school-age child.
9 Discuss the use of intelligence testing for school-age children.
10 Discuss the role of peer groups in the growth and development during middle childhood.
11 Discuss the sexual development of and education appropriate for school-age children.
12 List the major health teaching needs of school-age children.

KEY TERMS

Cognitive style
Corporal punishment
Discipline
Latchkey children
Middle childhood
Mnemonic technique
Moral behavior
Moral reasoning
Plaque
Social cognition

DEFINITION

Middle childhood includes children between 6 and 12 years. School-age children, between the ages of 6 and 12, differ from preschoolers because they focus more on fact rather than fantasy. School-age children interact with teachers and others outside the family who will have a significant impact on their growth, development, and education. One of the major developmental tasks of this age group is forming a positive self-esteem from internal sources rather than depending on feedback from elders. The ability to develop close peer relationships will affect the development of new ideas, skills, and tools that will enhance their advancement toward maturity. Other developmental tasks include changing from concrete thinking to abstract thinking, developing secondary sex characteristics, and accepting more responsibility.

PHYSIOLOGICAL CHANGES

Myelinization of the brain is complete by age 7, and by age 12 the head has reached its adult size. The bones continue to ossify and grow and the body develops a lower center of gravity than in preschool years, due in part to a shift in posture and an increase in leg length. Physical growth is slow during the school-age years until a growth spurt, which occurs just before puberty. The average gain in weight is 5.5 to 7.0 pounds (2.5 to 3.2 kg) per year, and the average height increase per year is about 2 inches (5 cm). Children who are taller than their peers may face an extra challenge because they are likely to be treated as if they are older or more mature. The self-concept may suffer if the tall child does not live up to these inflated expectations.

The loss of primary teeth begins at about age 6, with the lower central incisor the first tooth to be lost (Figure 8-1).

Parents often treat the loss of primary teeth as a sign of growing up, and many parents reward the child whenever a tooth falls out. About four permanent teeth erupt each year in the same order as deciduous teeth. Regular dental checkups should be a part of routine health care to screen for dental problems and have the teeth cleaned. Daily dental care should include tooth brushing with a fluoride toothpaste in the morning, after each meal, and before bedtime. Limiting intake of sticky sweets and chocolates and encouraging snacks such as apples, raw carrots, and sugarless gum can reduce plaque

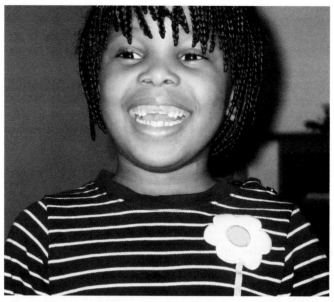

FIGURE 8–1 One of the most obvious physical changes of middle childhood is the loss of primary teeth. The loss of primary teeth starts at age 6, and about four permanent teeth erupt each year.

formation. **Plaque** is a sticky, transparent mass of bacteria that grows on the surface and spreads to the roots of the teeth. Plaque buildup can be prevented by regular tooth brushing and flossing. Flossing between the teeth can be modeled by the parents and quickly learned by the school-age child.

The gastrointestinal tract of the school-age child is more mature than that of the preschooler, and stomach capacity increases. The child requires less caloric intake than the preschooler and usually snacks less. Sensory organs mature and sharpen senses of taste, smell, and touch, and preferences for specific foods develop. Large-print books are no longer necessary, because visual maturity is achieved sometime between preschool age and age 6.

Newly developed fine and gross motor skills enhance their ability to play independently. Age-appropriate toys include bicycles, skates, swimming gear, and jump ropes. School-age children master coordination and control, allowing them to enjoy team sports such as baseball, play a musical instrument, or tap dance. Excess time spent with computer games and video games may contribute to a sedentary lifestyle and increase the risk for obesity or health problems in later life.

Childhood obesity also carries a risk of negatively affecting the child's self-image and social development.

Many schools have physical fitness programs, which promotes a healthy lifestyle consistent with the goals of *Healthy People 2010*.

Eight year olds take pride in mastering skills and in showing off their accomplishments. By age 9 or 10 physical strength is greatly increased and interest in specific sports or other activities develop. Increased understanding of rules and teamwork enable these children to participate in competitive games. School-age children often compare themselves according to their ability to master good grades or excel at sports. This affects the development of their self-esteem. Maintaining optimum nutrition and preventing injury are two more health challenges of the school-age years.

COGNITIVE DEVELOPMENT

According to Piaget, school-age children are concrete thinkers. They think logically and understand rules, although they learn best when they can see and handle objects. Hands-on learning is most effective for school-age children. Table 8-1 lists mastery of tasks and behaviors necessary for success in school and related parental guidance that can be offered.

Cognitive deficits must be assessed early so the child can be successful in school. See Table 8-2 for cognitive deficits and their effect on school performance.

Erikson refers to school age as the stage of industry. In this stage the child has a thirst for knowledge and a desire to master skills and emulate role models or heroes. If a parent intrudes on children's efforts at achieving a skill—perhaps by helping too much or doing it for them—a sense of inferiority can develop. Even if children receive an *A* for a project, they will not achieve a sense of industry if they know the work was not really the result of their own efforts.

School-age children can group similar items together and understand that words have more than one meaning. They may delight in telling jokes to each other and tell jokes to entertain friends or tease adults.

By age 7 egocentrism decreases. Children realize others may have valid opinions that differ from their own, and they may seek out another person's opinion concerning an issue. With a decrease in egocentrism, children become more cooperative and begin to understand how their actions may affect other people. This understanding, called **social cognition,** enables children to get along better with peers and can enhance their self-concept.

The development of **moral reasoning** happens as the child learns to understand rules and determine if an action is right or wrong. **Moral behaviors** are actions based on moral reasoning. In early childhood, rules are important. A 5-year-old child may show intense frustration if a peer breaks a rule. In later childhood the 10 year old may enjoy making his or her own rules for a game or bartering to change the rules. Culture or an environment such as poverty or war can influence moral behavior. Knowing what is culturally or morally right does not guarantee acting in accordance with that knowledge. Lying, stealing, and cheating behaviors are common in school-age children even as they learn moral behavior. Therefore adult modeling of honesty and fairness is essential as the child is learning moral behavior (Box 8-1).

Kohlberg was a theorist who suggested that moral reasoning develops as cognitive function matures, so the ability to think logically is related to moral behavior. Other theorists emphasize that moral behavior is learned through positive reinforcement. Parents teach by rewarding desired behavior. Punishment for undesirable behavior is less effective. Punished children may feel less motivated, less capable or confused or may focus on the punishment and its emotional consequences rather than the behavior.

TABLE **8-1**

MASTERY OF TASKS NECESSARY FOR SCHOOL SUCCESS

Child's Tasks	Parent's Tasks	Interventions
Adapt to differences in expectations of various teachers.	Communicate with teacher to maintain consistency in expectations and discipline.	School nurse can be contacted to facilitate parent-teacher-child interaction.
Compete with 30 or more peers for adult attention.	Praise child's accomplishments. Avoid comparisons to other children.	Observe parent-teacher interactions and provide guidance and positive support.
Learn to accept criticism from peers and teachers without losing self-esteem.	Supervise peer activities. Facilitate constructive communication.	Provide teacher-parent guidance. Teach constructive and positive feedback.
Assimilate peer values with family values.	Maintain open communication. Encourage peer activity. Introduce and accept other cultures in community.	Provide anticipatory guidance in dealing with behavior problems. Observe and deal with signs of prejudice.
Find satisfaction in school achievements.	Help children to achieve. Do not complete tasks for them.	Provide suggestions for identifying strengths and weaknesses. Build on strengths.
Participate in group activities.	Encourage child to join a group or club and actively participate as a member.	Refer to community agencies such as churches, organizations, and club activities as needed.
Learn behavioral self-control. Cope with negative treatment from others in a constructive way.	Encourage participation in activities away from home and with peers. Help build faith in child's problem-solving skills. Discuss coping with prejudices.	Encourage parents to let go and provide guidance while encouraging independence.

Modified from Leifer, G. (2003). *Introduction to maternity and pediatric nursing* (4th ed.). Philadelphia: W.B. Saunders.

In addition to using reward or punishment in guiding children's learning, modeling how a child's actions may affect others is also helpful in developing moral behavior.

Cognitive Styles

A school-age child must have an attention span of 45 minutes to process information and encode it into memory, so it can later be retrieved or remembered. Children approach learning and problem solving in various ways. A **cognitive style** refers to a

BOX 8-1	**Moral Behavior Includes Three Phases**
1 Knowledge (logic)	Knowing what is right
2 Emotion	Feeling good or bad about what is right
3 Action (behavior)	Behaving according to the rule of what is right

pattern of thought and reasoning. Some children take a cluster of knowledge and group it in a certain way to better remember the information. Some use **mnemonic techniques** such as the rhyme for remembering the number of days in each month.

The elementary school curriculum is designed to gradually increase cognitive demands on the school-age child. The first 2 years of elementary school focus on learning to read, write, and do basic math skills. By fourth grade the volume and complexity of the work increases. If basic skills were not learned well, the child may not progress smoothly. Other factors that affect success in school include the child's desire to please teachers and parents, compete with other children, work for delayed rewards, and take risks by trying new things. Feelings of success encourage the child to continue making efforts. Feelings of failure may lead to avoidance of risks or low self-confidence.

Communication Skills

School-age children are usually able to express themselves verbally, and they often use language as a tool in their relationships with others. They can tell jokes that tease and

TABLE 8-2
COGNITIVE DEFICITS AND THEIR EFFECT ON SCHOOL PERFORMANCE

Deficit	Related School Problem
Inability to understand spatial relationships by visual examination.	Repeatedly confuse letters *b*, *d*, and *g*. Difficulty with basic reading and writing.
Difficulty in sensing body position and programming movements.	Poor handwriting—tight grasp of pencil.
Inability to decipher similar sounding words.	Difficulty following directions, leading to short attention span and behavior problems.
Difficulty with long-term memory and recall.	Delayed mastery of counting and alphabet recital.
Easily distracted.	Difficulty following complex instructions.
Difficulty remembering items in order.	Difficulty in organizing assignments and planning completion.
Difficulty in receptive language.	Difficulty in following directions—attention cannot remain focused.
Impaired expressive language.	Difficulty with recall memory. Difficulty expressing feelings or talking spontaneously in a group.

Modified from Behrmann, R., Kleigman, R., & Jensen, H. (2004). *Nelson's textbook of pediatrics* (17th ed.). Philadelphia: W.B. Saunders.

express sarcasm. Adults should offer a model of clear and appropriate language usage. A child who has a language or other communication problem is at risk for social isolation and underachievement in school.

Bilingual education programs are offered to school-age children who speak English as their second language. However, if the teachers are not proficient in the child's primary language, the child may have to learn English by a total immersion technique, which means the child learns the language by hearing it used every day in the classroom. This may add stress socially, academically, and emotionally. It is important that the schools offer support programs for bilingual or language impaired children to reduce stress and associated behavior problems such as frustration, anger, and rebellion.

Intelligence Tests

The original version of the Stanford-Binet intelligence quotient (IQ) test was published in France in 1905 and then brought to the United States. This test assesses mental capabilities of the child and compares set norms or expectations for each age. To determine a score, the mental age is divided by the actual age in years and then multiplied by 100. For example, if a child performs on tests at a level expected for a 10 year old and the actual age in years of the child is 10, the IQ score would be $10/10 \times 100 = 100$.

David Wechsler developed the Wechsler Intelligence Scale for school-age children and adolescents ages 6 to 16 (WISC-III, 1991) and the Wechsler Preschool and Primary Scale of Intelligence (WPPSI-III, 1989) for 3 to 7 year olds. Both assess verbal and nonverbal intelligence. The tests are not meant to be an overall test of general intelligence. The test should be administered to each child by a licensed psychologist. They can be used to predict school performance and can identify children who may need extra help or additional challenges.

PSYCHOSOCIAL DEVELOPMENT
Task of Industry

Erikson was a theorist who believed the primary task for school-age children was to develop a sense of industry. A child can gain satisfaction from achieving even small goals. Praise is essential in this stage of development to build motivation to learn and achieve. Seven year olds may not have the attention span necessary to complete complex tasks. Nine year olds can usually work on a task to completion. By age 11, children are usually able to maintain work and motivation for a delayed reward. A child who does not receive praise for achievements may feel inferior.

Peer Relationships

School-age children begin to compare family values with values of others. Friendships with same-sex peers are very important for the school-age child. The reliance on and importance of the family decrease and sibling rivalry can cause some chaotic episodes. The child may become self-conscious about kisses and hugs from parents in public. Children who have difficulty separating from family and adjusting to school may be responding to the parents' difficulty in letting them go. Divorces, family violence, and other home problems can interfere with a child's achievement of age-appropriate developmental tasks with peers. The school-age child develops a close relationship with friends and shares precious toys and innermost thoughts and secrets with them. School-age children protect their possessions, value privacy, and should be given the responsibility of managing chores and money. However, allowances and family chores function best if they are kept separate. Regular home chores help children gain a sense of responsibility and achieve a feeling that they are a member of a family group. The home, the school, and the neighborhood each have an impact on the growth and development of the child. The culture of a school-age child involves memberships in groups of some kind. If parents do not find a socially acceptable group, such as Scouts or a religious group, children may find their own group—for example, a gang—and may be influenced by them to engage in socially unacceptable behavior to gain acceptance and achieve a sense of belonging. Conformity to most groups is rewarding and enables social success with peers. When a child is labeled or outcast by a peer, the identification may stay with the child and be incorporated into his or her self-image.

Play

Children between the ages of 5 and 7 engage in rough-and-tumble play. By age 7 children are able to engage in competitive play and use coping strategies to deal with team cooperation, conflict, losing, and winning. Competition is often a welcome challenge. Participation in organized sports can develop teamwork and physical fitness. High stress and excessive pressure to win are not helpful and should be avoided. In team sports, all children should be encouraged to participate without excluding those who are less physically talented.

The American Academy of Pediatrics Committee on Sports Medicine and School Health recommends teaching motor skills and fitness exercises in the school setting to develop skills and promote positive attitudes toward exercise that may lead to a lifelong health and fitness philosophy. The focus should be on mastery and enjoyment rather than only on winning. Punishment in the form of assigning extra running of laps or extra exercise promotes negative attitudes toward exercise.

Protective accessories should be worn by children who engage in high-impact sports such as football to prevent injury of the immature skeletal system (Figure 8-2).

Activities such as collecting things or playing board games are often enjoyed by the school-age child. Computer or video games can help develop hand-eye coordination and challenge intellect and are healthy outlets as long as they do not replace daily physical activity. Creativity should be encouraged because it helps to develop general thinking and problem-solving skills. Art and music lessons appropriately encouraged can help develop lifelong interests, appreciation, and talents.

Latchkey Children

In the United States, **latchkey children** are those who are left unsupervised after school because both parents work and extended family are not available to care for them. Some

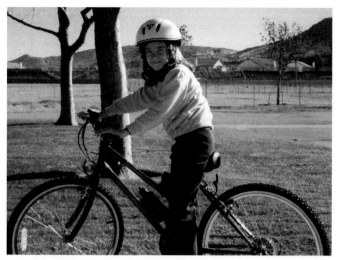

FIGURE 8–2 It is important to teach school-age children to use appropriate protective gear in sports activities. Wearing a helmet while bicycle riding can reduce serious injuries. (From Leifer, G. [2003]. *Introduction to maternity and pediatric nursing* [4th ed.]. Philadelphia: W.B. Saunders.)

children left home alone enjoy the independence and develop maturity and problem-solving skills. Other children are at higher risk for feeling isolated and may be at increased risk for accidents. A backup adult should be available in case of an emergency.

After-school programs with supervised activities may be available in some communities and can help the school-age child maintain contact and interaction with peer groups (Box 8-2).

SEXUALITY

According to Freud, the child is in a period of sexual latency during the middle childhood years and children often identify with same-sex parents. Both the family and the school can influence gender identity. Unisex play and clothes are available, but many families tend to dress boys and girls in traditional male or female styles and colors. Toys can also be gender specific. Dolls are often reserved for girls and trucks and tools for boys. Gender-specific toys may guide the development of self-expectations or likes and dislikes.

Between the ages of 4 and 7 children engage in play activities that may involve viewing or touching the genitals. It is the parents who place sexual meaning on the activity, not the children. A negative body image may develop if parents imply that a part of the body is dirty or bad. Children often ask questions related to sexuality and should be given honest and accurate answers. Ten to eleven year olds may be curious and are sensitive about developing secondary sex characteristics, and girls may eagerly await (or dread) signs of breast development. Interest in the opposite sex is often a sensitive topic and may be strongly denied. Ten to eleven year olds appreciate privacy and may be

---

| **BOX 8-2** | **Guidance for Latchkey Families** |

Teach Child About Safety

Do not enter the house if the door is ajar or anything looks unusual.

Do not leave the house or yard without permission.

Never admit a stranger into the house.

Never agree to meet with someone you met online.

Never respond to messages on the computer that sound weird.

Do not display keys; keep door locked.

Teach how to answer the telephone (parents are busy, not "out").

Do not take shortcuts to school through alleys or across train tracks.

Walk to and from school with friends.

Never accept rides with strangers.

Know how to reach a trusted adult.

Teach first aid techniques; know how to call 911.

Review fire safety rules and route of escape; walk through the procedure with the child.

Know and obey basic safety rules.

Teach Parents To

List emergency numbers and post them near the telephone.

Designate a neighbor who is usually home for help in emergencies.

Teach the child his or her own name, telephone number, address, and parents' name.

Leave work number with the child.

Lock up firearms or remove them from the house.

Prepare a first aid kit and designate its location.

Address street safety with the child when returning from school; include precautions with strangers.

Consider obtaining a pet for the child.

Be home on time or call the child.

Leave a tape-recorded message to decrease the child's loneliness; recommend specific activities rather than television.

Help the child to feel successful and appreciated.

Assess the home and neighborhood for hazards specific to their locale.

Modified from Leifer, G. (2003). *Introduction to maternity and pediatric nursing* (4th ed.). Philadelphia: W.B. Saunders. Data adapted from State of California Office of Criminal Justice Planning, Sacramento, California; and McClellan, M. (1984). On their own: latchkey children. *Pediatric Nursing, 10*, 2000.

---

embarrassed to show their bodies. However, many 9- to 11-year-old children are now rushed through their childhood (Elkind, 2002). As MTV fans, they enjoy pop and hip-hop music with sexually seductive lyrics. They enthusiastically accept adult-type activities and dress. Some preteens wear hip-huggers and halters to school, and some schools have had to adopt strict dress codes or school uniforms to counter this trend.

Sex education is a lifelong process and may begin earlier than many parents believe. Parents convey their attitudes toward sexuality to the growing child, and sometimes parents need guidance in understanding their child's sexual curiosity. School-age children may occasionally masturbate. This behavior is normal and does not cause acne, impotence, mental disease, or blindness. Young boys should be informed about the experience of wet dreams, and young girls should be prepared for menarche. Facts concerning sex and drugs are an important part of sex education in the school-age years. Sex education can be introduced in the context of normal anatomy and physiology. Values can be added and influenced by active parent and teacher participation and by encouraging questions and discussion. The Sex Information and Education Council of the United States (SIECUS), located in New York, advocates that sex education programs be taught from six basic aspects: biological, social, health, personal adjustment, interpersonal relationships, and developing values. Age-appropriate, culturally relevant, written information that treats sexuality as a healthy aspect of life should be included. Table 8-3 reviews the use of the nursing process in sex education for the school-age child.

TEACHING TECHNIQUES FOR THE SCHOOL-AGE CHILD

Most school-age children have a natural curiosity and therefore are ready and eager to learn. Because the extended attention span of the school-age child is limited to 45 minutes maximum, teaching sessions should be planned for no more than this amount of time. All information should be presented to the school-age child in a truthful, factual, and age-appropriate level. Step-by-step instructions are needed for children who are concrete thinkers. Encouraging verbal feedback from the child will ensure that the information given was not misinterpreted. During any teaching process, periods of praise and occasional rewards reinforce learning accomplishments. Teaching techniques should encourage the school-age child to accept responsibilities and should provide hands-on reinforcement whenever possible. Group instruction is effective in teaching positive health behaviors because peer attitudes can influence learning and enhance application of values taught.

TABLE 8-3

NURSING PROCESS IN SEX EDUCATION OF THE SCHOOL-AGE CHILD

Intervention	Observation/Goal
Data collection; history taking (Assess readiness to learn)	Readiness to learn is indicated by asking questions concerning sex, menstruation, "wet dreams," and pregnancy.
Analysis (Assess interactions)	Observe parent-child interactions and determine level of communication.
	Observe peer interaction to determine the child's self-image, self-confidence, and ability to communicate about sensitive issues.
(Assess parents)	Observe parents' knowledge and ability to discuss issues pertaining to sex education.
(Assess child)	Determine child's understanding of sexual development and body changes.
Planning/Implementation	Discuss growth and development with the parents and child.
	Reinforce teaching techniques and opportunities with parents.
Evaluation	With each clinic or home visit, reevaluate parent-child interaction concerning sex education.

Modified from Leifer, G. (2003). *Introduction to maternity and pediatric nursing* (4th ed.). Philadelphia: W.B. Saunders.

Health teaching needs of healthy school-age children include prevention of injury; maintenance of adequate nutrition; the importance of regular dental care; screening for scoliosis and vision and hearing deficits; and the need for immunizations.

Immunizations are reviewed in Appendix A.

School nurses can be a valuable resource for assisting preadolescents in how to make positive choices, develop interpersonal relationships, develop positive self-esteem, utilize problem-solving skills, and access community resources. School nurses should be aware that sometimes a school-age child will complain of minor health problems that have little evidence of pathology as a way of reaching out for help with psychosocial problems.

School-age children can understand the cause of illness and its consequences in terms of missing school and peer activities. They also understand that others will feel sorry for them. However, having to live with a long-term, chronic illness can slow cognitive learning. In most cases, illness causes more anxiety related to separation from peers, falling behind in school, and being left out of social activities than anxiety related to the illness itself. An important primary goal in the care of a school-age child is to foster normal growth and development even if some physical or intellectual disabilities are present. Teaching diabetic school-age children to test their own blood sugar and administer their own insulin is an example of age-appropriate teaching.

DISCIPLINE

The word **discipline** comes from the Latin word *disciplinare*, which means "to teach." Discipline should be thought of as providing age-appropriate positive reinforcement of good behavior that plays an important role in social and emotional development of children.

Punishment is only one aspect of discipline. Reward is another option. If punishment is used, it should be prompt, consistent, and fair. Parents often rely on culturally traditional discipline techniques. Some may shy away from asking for help due to fear that their parenting skills may be criticized. It is through appropriate discipline that children learn self-control and a sense of parental caring. Whenever misbehavior occurs, the motivation should be investigated. Misbehavior often occurs if the child is bored or needs attention or as a reflection of a larger problem at home. Sometimes punishment can reinforce bad behavior if it is the only way attention can be achieved. Negative attention is better than no attention at all in the minds of many children.

Certain temperaments may predispose the child to misbehave. Children with attention deficit disorders (ADD) are also likely to unintentionally misbehave. Harsh physical punishment can increase misbehavior (Herrenkohl et al, 2001). Discipline should combine reward and punishment, be based on age-appropriate behavior expectations, offer the child information on alternative choices of behavior, and teach respect of others. Because the school-age child understands cause-and-effect relationships, discipline needs to be immediate and consistent so that the child understands that the behavior resulted in the reward or punishment. The school-age child can understand and respect rules. Therefore rules, behavior standards, or social interactions can be guided and reinforced according to those rules. Involving the child in designing an appropriate mode of punishment can help develop moral judgment and autonomy.

Including positive reinforcement in disciplinary efforts is crucial to development of good behavior. Attention or praise from parents or teachers is an example of positive reinforcement. If misbehavior results in extra attention from the parent or teacher, this may reinforce bad behavior. That means in order to have effective discipline, attention should be given when behavior is good. Rewards for good behavior can be in the form of extra attention, a smile, a hug, a word of praise, extra privileges, or a token reward such as a sticker or star, which can be accumulated and cashed in later for a material reward. As punishment, stars can be removed after bad behavior.

Discipline should be used only for teaching and not for revenge, to vent anger, or to demand behavior that is beyond the child's ability. Time-outs (discussed in Chapter 7) are appropriate for the 18-month to 6-year-old age group. Removal of privileges such as television programs can be an effective punishment for the school-age child. Verbal punishment in the form of scolding can provide the needed correction for the child, but scolding can escalate into a shouting match or result in frustration or increased noncompliance.

Corporal punishment is spanking, hitting, or inflicting pain to stop or alter behavior. Acceptable spanking has been defined as "the use of an open hand on the buttocks with the intention of modifying behavior without causing injury" (American Academy of Pediatrics, 1998). There is a fine line between corporal punishment and child abuse. For this reason, child experts discourage the use of corporal punishment. Spanking may be initially effective because of its shock value to stop a dangerous situation, but it may not be effective as a long-term tool of discipline. Frequent spanking teaches violent behavior and can lead to decreased self-esteem, depression, and low educational achievement. There are many other forms of discipline that are more effective and clearly nonabusive. These include positive reinforcement (reward), removing privileges, or adding chores.

Parents benefit from guidance in formulating effective discipline techniques. Every well child visit should include a discussion of behavior management and discipline in the home. Teacher education programs also should include discipline techniques for classroom management. Discussion should include alternatives to corporal punishment, anger control skills, and discipline that matches the developmental and educational needs of school-age children. Community resources may include referral to parenting classes, support groups, or professional counselors.

HEALTH AND SAFETY NEEDS OF THE SCHOOL-AGE CHILD

A summary of growth and development during the school-age years and the child's health and safety needs are reviewed in Table 8-4.

TABLE 8-4

SUMMARY OF GROWTH AND DEVELOPMENT AND HEALTH MAINTENANCE OF SCHOOL-AGE CHILDREN

Age (Years)	Physical Competency	Intellectual Competency	Emotional-Social Competency	Nutrition	Play	Safety
General: 6 to 12 years	Gains an average of 2.5 to 3.2 kg/yr (5.0 to 7.0 lb/yr). Has overall height gains of 5.0 cm/yr (2 in/yr); growth occurs in spurts and mainly in the trunk and extremities. Loses deciduous teeth; most permanent teeth erupt. Progressively more coordinated in both gross and fine-motor skills. Caloric needs increase during growth spurts.	Masters concrete operations. Moves from egocentrism; learns that he/she is not always right. Learns grammar and expression of emotions and thoughts. Vocabulary increases to 3000 words or more. Handles complex sentences.	Central crisis; industry vs. inferiority; wants to do and make things. Progressive sex education needed. Wants to be like friends; competition is important. Fears body mutilation, alterations in body image; earlier phobias may recur; nightmares; fears death. Nervous habits are common.	Fluctuations in appetite because of uneven growth pattern and tendency to get involved in activities. Tendency to neglect breakfast in rush of getting to school. Although school lunch is provided in most schools, child does not always eat it.	Plays in groups, mostly of same sex; gang activities predominate. Books for all ages. Bicycles important. Sports equipment, cards, board and table games. Most play is active games requiring little or no equipment.	Enforce continued use of seat belts during car travel. Bicycle safety must be taught and enforced. Teach safety related to hobbies, handicrafts, mechanical equipment.

(Continued)

TABLE 8-4

SUMMARY OF GROWTH AND DEVELOPMENT AND HEALTH MAINTENANCE OF SCHOOL-AGE CHILDREN—cont'd

Age (Years)	Physical Competency	Intellectual Competency	Emotional-Social Competency	Nutrition	Play	Safety
6 to 7 years	Gross motor skill exceeds fine motor coordination Has good balance and rhythm—runs, skips, jumps, climbs, gallops Throws and catches ball. Dresses self with little or no help.	Has vocabulary of 2500 words. Learning to read and print. Begins concrete concepts of numbers, general classifications of items. Knows concepts of right and left; morning, afternoon, and evening, coinage. Has intuitive thought process. Is verbally aggressive, bossy, opinionated, argumentative.	Boisterous, outgoing, and a know-it-all. Whiny; parents should sidestep power struggles, offer choices. Becomes quiet and reflective during seventh year; very sensitive. Can use telephone Likes to make things; starts many project, finishes few. Give some responsibility for household duties.	Persistence of preschool food dislikes. Tendency for deficiencies in iron vitamin A and riboflavin, 100 ml/kg of water per day, 3g/kg protein daily.	Still enjoys dolls, cars, and trucks. Plays well alone but enjoys small groups of both sexes; begins to prefer same-sex peers during seventh year. Ready to learn how to ride a bicycle. Prefers imaginary, dramatic play with real costumes. Begins collecting for quantity, not quality. Enjoys active games such as hide-and-seek, tag.	Teach and reinforce traffic safety. Child needs adult supervision of play. Teach child to avoid strangers and never to take anything from strangers. Teach illness prevention and reinforce continued practice of other health habits. Restrict bicycle use to home ground and no traffic areas; teach bicycle safety. Child should wear helmet.

Age	Physical	Cognitive/Language	Social/Emotional	Nutrition	Play	Safety
					Likes simple games with basic rules.	
					jump rope, in-line skating, soccer.	Teach and set examples about harmful use of drugs, alcohol and smoking.
8 to 10 years	Myopia may appear. Secondary sex characteristics begin in girls. Hand-eye coordination and fine motor skills are well established. Movements are graceful, coordinated. Cares for own physical needs completely Is constantly on the move; plays and works hard.	Learning correct grammar and expression of feelings in words. Likes books he can read alone; will read funny papers and scan newspaper. Enjoys making detailed drawings. Mastering. classification, serialization, spatial, temporal, and numerical concepts. Uses language as a tool; likes riddles, jokes, changes, word games.	Strong preference for same-sex peers. Antagonizes opposite-sex peers. Self-assured and pragmatic at home; questions parental values and ideas. Has a strong sense of humor. Enjoys clubs, group projects, outings, large groups, camp. Modesty about own body increases over time; sex conscious. Works diligently to perfect the	Needs about 2100 calories/day; nutritious snacks. Tends to be too busy to bother to eat. Tendency for deficiencies in calcium, iron, and thiamine. Problem of obesity may begin now. Has good table manners. Able to help with food preparation.	Ready for lessons in dancing, gymnastics, music. Restrict television time to 1 to 2 hours each day. Likes hiking, sports. Enjoys cooking, woodworking, crafts. Enjoys cards and table games. Likes radio and CDs. Begins qualitative collecting.	Stress safety with firearms. Keep them out of reach and allow their use only with adult supervision. Know who the child's friends are; parents should still have some control over friend selection. Teach water safety; swimming should be supervised by an adult. Enforce balance in rest and activity.

(Continued)

TABLE 8-4

SUMMARY OF GROWTH AND DEVELOPMENT AND HEALTH MAINTENANCE OF SCHOOL-AGE CHILDREN—cont'd

Age (Years)	Physical Competency	Intellectual Competency	Emotional-Social Competency	Nutrition	Play	Safety
		Rules are a guiding force in life now. Very interested in how things work and what and how weather, seasons, and the like are made.	skills he/she does best. Happy, cooperative, relaxed and casual in relationships Increasingly courteous and well mannered with adults. Gang stage at a peak; secret codes and rituals prevail. Responds better to suggestion than to dictatorial approach.			
11 to 12 years	Vital signs approximate adult norms. Growth spurt for girls.	Able to think about social problems and prejudices; sees others	Intense team loyalty; boys begin teasing girls and girls flirt with boys	Male needs 2500 calories/day; female needs 2250 (70 calories/kg/day);	Enjoys projects and working with hands. Likes to do errands and jobs	Continue monitoring friends. Stress bicycle and in-line skate

Inequalities between sexes increasingly noticeable, with boys having greater physical strength. Eruption of permanent teeth complete except for third molars. Secondary sex characteristics begin in boys. Menstruation may begin.	points of view. Enjoys reading mysteries or love stories. Begins playing with abstract ideas. Interested in whys of health measures and understands human reproduction. Very moralistic; religious commitment often made during this time.	Wants unreasonable independence; is rebellious about routines; has wide mood swings; needs some time daily for privacy. Very critical of own work. Hero worship prevails. Facts-of-life chats with friends prevail. Masturbation increases. Appears under constant tension.	both need 75 ml/kg of water/day and 2g/kg protein daily.	to earn money. Very involved in sports, dancing, talking on phone. Enjoys all aspects of acting and drama.	safety on streets and in traffic and the use of helmets and other protective gear.

From Betz, C., Hunsberger, M. & Wright, S. (1994). *Family-centered nursing care of children* (2nd ed.). Philadelphia: W.B. Saunders.

KEY POINTS

- Middle childhood includes school-age children between 6 and 12 years of age.
- In the school-age child the body develops a lower center of gravity than it had in preschool years.
- The loss of primary teeth begins at about age 6, and approximately four permanent teeth erupt each year.
- Regular dental checkups are an important part of routine health care.
- Visual maturity is complete between preschool age and 6 years, and therefore large-print books are no longer necessary.
- Excessive time spent with computer and video games can contribute to a sedentary lifestyle, which may result in obesity, poor health, and poor social development.
- By age 9 to 10 an understanding of rules and teamwork enable the child to participate in competitive team games.
- School-age children, according to Piaget, are concrete thinkers, and hands-on learning is retained best.
- School-age children often tell jokes to entertain peers and tease elders.
- School-age children are less egocentric and can understand how their actions affect others.
- Moral behavior is based on logical understanding and feeling pride or guilt as a result of the behavior. Knowing a rule is right does not guarantee behavior according to that rule.
- In later childhood the 10 year old may enjoy creating new rules or changing the rules of a game.
- Kohlberg believed moral reasoning develops as cognitive skills mature.
- A school-age child may have a maximum attention span of 45 minutes.
- School-age children use language as a tool in relationships with others.
- Intelligence tests were designed to be used to predict school ability and future performance.
- The primary developmental task of the school-age child is developing a sense of industry by mastering skills and achieving goals.
- Belonging to a peer group is very important to a school-age child.
- The home, school, and neighborhood each affect the growth and development of a school-age child.
- Creativity should be encouraged because it helps develop problem-solving skills.
- Information concerning sexuality should be age-appropriate, culturally relevant, and treated as a healthy aspect of life.
- Discipline should be used for teaching and reinforcing good behavior, which plays an important role in social and emotional development.
- The major health teaching needs of the school-age child include prevention of injury; maintenance of adequate nutrition; providing regular dental care; screening for scoliosis, vision, and hearing problems; and developing an active lifestyle.

CRITICAL THINKING

A child is enrolled in public school for the first time. Discuss some advice a school nurse or health care worker can offer the child's parent to help this child be successful in school.

MULTIPLE-CHOICE
REVIEW QUESTIONS

1 Middle childhood includes children between the ages of:
  1 3 to 5 years
  2 6 to 12 years
  3 13 to 15 years
  4 16 to 19 years
2 A major developmental task of middle childhood includes:
  1 Developing a positive self-esteem and self-image
  2 Eruption of permanent teeth
  3 Ability to play video games
  4 Prevention of injury
3 The type of play activities typical in the middle-childhood age group include:
  1 Parallel play
  2 Competitive games
  3 Solitary play
  4 Reading and fantasy
4 The Wechsler intelligence test is used to determine:
  1 The overall intelligence of the child
  2 Verbal and nonverbal intelligence
  3 Presence of mental retardation
  4 Whether the child has college potential
5 Middle childhood includes Erikson's stage of:
  1 Trust
  2 Autonomy
  3 Industry
  4 Identity

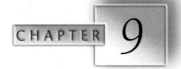

Adolescence

OBJECTIVES

Upon completion of this chapter, the student will be able to:

1 Define adolescence.
2 State the three phases of adolescence.
3 State the physiological changes that occur during adolescence.
4 Define puberty.
5 Identify the major developmental tasks of adolescence.
6 Discuss the adolescent's stage of development according to Erikson and Piaget.
7 Discuss how to determine the fertile period of a female adolescent.
8 Summarize the nutritional requirements during adolescence.
9 Identify how a person's cultural background might contribute to behavior.
10 Discuss the impact of peers, cliques, and best friends on the growth and development of the adolescent.
11 Discuss the role of dating in the development of cognitive and social behavior development.
12 Discuss the role of parents in fostering the positive growth and development of the adolescent.
13 State two specific health risks in the adolescent age group.

KEY TERMS

Abstinence
Adolescence
Asynchronous
Clique
Cultural competence
Ejaculation
Empathy
Menarche
Menstrual cycle
Nocturnal emissions
Ovulation
Puberty
Secondary sex characteristics
Spermatogenesis
Adolescence

DEFINITION

The origin of the word **adolescence** is from the Latin word *adolesere,* which means "to grow and mature." Adolescence is considered to be the bridge between childhood and adulthood. It is a unique stage of development characterized by many physiological, cognitive, psychosocial, and sexual changes. The health habits and coping skills formed during this period last for a lifetime, and mastery of developmental tasks during this period helps prepare the adolescent for adulthood.

The U.S. Department of Health and Human Services' *Healthy People 2010* (see Chapter 1) has developed specific national goals and objectives related to adolescent health. Since the start of the *Healthy People* initiative, adolescent and young adult mortality has been reduced by 26% (ASTHO, 1999).

DEVELOPMENTAL TASKS

Developmental tasks encountered during adolescence include establishing a stabilized sense of identity, separation from family, career planning, and establishing close peer relationships and intimacy.

Adolescence is often separated into three phases: early adolescence (10 to 13 years), middle adolescence (14 to 16 years), and late adolescence (17 to 20 years). The 13-year-old adolescent differs greatly from the 18-year-old adolescent. Each of these three distinct phases of adolescence has its own set of challenges (Table 9-1).

PHYSIOLOGICAL CHANGES

Early adolescence (also called preadolescence) is characterized by physical changes in the structure and function of various parts of the body. Weight gain is common, and the

TABLE 9-1

THREE PHASES IN THE GROWTH AND DEVELOPMENT OF THE ADOLESCENT

	Early (10 to 13 years)	Middle (14 to 16 years)	Late (17 to 20 years)
Physical growth	Appearance of secondary sex characteristics	Spurt in height growth	Growth slows
Body image	Self-conscious Adjusts to pubertal changes	Experiments with different images and looks	Accepts body image Personality emerges
Self-concept	Low self-esteem Denial of reality	Impulsive Impatient Identity confusion	Has positive self-image Empathetic Independent thinker
Behavior	Behaves for rewards	Behaves to conform	Shows responsible behavior
Sexual development	Sexual interest	Sexual experimentation	Sexual identity emerges Develops caring relationships
Peers	Unisex cliques of friends Has best friend Engages in hero worship Has adult crushes	Begins dating Has need to please significant peer Develops heterosexual peer group	Values individual relationships Begins partner selection
Family	Is ambivalent to family Strives for independence	Struggles for autonomy and acceptance Rebels/withdraws Demands privacy	Achieves independence Reestablishes family relationships
Cognitive development	Concrete thinking Here and now is important	Early abstract Daydreams, fantasizes Starts inductive and deductive reasoning	Abstract thinking Idealistic
Goals	Socializing is priority Goals may be unrealistic	Identifies skills/ interests Becomes a super-achiever or dropout	Identifies career goals Enters work or college
Health concerns	Concerned about normalcy	Concerned about experimenting with drugs or sex	Idealistic Decision making for lifestyle choice

TABLE 9-1

THREE PHASES IN THE GROWTH AND DEVELOPMENT OF THE ADOLESCENT—cont'd

	Early (10 to 13 years)	Middle (14 to 16 years)	Late (17 to 21 years)
Interventions	Convey limits Encourage verbalization	Help them solve problems from choices Use peer group sessions Provide privacy	Discuss goals Allow participation in decisions Provide confidentiality

Modified from Leifer, G. (2003). *Introduction to maternity and pediatric nursing* (4th ed.) Philadelphia: W.B. Saunders.

major cause is an increase in musculoskeletal mass. However, growth is **asynchronous,** which means different parts of the body mature at different times, possibly resulting in a temporary awkward appearance. A growth spurt occurs during adolescence, and adult height is reached by approximately age 18. Because the sweat glands are more active, various skin problems such as acne can occur, which may have social consequences and challenge teens' coping abilities. A facial pimple on the day of an important social event can cause chaos in the family.

During adolescence the stomach and intestines increase in size and volume, resulting in increased appetite and food consumption. The second and third molars, as well as wisdom teeth, erupt in early adolescence, and the jaw reaches adult size in mid- to late adolescence. Orthodontic tooth alignment with braces is often prescribed.

The weight and volume of the lungs increase, resulting in improvement of respiratory function. Improvements in eye-hand coordination and motor function enhance manual dexterity. Motor function also improves, and these factors contribute to the development of an interest and skill in sports activities and interactive computer games.

Puberty

The word **puberty** refers to sexual maturity or having the functional ability to reproduce. Puberty involves physical and psychological changes.

Boys

For boys, puberty begins between 10 and 13, with hormonal changes. **Secondary sex characteristics** are not involved in the reproductive process but appear at this time. Increases in androgens (testosterone and androsterone) are responsible for producing the male secondary sex characteristics. These include growth of pubic, facial, and body hair; enlargement and darkening in color of the scrotum; and an increase in penis size. The vocal cords also lengthen and thicken, resulting first in voice instability (voice cracking) and then in a deepening of the voice. An area in the brain, called the hypothalamus, secretes gonadotropin-releasing hormone (GnRH), which stimulates the anterior pituitary gland to secrete gonadotropins, follicle-stimulating hormone (FSH), and luteinizing hormone (LH). These gonadotropins stimulate the testes, which are located in the scrotum, to produce testosterone, and under normal conditions a stable level of testosterone is maintained in the blood throughout most of the lifespan. FSH and testosterone stimulate **spermatogenesis**, which is the production of sperm. Sperm production starts during mid-puberty and continues throughout the male lifespan. Sperm production requires a temperature of about 3° F below normal body temperature. This cooler temperature is possible because the testes are located outside the abdominal cavity, in the scrotum, which hangs between the legs. Males of all ages should be counseled against wearing tight undergarments or sitting on enclosed plastic or leather seats for prolonged times, because fertility can be reduced if the temperature around the testes is too high.

Ejaculation is the release of sperm during an orgasm. This ability indicates the testes are mature. Most boys experience **nocturnal emissions**, also known as "wet dreams," when they ejaculate semen during sleep. This experience is part of normal sexual development and is not necessarily related to sexual activity.

Because of the enlargement of the scrotum and the penis during puberty, an athletic scrotal support (jock strap) should be worn by boys participating in sporting events to prevent injury to these vulnerable organs. Good personal hygiene is necessary to prevent friction rashes (known as jock itch), which is a fungal infection. Sharing of athletic supporters creates a risk for spreading these infections and is strongly discouraged.

Girls

For girls during puberty, hormone secretions begin to establish a pattern within a monthly cycle. This pattern can typically be 28 to 32 days apart. Menstrual cycles begin at puberty and last about 40 years, when the hormone cycles stop and menopause begins.

The hypothalamus gland produces a gonadotropin-releasing hormone (GnRH), which stimulates the pituitary gland to release luteinizing hormone (LH) and follicle-stimulating hormone (FSH). In girls these hormones then stimulate the release of the female sex hormones (estrogen and progesterone) from the ovaries. Many thousands of eggs are present in the ovaries at birth. During ovulation, which typically happens once each menstrual cycle, one of the eggs finally matures and is released from the ovary (**ovulation**) into the fallopian tube, which leads to the uterus. As the egg travels in the fallopian tube toward the uterus, it can be fertilized if a sperm is present. If a sperm does not fertilize the egg, the egg enters the uterus and is expelled from the body with the blood and mucus that had thickened the walls of the uterus to prepare it for pregnancy. This blood, mucus, and unfertilized egg expelled from the body are called a menstrual flow (menstruation, or "period"). The very first menstrual period is called the **menarche**. The menarche usually occurs between ages 12 and 13 but can occur between 10 and 15. The **menstrual cycle** consists of (1) maturing the egg in the ovary, (2) formation of blood and mucus in the lining of the uterus, (3) ovulation, and (4) expelling the unfertilized egg with the blood and mucous lining from the uterus. This cycle lasts approximately 28 days and repeats until menopause. The menstrual flow typically lasts from 2 to 5 days, with a blood loss of about 1 ounce along with 1 to 2 ounces of serous fluid.

Ovulation occurs about 14 days before menstruation starts, and the egg lives for 1 day. Therefore this time is considered the most *fertile period* of a woman's cycle, when pregnancy can occur if sperm are present. Unwanted pregnancy can be prevented using one of several methods. The best way to prevent an unwanted pregnancy is to avoid sexual intercourse, referred to as **abstinence.** Daily birth control pills prevent ovulation but can have systemic side effects. Intrauterine devices (IUDs) prevent a fertilized egg from adhering to the wall of the uterus, and condoms, if used correctly, can prevent the sperm from entering the vagina. Condoms also have the benefit of preventing the spread of sexually transmitted diseases (STDs), such as chlamydia, gonorrhea, syphilis, and human immunodeficiency virus (HIV). In some research studies the term *sexually transmitted infections* (STIs) is replacing the term STDs. However, the Centers for Disease Control and Prevention (CDC) still uses the term *STD.* Condoms are best used in combination with other methods, such as spermicides, to increase protection against pregnancy. Various hormone shots, such as Depo-Provera, prevent ovulation from occurring but require repeated injections (Table 9-2).

In girls, secondary sex characteristics often become apparent before menarche. Hair develops in the pubic area and the axilla or underarms. Breasts begin to develop, fat begins to deposit more in the hips and thighs rather than being evenly distributed, and body contours change. At this time, adolescent girls are ready for their first bra to support their developing breasts. The bra straps should not fall from the shoulders but should not be too tight and the bra cup should support the fullness of the breasts near the underarms. Sports bras may be more desirable for girls who participate in athletics. A balance of diet and exercise is important for menstrual regularity and overall health.

Adolescence is the best time to teach preventative health measures such as testicular self-examination (TSE) for boys and breast self-examination (BSE) for girls. Sex education classes should include information about safe sex, family planning, and prevention of STDs. The school nurse can be a valuable resource person to help locate family planning services, such as Planned Parenthood, that may be available in the local community.

Adolescents often have emotional reactions and concerns about their changing bodies. Boys may have socially embarrassing erections, and comparison of penis size can be a normal part of social interaction and exploration. Girls are often concerned with their breast size and menstrual discomforts. Teen magazines often exploit the ideal female figure and the muscular male body with standards that are very difficult for the average teen to meet. The changing body plays an important role in the development of an adolescent's self-image. Research suggests that early developing males may enjoy more social success and positive self-esteem, whereas girls who develop early may be at more risk for lower self-esteem and a drop in school performance (Behrman et al, 2004).

Teen Pregnancy

By the twelfth grade (age 18) the teen pregnancy rate was 48.5 pregnancies per 1000 women between 15 and 19 years of age in the year 2000 (CDC, NCHS, 2002). Many

TABLE 9-2

BIRTH CONTROL OPTIONS*

Method	How Used	Protects Against HIV & Other STDs?
Most Effective		
Abstinence	Avoid sexual intercourse	Yes
Hormonal		
Oral contraceptive ("the Pill")	Usually taken once every day	No
Contraceptive injections (Depo-Provera)	Can take injection at specific intervals (e.g., every 3 months)	No
Norplant	Six matchstick-size capsules placed underneath skin of the arm provides contraception for up to 5 years. Can be removed by a health care provider at any time.	No
Vaginal ring	Inserted monthly; stays in for a 3-week period and removed for 1 week.	No
Skin patch	A new patch is applied to skin once a week for 3 weeks, not worn for 1 week (to allow for menstruation).	No
Nonhormonal		
Male condom	New condom must be applied before each act of coitus or sexual encounter.	Yes
Female condom	New condom must be inserted before each sexual encounter.	Yes
Spermicidal foams	Must be applied or inserted before each sexual encounter.	No
Cervical cap	Used with spermicide at every sexual encounter.	No
Copper IUD	Must be inserted by health care provider; lasts up to 10 years.	No
Permanent		
Vasectomy	One surgical procedure provides permanent prevention of pregnancy (in some cases, can be reversed).	No
Tubal ligation	One surgical procedure provides permanent prevention of pregnancy (in some cases, can be reversed).	No

*It is important to understand that a woman's fertile period (when pregnancy can occur if sperm is present) is 14 days *before* the beginning of the next menstrual period. This is not necessarily the same as 14 days after the last menstrual period if the cycle is less than or more than 28 days apart.

of these adolescents have had multiple partners. By high school graduation, 1 in 10 students has either been pregnant or fathered a pregnancy.

In many cultures a ritual rite of passage occurs at the onset of puberty. In the United States, sex in movies, television, and other media may influence the behavior of adolescents, who are beginning to explore dating.

Health care professionals, educators, parents, school nurses, and counselors are challenged to provide guidance and education that will promote healthy behaviors.

Sexual topics are a high priority for the adolescent. Boys may seek sexual experience because of social role expectations. Girls and boys seek sexual activity because of coercion, peer pressure, or curiosity. For these reasons, sex education is important *before* adolescence and must continue throughout adolescence. Accurate information about prevention of pregnancy and STDs from an authoritative source can help teens make responsible and informed choices related to sexual matters. Too often, teens obtain misinformation from peers or other unreliable sources and become vulnerable to unsafe practices or abuse. For example, many young girls are told they cannot become pregnant the first time they have sexual intercourse. This is not true.

Young teens who become pregnant must deal with their own developmental tasks, as well as the tasks of parenthood. Counseling concerning their options and close health supervision are essential for a positive outcome in a teen pregnancy. Teens are at high risk for date rape and other sexual abuses, and therefore education concerning safe practices and preventative strategies is essential. Community resources that provide special programs for sexually active or pregnant teens are available, and school-based resources, such as education programs, provide opportunities for individual counseling.

COGNITIVE DEVELOPMENT

According to Piaget, young adolescents are in the *concrete phase* of thinking, which means they interpret words and concepts literally. By middle adolescence they begin to think more abstractly. This stage of cognitive development is called the *formal operation stage*. Adolescents in this stage can process information quickly and efficiently, and their thinking becomes more complex. Adolescents can be self-absorbed and self-conscious. They may feel that everyone is looking at them and worry that others may notice even slight blemishes on their skin. They can spend hours examining and experimenting with hairstyles and dress, feeling they are on a stage with all the world as their audience (Figure 9-1).

At times adolescents can also see themselves as unique and powerful. They may try to manipulate rules, engage in risky behaviors, or deny their own mortality. Some adolescents admire "idols" and can be disappointed or confused if they find out that their

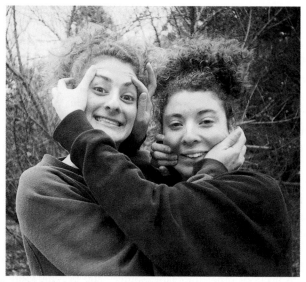

FIGURE 9-1 Best friends experiment with hairstyles, expressions, and makeup. Best friend interaction supports growth and development. From (Leifer, G. [2003]. *Introduction to maternity and pediatric nursing* [4th ed.]. Philadelphia: W.B. Saunders.)

idol is not perfect. It is healthy for adolescents to discover their own uniqueness and separate from their family. However, sometimes teens can become isolated, which may raise the risk of depression or self-harming behavior when a problem arises.

Debate is a healthy mental exercise that can sharpen cognitive and social skills and defuse intense emotions for most adolescents. School debate teams help teens express varying views in socially acceptable ways. Debate is often interpreted as argumentative by parents and teachers, who may find challenging teenagers difficult to get along with. Teenagers often daydream, which may be an imaginary acting out of what would be said or done in various situations. Daydreams help the adolescent think through how they might respond in situations and can be a safety valve for strong emotions. Daydreams in the adolescent are harmless unless they interfere with functioning in school or relationships. Young adolescents fantasize about unrealistic career ideas, but by middle adolescence they may realize their true strengths and limitations and thus may set more realistic goals.

Kohlberg described the adolescent as moving toward the postconventional stage of moral judgment (see Chapter 4). The early adolescent is motivated by the need to conform and please others. As later adolescence approaches, moral principles are based on one's own individual thinking and beliefs.

PSYCHOSOCIAL DEVELOPMENT

According to Erikson, one of the major tasks of adolescence is achieving a stable self-identity (see Chapter 4). Adolescents may try out various temporary styles and social roles in the process of finding their own individual identity. This process of identity exploration can lead to role confusion. In role confusion the adolescent can overcommit to many causes and appear to go through personality changes. To achieve a sense of their own identity, adolescents must believe their identities are separate from their role as a child in their family. The family can help secure a positive outcome in achievement of this task by offering support and guidance and by giving adolescents freedom to discover their own interests. Close relationships with peers are helpful for adolescents exploring different roles and ideas. Close friendships develop mainly with same-sex friends in the early adolescent phase. They validate each other's thoughts and actions and may imitate each other's traits and habits. Middle adolescents (14 to 17 years) are concerned with how they look and whom they date. Experimentation with sex and other social behaviors often occurs at this age, and a sense of omnipotence combined with curiosity may lead to risk-taking behaviors. As teens approach late adolescence, school performance, interaction with teachers and counselors, and participation in extracurricular activities can influence their successful achievement of career goals.

Problem-solving approaches are utilized in the task of establishing a first date. Social skills and cognitive reasoning are aided by good coping skills to meet the challenges of achieving many developmental tasks of adolescence. There may be some subtle gender differences in initiating a date. Boys typically take a more active role, but girls may use techniques to attract attention and encourage a boy to ask for a date. Not having a boyfriend or girlfriend may be considered as stressful as the stress of initiating a relationship. In later adolescence, relationships may become less experimental, more affectionate, and longer lasting. A feeling of abandonment may occur in early adolescence if one of two best friends leaves the other for a dating relationship. Feeling left out or guilty is common in early adolescence despite the understanding that a relationship with a significant other need not be exclusive of other friends.

Teen Violence

The United States rates highest in the industrial world in violent death rates. Violent crimes involving teenagers are an increasing problem in our society, with violence among adolescents occurring twice as often as among the general population (USD-HHS, 2000). Children and adolescents often use violence to handle conflicts (CDC, 1999). They may not have been effectively taught nonviolent techniques of managing conflicts during the formative years of developing socialization skills. Many children also witness their parents using physical violence at home to settle disputes. Both parents working and thus absent from the home after school hours and the increasing availability of guns and drugs on school campuses contribute to the occurrence of violence in the schools. Episodes of fighting often precede homicides. The impulsive nature of teenagers, their feelings of invincibility and immortality, their immaturity, and their exposure to violence on television and in interactive computer and video games and other media forms all combine to form a deadly vulnerability, which includes violence in their lifestyles.

Adolescents who are homeless, abused, or disadvantaged may not be able to deal with the other developmental tasks of adolescence, such as dating, social and identity development, and may act out in socially unacceptable ways. They may abuse drugs, show violent behavior, engage in risky sexual practices, or even attempt suicide.

CULTURE AND THE ADOLESCENT

Culture plays a role in how adolescents think and interact. In some cultures, body piercing and tattoos are an accepted or expected practice, whereas other cultures view them as inappropriate or deviant. Nurses and health care workers who work with teens must be culturally competent. **Cultural competence** involves recognizing how your own values differ from those of other cultures and respecting the values and practices of others. Focusing on the cultural values and individual strengths of the adolescent, rather than the differences or variances, can help establish relationships that will help achieve positive health teaching outcomes. Culture affects health care practices and modes of communication. In most cases the adolescent requires strict confidentiality. Maintaining this confidentiality can be a challenge when parents pay for the health insurance and control transportation access. It is important for nurses, health care workers, and educators to be truthful, keep promises, and provide privacy for the adolescent. Cultural and religious traditions can help stabilize identity and involve rituals that celebrate movement from childhood to the adult phase of life (Figure 9-2 and Appendix B).

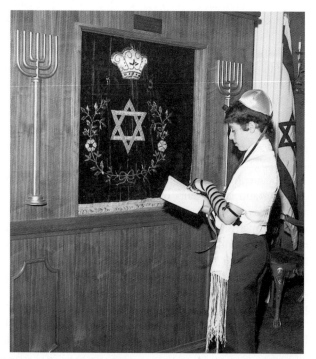

FIGURE 9–2 Many cultural and religious traditions involve rituals that celebrate movement from childhood to the adult phase of life. Here a boy participates in the bar mitzvah ceremony marking his thirteenth birthday, when he is considered to be entering adulthood. (From Leifer, G. [2003]. *Introduction to maternity and pediatric nursing* [4th ed.]. Philadelphia: W.B. Saunders.)

DEVELOPMENT OF RESPONSIBILITY

Adolescents look forward to challenges and often feel humiliated when placed in the dependent role. Independence in transportation can be achieved by riding a bicycle or driving a car. Babysitting or routine jobs to earn and manage money is important to the teenager. Using their own savings account or checkbook to purchase some of their own clothes and supplies are important personal management skills for adolescents to learn.

It is important for the adolescent to be responsible for making decisions, especially those relative to career, politics, and religion. The role of parents should be listening and guiding the adolescent rather than mandating behavior. According to the behaviorist B.F. Skinner, teens will repeat behavior that is positively reinforced (see Chapter 4). Bandura, a social cognitive theorist, suggests that setting an example for the teen will motivate positive behavior (see Chapter 4).

PEER RELATIONSHIPS

Peer group affiliation has a major impact on adolescent growth and development. School plays an important role in psychosocial development because it provides the opportunity for social interaction, peer group association, and clique formation. A **clique** is a social group with a fixed exclusive membership, sharing similar interests, values, and tastes. Belonging to a group is of utmost importance to adolescents. From this social group, the adolescent chooses a best friend, who enables the teen to experience mutual sharing of private thoughts and feelings. This may be helpful in normalizing and validating experiences and in forming successful relationships later in life. During this period in adolescence it is normal for openness and time spent with peers to increase and contacts with family to decrease. The teen may feel compelled to conform to peer pressures, which can cause problems and conflicts with family if the values of the peer group conflict with family values or traditions. If the adolescent and the family relocate to a new neighborhood or new state during this phase of the life cycle, the adolescent may have more difficulty joining an exclusive clique or group of friends in the new school. Failure to connect in a clique or peer group can cause feelings of loneliness, loss, and interpersonal failure. This may contribute to a lowered self-esteem or feelings of inadequacy. School performance may decrease due to social difficulty, independent of academic ability, and the adolescent may become vulnerable to risky behaviors such as self-soothing with illegal substances or cutting classes. The dynamics of peer interaction are essential for the adolescent. Parents who accept and welcome peers into their home can help encourage formation of healthy peer relationships and may have less conflict in their relationships with their adolescent. Peer counselors can be helpful in redirecting a troubled teen.

Erikson's sixth stage of psychosocial development, Intimacy versus Isolation, starts in late adolescence. After the middle adolescent establishes a fairly stable identity, the next developmental challenge is to share with another and develop a sense of intimacy. **Empathy** (understanding how others feel) is a quality essential to establishing a meaningful relationship with another person. This intimate relationship can be sexual, intellectual, or social. In late adolescence, a childlike dependence on the family is sometimes seen in times of illness or stress, but relating to the adolescent as a young adult is most supportive of adolescent development.

SEXUALITY

Developing a sexual identity is an important part of the adolescent's sense of self. Masturbation is one way for an individual to explore and learn about his or her body. Petting, or mutual masturbation, is a form of physical, erotic, and genital stimulation that teens engage in with each other and often does not include sexual intercourse (coitus). Petting or groping can lead to orgasm and is a common sexual outlet for young teens. This type of experimental behavior helps the adolescent learn about sexual responses that are pleasurable and behavior patterns that may contribute to later relationships. Sexually active and exclusive relationships often develop during later adolescence. Statistics show that approximately 70% of females have had sexual intercourse by age 18 and 20% of STDs occur in the adolescent age group (NCHS, 2000). The nurse must be aware that oral sex may not be considered a sexual act by many teenagers, but the risk of STD transmission in oral sex is high. Information concerning the risks of oral sex should be included in sex education programs.

The adolescent's sexual exploration creates risk for unplanned or unprotected sexual activity, which increases vulnerability to developing sexually transmitted diseases. In cases of extreme poverty, poor problem-solving skills, or drug dependence, an exchange of sex for food or drugs may occur, increasing the risk for HIV or acquired immunodeficiency syndrome (AIDS) infection. Adults must remember that sexually abused adolescents or those who are victims of rape do not consider themselves sexually active and thus may need appropriate interventions after such events to educate and protect them.

Sexual fantasy and experimentation is normal for both heterosexual and homosexual individuals. Homosexual behavior in adolescence is common. Sometimes experimentation with homosexual behavior has a relationship to future sexual identification and behavior, but it also may simply be part of an exploration of identity and lifestyle options. Homosexual behavior is reported in about 5% of adolescent boys and girls (Behrman et al, 2004). Homosexuality is no longer considered a sexual deviance or mental disorder by the American Psychiatric Association (APA, 2000). The role of the nurse and health care worker is to help the adolescent understand how to cope with confused or prejudiced reactions of others rather than to make attempts at changing behaviors.

TEACHING TECHNIQUES FOR THE ADOLESCENT

Teaching adolescents can be a challenge. There is enormous variability in the rates of physical, cognitive, and psychosocial maturity between early, middle, and late adolescence. Some adolescents pass slowly through the changes of puberty and cognitive development, yet may be advanced in physical development. The adolescent who appears physically mature but is not yet an abstract thinker does not learn or interact in the same way as an adolescent who is cognitively or emotionally mature and may be at high risk for destructive peer influences. Often adolescents who are physically mature before they are cognitively mature may be lured into an older peer group that engages in risky behaviors, and the teens may not be able to make responsible decisions concerning these actions.

The nurse or health care worker who understands the characteristics of each adolescent phase of development can be a very effective teacher or source of information for teens and their parents.

Identifying health risks of the adolescent is essential to plan teaching relevant to preventative health care. Rapid body changes can result in poor coordination that can result in sports injuries. Adolescents are capable of logical thought and abstract reasoning. They can understand cause and effect, health and illness, and disease prevention. However, healthy teens may have difficulty picturing themselves as sick or injured and may engage in high-risk behavior. They may have an "it will never happen to me" attitude toward illness or injury. Many adolescents have at least one serious health problem, such as asthma, allergies, or diabetes. Health conditions that benefit from preventative measures and early intervention include pregnancy, STDs, substances abuse, and depression. Motor vehicle accidents (MVAs) continue to be the leading cause of teen morbidity and mortality and are preventable with appropriate education and training.

The first step in effectively teaching adolescents involves establishing a trusting relationship. Communication must be supportive and not threaten their sense of independence or autonomy. If they are informed in a respectful way and understand the value of healthy behavior, they are more likely to use the information wisely. This approach is better than just telling them what they need to do. Providing privacy and one-to-one consultation can open up communication and reduce defenses. However, peer group teaching sessions may be more helpful and practical in discussing common problems such as smoking, sexual activity, substance abuse, and other health-related challenges. Discussion of options and decision making must be shared, and options that support the adolescent in thinking and acting as an adult and staying open to learning should be offered. Confrontation should be avoided. Often the health care worker, counselor, or nurse can help guide the family concerning parenting strategies relating to their teens. Setting realistic limits without damaging the sense of independence is a delicate balance and a learned skill for most parents.

The Society for Adolescent Medicine identified seven characteristics critical to providing effective health education and care for adolescents: availability, visibility, quality, confidentiality, affordability, flexibility, and coordination (Behrman et al, 2004). One of the goals of *Healthy People 2010* is to provide community resources with these characteristics to increase access to health care and education for all adolescents.

KEY POINTS

- Adolescence is the bridge between childhood and adulthood.
- Adolescence is divided into three phases: early adolescence (10 to 13 years of age); middle adolescence (14 to 16 years of age); and late adolescence (17 to 20 years of age).
- The major tasks of adolescence include establishing a sense of identity, separation from family, establishing intimacy and peer relationships, and career planning.
- The physical, psychological, cognitive, and emotional aspects of development may mature at different rates.
- *Puberty* refers to sexual maturity.
- The reproductive system is controlled by hormones regulated by the hypothalamus and secreted by the anterior pituitary glands and the ovaries or testes.
- By the twelfth grade, 66% of students report having had a sexually intimate experience.
- Ovulation occurs 14 days before the menstrual period begins.
- The changing body plays a role in the adolescent's development of self-image, self-esteem, and social interactions.
- Young adolescents are in the concrete phase of thinking.
- Daydreaming can be developmentally appropriate and a useful safety valve for strong emotions.
- By middle adolescence, career goals may become more practical and realistic.
- In late adolescence, moral principles are based on the adolescent's own beliefs.
- Culture plays a role in how adolescents think and interact, and traditions can help stabilize identity.
- It is important to allow adolescents to begin to behave independently and make their own decisions.
- Peer groups have a major impact on adolescent social and emotional growth and development.
- In late adolescence, intimacy with a peer can be sexual, intellectual, or social.
- Effective health education and care include availability, visibility, high quality, confidentiality, affordability, and flexibility.

CRITICAL THINKING

Sexual topics are a very important part of adolescent teaching. Outline a plan that will discuss menstrual health, help the adolescent girl understand her "fertile period," and create an awareness of birth control options.

MULTIPLE-CHOICE
REVIEW QUESTIONS

1 A developmental task of adolescence includes:
   1 Concrete thinking
   2 Stabilizing identity
   3 Accepting competition
   4 Social interaction
2 The definition of *puberty* is:
   1 Exhibiting secondary sex characteristics
   2 Having the ability to reproduce
   3 The decrease of gonadotropic hormones
   4 Becoming fertile
3 Which of the following, if used properly, can prevent the transmission of sexually transmitted diseases:
   1 Condoms
   2 Birth control pills
   3 Intrauterine device
   4 Spermicides
4 A women's fertile period occurs:
   1 14 days after the last menstruation
   2 14 days before the beginning the next menstruation
   3 Midway between menstrual periods
   4 Right after menstruation ceases
5 Which of the following social group forms is typical during the teenage years:
   1 Cliques
   2 Same-sex peers
   3 Heterosexual peers
   4 Parallel groups

CHAPTER *10*

Young Adulthood

O B J E C T I V E S

1 Define young adulthood.
2 State the developmental tasks of young adulthood.
3 Name the physiological changes that occur in young adulthood.
4 State at least four priority health issues related to the young adult stage of the life cycle.
5 List the reproductive health issues of young adulthood.
6 Utilize knowledge of men's health needs in applying gender-appropriate care and guidance.
7 State two health screening preventative programs important during young adulthood.
8 Discuss the role of schools in helping individuals adjust and cope with tasks and challenges of young adulthood.
9 Describe the psychosocial tasks of young adulthood as described by Erikson.
10 Explain Piaget's theory of cognitive thinking in young adulthood.
11 Describe Kohlberg's theory of moral development in the young adult.
12 Discuss Piaget's formal operational thinking as it applies to the young adult.

13 Trace the growth and development of a parent.
14 Design teaching techniques that will contribute to successful learning in the young adult.

KEY TERMS

Ectopic pregnancy
Hysterectomy
Intimacy
Intimate partner violence (IPV)
Pelvic inflammatory disease (PID)
Postformal operational thought
Sexually transmitted disease (STD)
Structure
Testicular self-examination (TSE)
Transitional phase
Vaginal birth after cesarean (VBAC)

DEFINITION

Young adulthood is most often defined as the age between 20 and 40 years. The stage may also be referred to as *early adulthood*. The legal age of adulthood is 18 years, when the individual can vote, be drafted into the military, and enter into marital relationships without parental consent. However, until an individual reaches age 21, there may still be legal limitations on some activities, such as the use of alcohol.

DEVELOPMENTAL TASKS OF YOUNG ADULTHOOD

The major developmental task or crisis of young adulthood is intimacy versus isolation. The young adult makes the transition from the safety of the parents' home and the structure of the high school to achieve the tasks of self-support; independence, developing intimate relationships, and establishing a stable family and lifestyle. By age 21, some adults live separately from parents, establish a commitment to a work identity, and develop an adult social role of their own design. Others do not take on these adult roles and responsibilities until after they pursue a college education to achieve a career goal. In some cases, social and political events such as war or an economic crash can interrupt the progress toward career goals or financial or social independence due to military service or the need to support family members through a financial struggle. The developmental process from adolescence to adulthood is most often a gradual one, but in many cultures there are traditional expectations during this transition.

PHYSIOLOGICAL CHANGES

Physical growth in height and weight and organ and sexual maturation are generally complete by young adulthood. Physical health, motor coordination, and physiological performance typically peak between ages 20 and 30 (Figure 10-1). The epiphyses of the long bones fuse by the early twenties, and muscular strength is at its peak.

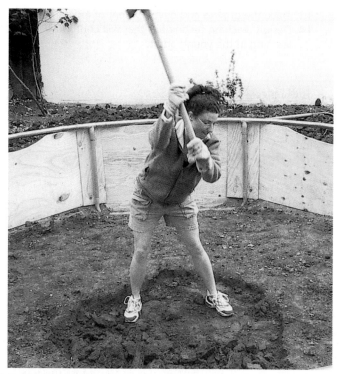

FIGURE 10–1 Physical health, motor coordination, and physiological performance are at their peak in young adulthood. Hard physical work and exercises are often enjoyed and are productive.

By age 30, muscle mass and body water may naturally decrease and fatty tissue increases, resulting in increased vulnerability to injuries. Efforts toward maintaining good physical fitness can prolong peak functioning or reestablish good health and fitness at an older age. Poor health habits can compromise health at any age.

The heart and lungs are also at their peak capacity during young adulthood. Lifestyle choices made during the young adult years will dramatically affect heart and lung health in middle age and beyond.

Wise food choices provide optimum nutrition, and regular exercise can help maintain health and prevent obesity or cardiovascular disease (Figure 10-2 and Table 10-1). The Food Pyramid was developed by the U.S. Department of Agriculture (USDA) as a guide for healthy daily food choices. Other food choice guides are being developed that propose fewer pastas and bread food groups and place certain oils, fruits, and vegetables at the base of the pyramid and red meat at the very top of the pyramid. Research is ongoing. Most health professionals agree either structure of the Food Pyramid reflects healthy food choices and is preferable to foods that supply empty calories such as cookies, cakes, sugary drinks, and many fast foods. Smoking or substance abuse can contribute to a more rapid decline in health, beginning when the habit starts and extending throughout the lifespan. The eruption of the wisdom teeth and development of gum disease are potential dental problems that commonly arise in this age group and must be dealt with during the young adult years. Conscientious brushing, flossing, and regular preventive dental care can help ensure dental health. As the individual approaches age 30, gastric secretions may decrease, resulting in increased gastric discomforts. Junk foods, highly spiced foods, food high in fat, and irregular eating habits established in adolescence may be more difficult to tolerate as a young adult progresses toward middle age. Visual acuity may begin to decline as the individual approaches middle age, and corrective lenses may be needed for reading or driving. Visual habits such as taking breaks from reading to focus eyes on a distant point can minimize visual decline associated with reading and frequent computer work.

Healthy People 2010 (see Chapter 1) has identified priority areas for health promotion during the young adulthood years. The priority areas include maintaining physical activity, fitness, and nutrition; decrease in use of tobacco and alcohol; positive mental health practices; and adequate information concerning family planning options. It is easier to develop positive health habits at a young age than to change or compensate for bad habits later in life. Most lifestyle choices and health habits are made during the young adult years.

Often, entrance into college provides the final opportunity for parents to initiate a health checkup and education concerning lifestyle choices. After the precollege physical examination, the young adult often does not seek health assessment unless a problem arises. The major causes of death in young adulthood are most often related to accidents or violence, and both are preventable.

WOMEN'S HEALTH ISSUES

Women have a great influence on childrearing and early learning. Maintaining women's health, therefore, may enable them to influence a generation of children to practice good health habits and choose healthy lifestyles. Education concerning women's health issues and access to care has increased dramatically in the past few years. Women's health clinics and women's health specialists are available at most health care facilities.

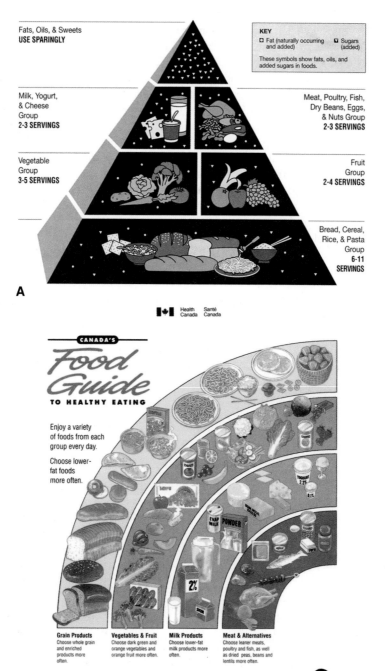

FIGURE 10–2 A, Food Pyramid. **B,** Canadian Food Guide to Healthy Eating. (**A** from Mahan, L.K., & Escott-Stump, S. [2000]. *Krause's food, nutrition, and diet therapy* [10th ed.]. Philadelphia: W.B. Saunders; **B** From Health Canada, 1993. Reproduced with the permission of the Minister of Public Works and Government Services Canada, 2003.)

TABLE **10-1**

APPROXIMATE ENERGY EXPENDITURE FOR LEVELS OF ACTIVITY EXPRESSED AS MULTIPLES OF RESTING ENERGY EXPENDITURE (REE)

Activity Category	Energy as Multiple of Ree	KCAL/MIN
Resting Sleeping, reclining	REE × 1.0	1–1.2
Very light Seated and standing activities, painting trades, driving, laboratory work, typing, sewing, ironing, cooking, playing cards, playing a musical instrument	REE × 1.5	Up to 2.5
Light Walking on a level surface at 2.5 to 3 mph, garage work, electrical trades, carpentry, restaurant trades, house cleaning, child care, golf, sailing, table tennis	REE × 2.5	2.5–4.9
Moderate Walking 3.5 to 4 mph, weeding and hoeing, carrying a load, cycling, skiing, tennis, dancing	REE × 5.0	5.0–7.4
Heavy Walking with load uphill, tree felling, heavy manual digging, basketball, climbing, football, soccer	REE × 7.0	7.5–12.0

From Food and Nutrition Board, National Research Council, National Academy of Sciences (1989). *Recommended Dietary Allowances* (10th ed.) Washington, DC: National Academy Press.

Wide variations exist in cultural practices related to women's health issues. Nurses must be alert to individual differences within a cultural group and avoid stereotyping patients from specific cultural backgrounds. A strong belief in fate may prevent some women from seeking early health care. Diet, religious objects, and use of folk medicine also play a role in preventing illness in some cultural groups. Modesty can influence the desire to avoid genital examinations, and so maintaining privacy is very important. Communication techniques between the nurse and patient are important because eye contact, touch, and use of personal space influence rapport between patient and caregiver. Some women prefer receiving health care from female providers. Cultural response to a change in gender function may influence a women's acceptance of contraception or sterilization practices. In some cultures, women who are menstruating are considered unclean and are isolated and forbidden to have contact with males. In other cultures, women consider menopause a nonevent and do not suffer from anxieties related to aging (see Appendix B). Cultural issues concerning the marriage of a person to a mate who is outside the cultural group can cause family disruption and conflict.

Cultural beliefs influence preferred labor management, position for birth, location of delivery, and the role of family members during labor and delivery. Ethical issues also influence women's health care. Ethical issues include abortion, surrogate parenting, infertility treatment techniques, adoption, stem cell research, gene therapy, cord blood

Because a unique risk to health occurs during pregnancy, providing family planning services for the young adult is essential (see Table 9-2). Maternal mortality rates have continued to decline over the past decade due to the availability of health care. The major risk factors contributing to the mortality rate include lack of prenatal care, inadequate knowledge of health needs, and poor nutrition. The death rate for young mothers obtaining legal abortions in the United States is low, but those performed outside an accredited facility often have negative outcomes. Therefore the nurse or health care worker can play an important role in referring the young adult to available community resources. The rate of ectopic pregnancy (pregnancy in the fallopian tube instead of the uterus) is 11.3 per 1000 pregnancies among women 15 to 44 years (CDC, 1999). Ectopic pregnancies can be the result of fallopian tube malformation or from damage caused by **pelvic inflammatory disease** (PID). **Sexually transmitted diseases** (STDs) are the major causes of PID. Therefore promoting healthy behaviors related to safe sex practices during adolescence and young adulthood can reduce maternal morbidity and mortality. Annual Papanicolaou (Pap) smears are encouraged for sexually active young women because human papillomavirus (HPV) is also known to be a cause of cervical cancer and both tests are done at the same time. HPV tests may soon be replacing the traditional Pap test because the results are more sensitive and accurate (Kulasingam et al, 2002). Encouraging breast self-examinations and mammograms at appropriate intervals can lead to early detection and early intervention for breast cancer (Figure 10-3).

banking, and organ transplantation. Social issues such as homelessness, access to health care, and poverty also need to be considered issues in women's health care.

Hysterectomy (removal of the uterus) is the most common surgery performed on women during the reproductive years, with the mean age for hysterectomy being 40.9 years (Ravnikar, 1994). The increasing use of laser techniques to treat uterine fibroids

The practice trial of **vaginal birth after cesarean** (VBAC) remains controversial, but *Healthy People 2010* goals include reducing the rate of cesarean births by the year 2010.

may decrease the need for this surgery. Cesarean section births contribute to the high rate of surgical procedures in young adult women.

The multiple roles of women in the young adult phase of life can contribute to stress and the potential development of depression or anxiety. A single working mother may have combined responsibilities of running a household, earning enough money to cover basic expenses, finding adequate affordable day care for young children, and car-

Perform breast self-examination monthly. If you are menstruating, do the examination 1 week after the beginning of your period because your breasts are less tender at this time. If you are not menstruating, choose any day that you can easily remember, such as the first day of each month. Examine your breasts three ways: before a mirror, lying down, and in the shower.

BEFORE A MIRROR

Inspect your breasts in four steps: (1) arms at your sides; (2) arms over your head; (3) with your hands on your hips, pressing them firmly to flex your chest muscles; (4) and bending forward. At each step, note any change in the shape or appearance of your breasts. Note skin or nipple changes such as dimpling of the skin. Squeeze each nipple gently to identify any discharge.

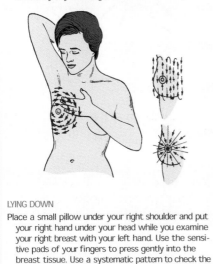

LYING DOWN

Place a small pillow under your right shoulder and put your right hand under your head while you examine your right breast with your left hand. Use the sensitive pads of your fingers to press gently into the breast tissue. Use a systematic pattern to check the entire breast. One pattern is to feel the tissue in a circular pattern, spiraling inward toward the nipple.

Another method is to use an up-and-down pattern. Use the same systematic pattern to examine the underarm area because breast tissue is also present here. Repeat for the other breast.

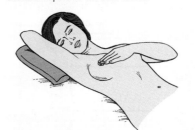

IN THE SHOWER

Raise your right arm. Use your soapy fingers to feel the breast tissue in the same systematic pattern described under Lying Down.

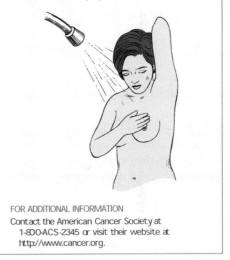

FOR ADDITIONAL INFORMATION

Contact the American Cancer Society at 1-800-ACS-2345 or visit their website at http://www.cancer.org.

FIGURE 10–3 Breast self-examination. (From Leifer, G. [2003]. *Introduction to maternity and pediatric nursing* [4th ed.]. Philadelphia: W.B. Saunders; illustrations from Lowdermilk, D.L., Perry, S.E., & Bobak, I.M. [2000]. *Maternity and Women's Health Care* [7th ed.]. St.Louis: Mosby.

ing for an elderly parent. These responsibilities may cause the young woman to delay seeking health care for herself, which can lead to devastating results.

Violent behavior against women is an epidemic and contributes to the morbidity and mortality statistics of young adult women (Figure 10-4). Domestic violence can include psychological, physical, sexual, financial, and social abuses between intimate partners. The result is often social isolation and physical trauma. The CDC now refers to domestic violence as **intimate partner violence** (IPV). More than 1 million incidences of IPV occur each year (CDC, 2000) and involve all ethnic, racial, socioeconomic, and educational levels of the population (Box 10-1).

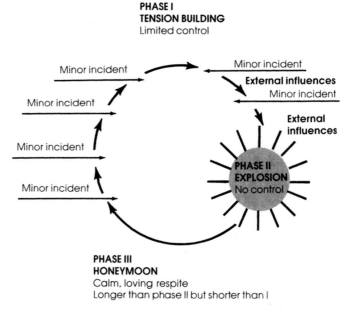

PHASE I
TENSION BUILDING
Limited control

Minor incident

Minor incident

Minor incident

Minor incident

Minor incident

Minor incident

External influences
Minor incident

External influences

PHASE II
EXPLOSION
No control

PHASE III
HONEYMOON
Calm, loving respite
Longer than phase II but shorter than I

FIGURE 10–4 Cycle of violence. (From Rawlins, P., Williams, S., & Beck, C. [1993]. *Mental Health Psychiatric Nursing.* St. Louis: Mosby.

Many communities have programs to deal with domestic violence and other crimes targeting women. *Healthy People 2010* lists specific objectives related to prevention and treatment programs (see Chapter 1).

MEN'S HEALTH ISSUES

Men currently do not have gender-specific health care providers as women do. Men's health as a specialty may be a future trend but is not yet established in most health care facilities. Young male adults appear to seek health care or guidance less often than women within this age group. Although they may accompany their pregnant partner to the obstetrician, unless they have fertility issues, men rarely seek medical assistance until a specific problem presents itself (Benson et al, 1994).

BOX 10-1 **Signs of Intimate Partner Violence**

- Erratic prenatal care
- Erratic child health care appointments
- Bruises and lacerations in various stages of healing
- Self-blame for marital or relationship problems
- History of alcohol or drug abuse in partner
- History of abuse as a child (cycle of violence)
- History of minor battering incidents

The high testosterone levels in males may contribute to a lower cholesterol level than in women. Statistically, men may be at a higher risk for injury due to their work environment. Men may also smoke and drink alcohol more often, as compared with women, contributing to the development of many health problems.

Some men may resist seeking health care even when a health problem is present or do not seek preventative screening programs (Gotchman, 1995). However, recent public education has increased the awareness of the need for testicular self-examination (TSE) by all young adult males as part of a preventative program. The highest rate of testicular cancer is within the 17- to 35-year-old age group; thus TSE is an important aspect of preventive health care. Free clinics are available within many communities for STD testing and treatment and human immunodeficiency virus/acquired immunodeficiency syndrome (HIV/AIDS) counseling. Physical examinations have become routine requirements at colleges before a student can enter sports programs and can be the initial access route to health care. Education concerning the harmful effects of smoking, alcohol, substance abuse, and obesity and ways to reduce these problems has increased awareness of health in men. Health and fitness clubs have become a popular and lucrative business and have led to improvements in the health status of men and women. However, nurses and health care workers must caution men concerning the adverse effects of overtraining.

Increasing access within the community and workplace to health education and screening can be very advantageous. Studies have shown that community education and federal intervention concerning issues such as the need for seat belt use, the dangers of smoking and drinking, and the use of condoms may have contributed significantly to more healthy behavior choices. Many colleges and community groups host health fairs where blood pressure checks and education concerning various lifestyle choices are offered.

PSYCHOSOCIAL DEVELOPMENT

Schools play a significant role in helping the adolescent prepare for the developmental tasks and challenges of young adulthood. Parenting and family life classes and money management workshops are examples of courses that can help prepare for the transition into adult life. Students who plan on attending college often do not experience these preparatory courses because their focus is on college prerequisite courses. Some colleges have designed survival programs that help freshman students adjust to their new environments and adult responsibilities. Most colleges also offer career counseling and support services for young adults to help them achieve their educational goals. Work-study courses introduce young adults to the work environment and help them adapt to a work milieu.

There are many developmental tasks and challenges that occur during the young adult years. These tasks include developing a mature sense of right and wrong, successful separation from family control, initiating a lifestyle practice, establishing friends and intimate relationships, deciding on marriage and career goals, and developing parenting skills (Figure 10-5). The sense of identity should be formed and stable by young adulthood and will start the individual on a path toward specific goals. These specific goals can change in later stages of the lifespan, when unexpected events, further self-learning, or periods of transition allow time for reflection and reevaluation of accomplishments and new goals can be formulated.

Intimacy

Erikson described establishing **intimacy** as one of the major tasks of young adulthood (see Chapter 4). Intimacy involves more than sexual behavior. It includes the ability to develop a warm, trusting, honest relationship with another person with whom it is safe to be open and express and share private thoughts. If a clear sense of identity has not been achieved during adolescence, then the young adult may feel guarded and only form casual relationships. Eventually this may contribute to isolation or difficulty in forming deep long-term commitments.

Cognitive Ability

Intellectual and creative skills and abilities peak during young adulthood and improve with expanded education and experience. Piaget was a theorist (see Chapter 4) who believed that development of the formal operation as a method of thinking begins in adolescence and extends into young adulthood. The level of abstract thinking and logical reasoning is enhanced by the technology that is available in everyday life. The formal operation type of thinking is necessary in the use of effective problem-solving techniques.

The young adult's cognitive process involves realizing that knowledge is the integration of multiple points of view. This process of integrating various points of view to develop knowledge and understanding is sometimes referred to as **postformal opera-**

FIGURE 10–5 Establishing friendships and deciding on marriage and career goals are tasks of young adulthood.

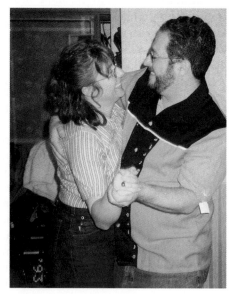

tional thought (Commons et al, 1982). Individuals who have a well-developed post-formal thought process are best able to problem solve in general, including choosing between multiple-choice answers on a test. Therefore school performance may be best in the young adult age group.

Levinson was a psychologist who described four seasons of life (see Chapter 4). He believed that each season had a structure that is separated by transitional periods. During the period of **structure** in the young adult season of life, choices are made such as a marriage partner and commitment to a career. During the following **transitional phase** those choices are reviewed and reevaluated and changes may be made. During one of the later transitional phases, individuals may reflect on past activities and may become unhappy because of missed opportunities or what they perceive as wrong choices. This may contribute to a midlife crisis experience.

Moral Reasoning

Kohlberg was a theorist who believed that the individual must be capable of the formal operational level of thought before achieving mature moral reasoning. Life experiences in an adult role or a college milieu can enhance the development of moral reasoning. Taking responsibility for the care of others, dealing with differing points of view of others, and understanding how their own actions affect others all contribute to the development of mature moral reasoning.

Sexuality

Young adults who are significant in a child's life can role model positive displays of affection. Having young children see loving and joyous contact, such as hugging and kissing between parental role models and close family members, can help a child understand caring behaviors. Although allowing nudity in the home is a personal choice for parents, the concept of demonstrating comfort with their own bodies helps children to develop a positive body image. Treating one part of the body as dirty or naughty may result in having to readjust these beliefs when the child reaches maturity in order to achieve a sense of comfort in intimacy, and therefore their mastery of this task may be delayed.

Sexual intimacy in young adulthood differs from that in adolescence. By young adulthood, identity and cognitive function have reached the level that allows intimate sharing, controlled but honest emotional expression, caring about the partner, and the ability to make compromises and commitments. Sexual behavior and expectations are influenced by culture, customs, and environment. However, the ability to develop a sense of intimacy and attachment required for a long-term commitment is closely related to the individual's experience as an infant concerning attachment with a parent. Healthy parent-child bonding produces a sense of security and trust. If relationships with parents in the early years did not produce a healthy secure attachment, then achievement of a secure and stable intimacy with others in the young adulthood phase of life may be more difficult or delayed.

Marriage

Many young adults who pursue higher education in college either postpone marriage or choose careful family planning or child care arrangements that allow them to continue to pursue their goals. Table 9-2 reviews contraceptive options available for effective family planning. Marriage most often occurs during the young adult phase of the life cycle. However, many delay marriage to later life, until they are established in their careers. Today childbearing can be achieved at a later age due in large part to the advances in research and technology. People often select partners who are similar to themselves in interests, values, religious beliefs, and education. Family pressures or cultural traditions may also play a role in choosing a marriage partner.

Partner choice is thought to be based on a three-stage process (Murstein, 1982). The first stage is the *stimulus stage*, which involves initial impressions and awareness of characteristics that attract the couple to each other. The *value-comparison stage* follows and involves getting to know each other better. The third, the *role stage*, involves evaluating long-term compatibility and deciding on a long-term commitment.

Gender roles and career issues play an important part in early adjustment to marriage. Balancing work, marriage, family, and parental roles is a challenge for young adults. This period is known as the beginning task of *generativity*, as described by Erikson (see Chapter 4). It should be noted that generativity can be achieved by means other than parenting, such as involvement in a career, close interactions with family, or active community activities.

Parenting

In today's society, not all adults achieve or desire marriage and family. Some pursue careers that are fulfilling, thereby leaving little time for the responsibilities that marriage and parenthood require. Others choose to be in long-term, committed relationships without children, and some choose to delay marriage and childrearing until later life stages. However, this chapter will include the development of parenting skills as one of the tasks of young adulthood.

The development of a parent begins at the time conception is confirmed (Table 10-2). When parents learn they are to have a baby, both positive and negative feelings are evoked. They may want the baby and want to be perfect parents. However, they may worry about being inadequately prepared for the parental role, the time commitment, and the impact on their careers and lifestyle. In the second trimester of pregnancy, when parents can feel the fetus move, their focus turns to the baby and what it might be. By the beginning of the third trimester of pregnancy, parents ascribe personality traits to the fetus and are receptive to teachings about parenting and child care. If the newborn arrives as a welcomed guest in the home and the parents are supportive of each other, healthy parenting styles can be easily learned. At least 6 months of maternity leave may be ideal in fostering attachment between parent and child, but often financial or career pressures require a shorter adjustment time. Close parent-child interactions during the early months of life can help in the formation of healthy attachments and positive parenting styles. Stepparents or parents who adopt older children may need extra time and effort to develop parent-child attachment and relationships.

The infant soon learns to associate the presence of the mother with feeding and relief of hunger and discomfort and soon calms whenever the mother is present. This behavior in turn strengthens the mother's sense of adequacy and effectiveness as a parent. Parent-infant attachment is best observed during a feeding, when both mother and

TABLE 10-2

GROWTH AND DEVELOPMENT OF PARENTS

Child's Task (Erikson's Stages)	Parents' Task	Intervention
First Prenatal Trimester		
Growth	Develop attitude toward newborn. "Happy" about child? Parent of one disabled child? Unwed mother? These factors and others will affect the developing attitude of the mother.	Develop positive attitude in both parents concerning expected birth of child. Use referrals and agencies as needed.
Second Prenatal Trimester		
Growth	Mother focuses on infant because of fetal movements felt. Parents picture what infant will look like, what future he/she will have, and other ideas.	Parents' focus is on child care and needs and providing physical environment for expected infant. Therefore information concerning care of the newborn should be given at this time.
Third Prenatal Trimester		
Growth	Mother feels large. Attention focuses on how fetus is going to get out.	Detailed information should be presented at this time concerning the birth process, preparation for birth, breastfeeding, and care of sibling at home.
Birth		
Adjustment to external environment	Elicit positive responses from child and respond by meeting child's need for food and closeness; if parents receive only negative responses (e.g., sleepy infant, crying infant, difficult feeder, congenital anomaly), development of the parent will be inhibited.	Encourage early touch, feeding, and other practices. Explain behavior and appearance of newborn to allay fears. Help parents to identify positive responses. (Use infant's reflexes, such as grasp reflex, to identify a positive response by placing mother's finger into infant's hand.)
Infant		
Trust	Learn "cues" presented by infant to determine individual needs of infant.	Help parents assess and interpret needs of infant (avoid feelings of helplessness or incompetence). Do not let in-laws take over parental tasks. Help parents cope with problems such as colic.

(Continued)

TABLE 10-2

GROWTH AND DEVELOPMENT OF PARENTS—cont'd

Child's Task (Erikson's Stages)	Parents' Task	Intervention
Toddler Autonomy	Try to accept the pattern of growth and development. Accept some loss of control but maintain some limits for safety.	Help parents cope with transient independence of child (e.g., allow child to go on tricycle but don't yell "Don't fall" or anxiety will be radiated.)
Preschool Initiative	Learn to separate from child.	Help parents show standards but let go so child can develop some independence. A preschool experience may be helpful.
School Age Industry	Accept importance of child's peers. Parents must learn to accept some rejection from child at times. Patience is needed to allow children to do for themselves, even if it takes longer. Do not do the school project for the child. Provide chores for child appropriate to his/her age level.	Help parents to understand that child is developing his/her own limits and self-discipline. Be there to guide child but do not constantly intrude. Help child get results from his/her own efforts at performance.
Adolescent Establishment of identity Acceptance of pubertal changes Development of abstract reasoning Examination of career choices Investigation of lifestyles Controlling of feelings	Parents must learn to let child live his/her own life and not expect total control over the child. Expect at times to be discredited by teenager. Expect differences in opinion and respect them. Guide but do not push.	Help parents adjust to changing role and relationship with adolescent (e.g., as child develops his/her own identity, child may become a Democrat if parents are Republican). Expose child to varied career fields and life experiences. Help child to understand emerging emotions and feelings brought about by puberty.

Modified from Leifer, G. (2003). *Introduction to maternity and pediatric nursing* (4th ed.). Philadelphia: W.B. Saunders.

infant should be focused on each other. If either is preoccupied or inattentive, parent-infant bonding may not be successful. If the parent is an adolescent, some developmental tasks of adolescence may interfere with the developmental tasks of parenthood. Special interventions by the nurse or health care worker can be helpful in prioritizing behaviors and meeting the major needs of the infant and adolescent parent. Refer to Chapter 9 for more information on the adolescent stage of development.

TEACHING TECHNIQUES FOR THE YOUNG ADULT

Successful adult learning always involves relating the information to the appropriate developmental tasks they are experiencing. For example, a new parent will most likely be very receptive to information concerning parenting skills. An adult in a managerial position at work may be most receptive to learning about managing styles and techniques. The knowledge and skills learned should be applicable to the learner, be realistic, and help solve current problems encountered by the learner. Concepts presented to young adults should build on their previous knowledge and skills, rather than beginning below their level of understanding, or they will be turned off. Teaching goals should be made clear, outlining how the new knowledge can be applied and how it will benefit their current life roles. Learning is a lifelong process. Teaching techniques for young adults should be interactive, problem oriented, and related to daily psychosocial tasks at work, home, or school.

KEY POINTS

- Young adulthood is most often defined as 20 to 40 years of age.
- Physiological performance has a natural peak between 20 and 30 years of age.
- Proper nutrition and exercise can prevent obesity and contribute to health during the young adult years and beyond.
- Most lifestyle patterns are established during the young adult years.
- It is easier to develop positive health habits as a young adult than to change habits later in life to achieve a positive health status.
- The major causes of death in the young adult age group are related to accidents and violence, and both are preventable.
- Promoting healthy behaviors relating to safe sex practices during adolescence and young adulthood can reduce the incidence of sexually transmitted diseases.
- Recent public education efforts have increased awareness of the need for testicular self-examination (TSE) and breast self-examination (BSE) as part of gender-specific preventive health programs.
- Health and fitness spas have become a lucrative business that help improve the health status of men and women. However, overtraining may adversely affect reproductive health and should be avoided.
- Developmental tasks of young adulthood include developing a stable sense of identity and a mature sense of right and wrong, successful separation from family control, establishing adult friendships and intimate relationships,

choosing marriage partners and career goals, developing parenting skills, and initiating a lifestyle.
- Piaget's formal operational thinking begins in adolescence and extends into young adulthood.
- Formal operational thinking is necessary for effective problem-solving skills.
- Postformal operational thought involves integrating various points of view.
- In most cultures there are established expectations of adulthood.
- The task of generativity can be achieved by a means other than parenting.
- Development of a parent begins when conception is confirmed.
- When teaching young adults, the goals and how the new knowledge can be applied in the lives of the learners should be made clear.

CRITICAL THINKING

Using Erikson's stages of growth and development, discuss how parents can apply positive parenting styles to help their children successfully achieve developmental tasks.

MULTIPLE-CHOICE REVIEW QUESTIONS

1 Young adulthood includes the ages between:
   1 12 to 16 years
   2 17 to 19 years
   3 20 to 40 years
   4 41 to 60 years
2 The young adult is in Erikson's stage of:
   1 Industry
   2 Autonomy
   3 Intimacy
   4 Identity
3 An ectopic pregnancy is:
   1 An unplanned pregnancy
   2 A pregnancy occurring outside the uterus
   3 A pregnancy occurring in early adulthood
   4 A pregnancy consisting of twins
4 Effective teaching techniques for the young adult should include:
   1 Information that is realistic and helps solve problems
   2 Information that is exciting and dramatic
   3 Information that relates to world problems
   4 Information that is already understood
5 The major cause of death in the young adult age group is:
   1 Congenital malformation
   2 Preventable accidents
   3 Heart disease
   4 Sedentary lifestyle

Middle Adulthood

OUTLINE

OBJECTIVES

Upon completion of this chapter, the student will be able to:

1 Define middle adulthood.
2 List the physiological changes that occur during middle adulthood.
3 Define the major developmental tasks and challenges of middle adulthood.
4 State the complexities of the menopausal experience in women.
5 Discuss the male climacteric.
6 Define midlife crisis.
7 Discuss sexuality in the middle adulthood phase of the life cycle.
8 List preventative health care measures appropriate for middle adulthood.
9 Define the "sandwich generation."
10 List teaching strategies that may be effective for the patient in the middle-adult phase of the life cycle.

KEY TERMS

Climacteric
"Empty nest" syndrome
Generativity
Hot flashes
Identity accommodation
Menopause

Midlife crises
Reproductive health
Sandwich generation
Sexuality
Stagnation

DEFINITION

Middle adulthood is currently defined as the period of development after the early adult years but before retirement (Skolnick, 1991). Middle adulthood is often referred to as the period between 40 and 60 years of age. It is influenced by genetics and the environment. An interaction of biological, psychological, and social changes occur. By middle age the adult has established roots in a community, with ties to culture, religious groups, schools, neighborhood centers, and friends. Some culture-specific influences affect development, but the greatest current environmental influence is the worldwide political dynamic that reaches across oceans to influence life and lifestyles in the United States.

Some theorists suggest that developmental changes are gradual and progressive, but others express the concept of passing through distinct stages (see Chapter 4).

PHYSIOLOGICAL CHANGES

Metabolic needs decrease during middle adulthood, and if diet and exercise are not part of a healthy lifestyle, excess weight begins to accumulate. A decrease in energy and perceived physical attractiveness may occur. A loss of muscle tone and skin elasticity may result in a less firm appearance of body contours. Body fat may redistribute to the hip area. Impacted wisdom teeth may require extraction, and periodontal disease is a risk if oral care is not meticulous. Hair may begin to gray and thin. Eye changes common to middle age can be easily corrected with glasses, contact lenses, or laser surgery. Diet, smoking, and lack of exercise influence cardiovascular changes that occur during midlife, but hormonal changes also influence risk factors for cardiovascular disease.

DEVELOPMENTAL TASKS

The main task or crisis of middle adulthood is **generativity** versus **stagnation** (Erikson, 1994). *Generativity* has been defined as contributing in a positive way to family or community. This contribution improves self-image and promotes subjective well-being. Failure to achieve generativity results in *stagnation*, which is total concern for self and denial of the developmental process. Generativity can be achieved in many ways and is not necessarily limited to having children and a family of one's own. There are many opportunities to achieve generativity through career and personal activities and achievements. Other developmental tasks of middle adulthood include managing a career and finances, managing a household, and nurturing marriage and family relationships. Maintaining a positive self-image is important to the middle-aged adult. When individuals deny they are aging and cannot view themselves as middle aged, they often find difficulty in adjusting to necessary changes and depression may develop. Maintaining a positive self-image is a challenge when society and the media place high importance on looking and acting young. An example of another important task of middle age is **identity accommodation,** which is changing the concept of one's own identity to fit what is real, rather than what was dreamed.

The affect of the spouse or significant other on continued development and life stability is important. The feedback of a spouse or significant other influences self-image in the midlife stage. New social experiences challenge the middle-aged adult. Involvement with child care, athletic events, parents of school friends, and parent-child relationships can also influence psychological well-being (Figure 11-1).

CHALLENGES

Maintaining optimum cognitive functioning is necessary to prevent a decrease in problem-solving skills. Adjusting to changes in relationships with co-workers, friends, and family are also important to maintaining psychological well-being. Many middle-aged adults find time to continue their education, which may have been interrupted by marriage and childrearing. The middle-aged adult may need more time to learn and assimilate new material, but once learned, the content is remembered with more accuracy. Perseverance and patience may be needed to succeed in school.

Women at midlife are at high risk for social isolation due to divorce, separation, or widowhood. The **"empty nest" syndrome** that can occur when grown children start to leave home for the first time may increase the feelings of isolation.

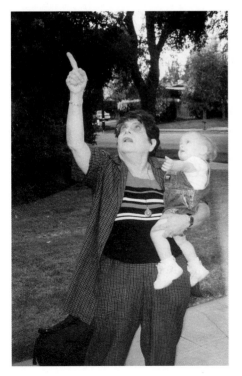

FIGURE 11–1 A grandmother enjoys teaching her grandchild about the world and remains involved in family activities. (From Sheick, D. [2002]. Mastering Group Leadership. *Psychosocial nursing and mental health services,* 40(9), 35.)

SEXUALITY

Sexuality is a part of every phase of the life cycle, beginning in infancy. However, sexuality is not limited to the sex act. Sexuality involves beliefs and behaviors that surround physiological responses, emotions, and sociocultural values. Communication, a sense of closeness, and mutual comfort are key aspects of sexuality. Middle adulthood is a time when the adult is often focused on career goals and financial stability, and so little time or energy may be set aside to fulfill sexual needs. Yet the middle-aged woman is at the peak of sexual desire and sexual pleasure because the pressures of pregnancy prevention are often relieved by the approach of menopause.

A significant percentage of the population in the United States is living as single adults. The reasons can include postponing marriage for a career, divorces, or never entering into a long-term relationship. Remaining single is an option in U.S. culture today that is not frowned on or considered abnormal. Options for sexual lifestyles for the single person can include celibacy, a sexually exclusive companion, or a long-term relationship with one or more partners. People may also live together without marriage for a variety of reasons, including the widow or divorcée who would have to give up monetary benefits if they were to remarry. Open marriages, extramarital affairs, group marriage, and "swinging" are other options for sexual pleasure in the adult phase of the life cycle (Masters et al, 1986).

Gradual hormonal changes occur before menopause, and these changes may start as early as age 35, although the age for actual menopause is closer to 50. Each woman responds to subtle menopausal changes in a unique way, and sexuality can be affected by these changes. Estrogen-sensitive skin can lead to dry skin. Breasts flatten and hair thins as estrogen-to-androgen ratios change.

The absence of children in the home, who may have left for college or marriage, may provide time to renew relationships between partners. A self-assured attitude, developed due to experience and age, may limit inhibitions and can create many enjoyable close moments with partners at this stage of life.

MIDLIFE CRISIS

Middle adulthood is a time of self-reflection, reevaluation, and prioritization. Looking back, the adult may grieve lost youth and missed opportunities. Looking ahead, adults may fear the inevitability of their own mortality. This may lead to despair. Sometimes reflection and reinterpretation of past experiences bring new insights and might serve as a turning point in self-perception.

Sometimes during this stage of the **midlife crisis** adults try to make up for lost opportunities of the past or challenge the inevitability of the future. They may start to engage in behaviors that are atypical for their character (Figure 11-2).

The Sandwich Generation

Middle adults are known to be in the **sandwich generation.** That means they must deal with increased financial and emotional responsibilities related to their children in addition to increased demands placed on them by their older and possibly dependent parents. These stressors contribute to the challenges of middle adulthood.

The family influences the adjustment to middle adulthood. A fulfilling marriage will help validate positive self-esteem, while divorce, separation, conflicts with adult chil-

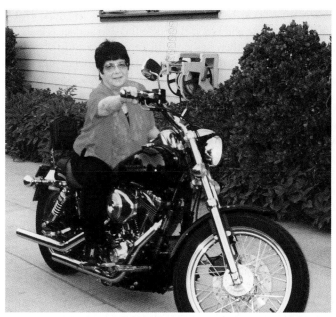

FIGURE 11–2 It is never too late to learn and enjoy skills of a new activity.

dren, or aging parents may impact the psychological functioning of middle-aged adults in a negative way.

REPRODUCTIVE HEALTH

Reproductive health is a term used to describe the health of the reproductive organs in all persons. The **climacteric** refers to the time in life in which hormonal changes result in cessation the reproductive ability in the female and a corresponding decrease in sexual activity in the male. Complex interactions exist among sex hormones, physiology, and physical and emotional well-being.

Structural differences in the male and female central nervous system begin in the embryonic stage of development and are influenced by hormones (Goldman et al, 2000). The reproductive years in the female involve a unique group of health issues. Sex hormones such as estrogen protect women from some illnesses that often affect men. As they age and sex hormones decrease with menopause, women develop risks for disease that are similar to men. Most clinical research concerning health has been conducted with male subjects, and these same research findings were applied to women. Application was not always accurate. Today women make up 40% of students in medical schools and more than 50% of minority graduates from medical schools. Women increasingly are influencing the direction of research and the delivery of health care.

Women's Health

Menopause is the cessation of the menstrual period due to hormonal changes in the body. Menopause usually begins between 45 and 55 years of age and is genetically controlled. The menstrual cycle becomes shorter and more irregular. **Hot flashes** may result when capillaries dilate and blood rushes to the skin surface. The body feels warm, the woman may sweat, and then vasoconstriction occurs and the woman feels cold. This can occur several times a day and is very uncomfortable and distracting to the woman. Hormone replacement therapy (HRT) may be prescribed but is not appropriate for all women due to risks for developing blood clots and other complications. Complementary and alternative medicine (CAM) therapy is popular with many women during menopause. The nurse and health care worker must assess any interactions between CAM therapy used by the woman and any prescribed medicines or treatments.

The onset and experience of menopause is unique to each woman. One specific approach to the onset of menopause will not be appropriate for all women. A detailed and accurate personal health interview can reveal problems that require interventions. (See Box 11-1 and Chapter 12 for more details in postmenopausal care.)

Recent medical advances have prolonged the physical reproductive capabilities of some women. The psychosocial issues involved in childbearing at a later age and the advantages and disadvantages of the middle-aged or older adult as a new parent present new challenges to the parents, child, and nurse.

Men's Health

Although women's health has become a specialty in medicine, a specialty in men's health is rarely seen. Sexual concerns of men are typically related to role changes, work-related stress, decreased physical fitness, and sexual performance anxiety. Indicators of health, as outlined in *Healthy People 2010*, include rates of longevity, morbidity, and mortality.

Although longevity rates have increased for both men and women, women still generally live longer than men. In each leading cause of death in adults, men have a higher rate of mortality. The morbidity rate is generally higher for women in both acute and chronic conditions. A contributory factor may be that men perceive themselves as healthy and therefore delay seeking medical care and preventative care. There may also be gender differences in health and illness. Research has shown that there are explanations for gender differences in health and illness (Waldron, 1997). Testosterone levels may lower high-density lipoprotein (HDL, lipid) levels, and body fat distribution in men may predispose them to heart disease. The male climacteric involves a gradual decline in the blood concentration of testosterone and other hormones. This results in a decrease in muscle mass and strength, a decrease in sex drive, and a decrease in a sense of well-being. Testosterone replacement therapy has recently been studied and found to have positive influences on

---

BOX 11-1   **Signs of Menopausal Changes in Women**
• Hot flashes
• Heart palpitations
• Headache
• Decreased vaginal lubrication
• Fatigue
• Insomnia
• Emotional lability (happy one minute, crying the next)

improving strength, decreasing fat accumulation, and increasing libido and a sense of well-being. Testosterone replacement therapy does not increase erectile function because blood circulation plays a major role in erectile function. Some nonprescription medications have recently become available for use for specific symptoms related to the male climacteric. Many drugs decrease testosterone levels in the male, such as chemotherapy, ingestion of lead and exposure to certain insecticides, ethanol, and many illicit drugs. Disease such as cystic fibrosis, sickle cell anemia, anorexia nervosa, liver disease, and renal failure also decrease testosterone levels in men. Androgen therapy is used with caution in older men with enlarged prostates and urinary symptoms.

Generally, men remain in the workforce longer than women and may partake in activities that pose a higher potential for injuries. Men engage in sports and leisure activities that also have a high risk for injury, and some may use illegal substances to prove their masculinity. Young boys are often socialized to ignore symptoms of illness and "not be a sissy," and so to avoid being labeled as sickly, men may postpone seeking medical advice until the problem is more advanced.

It is well known that strenuous exercise suppresses ovarian function in women, and many champion athletes have *amenorrhea* (absence of menstrual periods). Strenuous exercise can also affect men by decreasing testosterone levels and decreasing the sperm count; this effect can last for several months. Middle-aged men who fear the aging process may begin to experience alteration in sexual performance, but the ability to procreate, or father children, remains intact.

Gender-appropriate health education is important to provide vital information without damaging sex role–stereotyped self-images. Men typically contact the health care system via a pediatrician when young, a school nurse when school age, and a military doctor or company physician when a young adult and often do not choose a personal doctor until middle age. Recently, preventative care for men, in the form of testicular self-examination for testicular cancer and screening for prostate cancer, has been marketed and is included in routine health examinations. Men should be counseled concerning healthy lifestyles, sexually transmitted disease prevention, anticipated role changes, and job retraining when necessary. Expanded health promotion and early detection activities help achieve the goals of *Healthy People 2010* for men and women (Box 11-2). The recommended immunization schedule for adults is listed in Appendix A.

TEACHING TECHNIQUES FOR THE MIDDLE-AGED ADULT

Successfully teaching middle-aged adults depends on having an understanding of their typical concerns and potential sources of stress. Stress can inhibit learning or be the motivational force for learning. Misconceptions concerning menopause are common, and many adults want information related to preventing chronic illnesses. Content of teaching plans should be related to the problems and concerns of the individual and the age group.

Middle-aged adults may be concerned about the lives of their grown children, want help adjusting to the role of grandparent, or need help with designing strategies to care for their own older, frail parents. Middle-aged adults receive great personal satisfaction

---

| **BOX 11-2** | **Essential Health Screening for Middle-Aged Women and Men** |

Healthy, middle-aged women and men should have the following screening tests performed at regular intervals:
- Vision testing
- Dental checkups
- Blood pressure monitoring
- Lipid screening (cholesterol, triglycerides)
- Cardiovascular screening
- Colorectal cancer screening

Women:
- Breast examination and mammogram
- Papanicolaou (Pap) testing

Men:
- Testicular examination
- Prostate cancer screening

---

from contributing to the community and may start to plan their alternative lifestyles for retirement (Figure 11-3).

Middle-aged adults are often interested in learning about menopause and the teaching of coping styles that will help maintain a positive health status. Teaching strategies should incorporate the independence and competencies of the adult learner and provide information that coincides with concerns and stresses common to the age group. As with all age groups, a simple compliment (validation) concerning their learning competencies can also provide the reward needed to support motivation for further learning. An example of a creative group exercise related to helping the middle-aged adult accept the aging process in a positive way and build self-esteem is reviewed in Table 11-1. Similar group exercises are helpful for the older adult who may be having difficulty coping with mental health problems or the stresses of losing a spouse or partner.

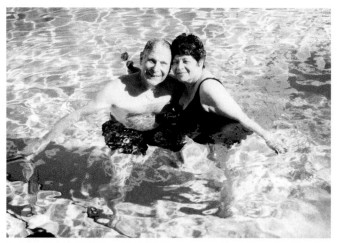

FIGURE 11–3 Retirement lifestyles can include many enjoyable and active leisure activities.

TABLE 11-1

CREATIVE STRUCTURED GROUP EXERCISES AND PROCESSING SUGGESTIONS

Structured Activity	Processing Focus
CRAFT PROJECTS: Adapt project and level of supervision to person's skill level and safety needs. Use theme of craft as an object lesson. Link symbolically to mental health and healthy living.	

Foam or Felt Leaves.

Structured Activity	Processing Focus
1. Use foam or felt to craft individual leaves to serve as name tags, decorate with sequins or glitter.	Discuss how, like each leaf, each person is distinctive. Link this concept to the value of each person in the group as special. However, like a torn or crinkled leaf no person is perfect. parts, positive or negative, contribute to each unique self. Link this concept to the acceptance of self and disorder as the first step to taking charge and preventing relapse.
2. Make a plaque showing progression of seasons using varying shades of leaves.	Link seasons with turning points in life. Like seasons, people go through changes and losses. Change is a chance to start over. Link this concept to clients situations (e.g., release from the hospital, change in living status). Process ways to cope with losses, holiday blues, or intense feeling experienced on the anniversary of a major change or crisis.

3. Piece together several leaves to
  a. Make a frame for each person's photograph.
  b. Make a wall hanging using a branch of a tree to form a tree trunk, with each person attaching his or her individualized leaves.
	Discuss that many leaves together are needed to frame the portrait or complete the tree.
	Likewise, each person may need to give or receive support by joining with others. Discuss deciding when to stand alone, "Branch" out, or join together in a group.

4. Fashion leaves into a Full wreath using the rim of a paper plate as a foundation. Decorate with items such as buttons, raffia, bows and pumpkin cutouts.	Like a wreath, life can be a circle, having continuity. Link this concept with decisions to continue to persevere despite having a mental illness (e.g., ability to choose each day to take medications, adhere to treatment, attend the group). Discuss crisis events and risks of staying in the circle (e.g., suicide attempts, stopping medications). Focus on using support systems, healthy self talk and healthy coping mechanisms.

(Continued)

TABLE **11-1**

CREATIVE STRUCTURED GROUP EXERCISES AND PROCESSING SUGGESTIONS—cont'd

Structured Activity	Processing Focus
Collage	
1. Using pictures and words from magazines or old greeting cards, paste together overlapping pictures and words representative of patients' qualities, favorite things, memories or values.	Relate pictures to person's strength and self-esteem. Discuss being different as associated with positive unique qualities versus the perception of being different due to the stigma of mental illness. Link this concept to assertiveness skills and the need for advocacy.
2. Create a group mural representing the treatment group. Each member contributes pictures to form the whole.	Use the group collage to highlight commonalities and the group's shared history, present and future. Link this concept to those of cohesion and support, as well as the need for separateness and skills to manage conflict. Discuss ways to manage on one's own during holidays or other times of separation.
3. Develop a collage depicting stressor and stress relievers.	Discuss what affects patient's perception of stressors. Discuss what can and cannot be changed, cognitive reframing, and healthy and unhealthy coping (e.g., addictions).

GAMES: Use innovative and traditional games adapted to highlight mental health concepts. Adapt complexity to client functioning and safety needs.

Noncompetitive Games	
1. Fishing for feelings: Write "feeling" words (e.g., lonely, joyous, jealous, peaceful) on colored paper "fish". Attach a large paper clip to each fish. Place fish on the floor with some fish face up (with the feeling word visible) and save face down. With clients sitting around the "pond," have them use a fishing pole with a magnet attached to fish for a feeling.	Link fishing to recreation and discuss family times, both positive and negative. Ask clients to talk about a time when the feeling they "caught" was experienced. When a client "catches" a fish that is down, link that concept with facing the unknown and discussing the risk taking and growth.
2. Stress Balloons: inflate balloons. Have patients use felt-tip markers to write a number of stressors on his or her balloon. Ask patients to bounce their balloons in the air and try to keep all the balloons off the ground. Inevitably, the balloons will fall. Let all patients stomp stress away by stepping on the balloons.	Teach patient about physical and emotional signs of stress. Discuss how laughter releases stress. Link this concept to how it is easier for many hands to juggle the stressors than for one person to strive alone. When all the balloons finally fall, discuss patients' choices to let some things go (e.g., forgive, move on).

TABLE 11-1

CREATIVE STRUCTURED GROUP EXERCISES AND PROCESSING SUGGESTIONS—cont'd

Structured Activity	Processing Focus
	Ask patient to name one way they will take care of themselves (e.g., relax) in the coming week

Competitive Games (divide patients into team)

1. Using a quiz show format, create six categories with five questions in each category. The question should be more difficult as the dollar value linked to each question increases. Use play money and a banker to add another arena for patient processing. Categories can focus on healthy living and self-care practices, signs and coping strategies associated with mental illness, or psychotropic medications and managing side effects.

Discuss competition versus cooperation, taking turns, and winning and losing. Discuss ways life is a game with rules. Discuss how one decides, when to obey or to step outside the rules. Link the concept of changing rules with the need to re-examine some of the rules learned in childhood (e.g. giving oneself permission to succeed, choosing wellness).

2. Write a word or phrase on a sign. Cover each letter individually. Patient teams take turns guessing letters until the word or phrase is discovered. For example, phrases can center around holiday themes and traditions, medications, stress and coping mechanisms, type of mental illnesses, or signs of decompensation.

Discuss the specific content highlighted by the game (e.g. managing medication side effects, recognizing signs of decompensation and met and unmet needs). Reinforce patients' personal power to choose how to view themselves or stressors, how to adapt and how to ask for, receive, and provide support.

3. Using a bingo format, create six-inch square boards on sheets of paper, with answers printed in each of 25 squares. The space in the middle of each sheet is a free space. Hand out bingo "cards" to teams. When an answer on the sheets is called, teams mark an x in that square. The first team to have five Xs in a row vertically, horizontally, or diagonally wins the game. Center the bingo games around themes, such as feelings, human needs, or communication tasks (e.g., shaking hands, saying one thing patients admire about the person to their right).

Like a printed bingo card, each person is given a genetic "bingo" card at birth, with some characteristics unchangeable (e.g. race, family of origin, gender, eye color, bone structure). Talk about patients' family roots, genetic "givens," body image or gender commonalities and differences, as well as the genetic component of some types of mental illnesses. Discuss feelings and what aspects of self-care are within one's capacity to change. Share ways to empower oneself to gain control over how each patient chooses to play life's bingo card.

From Scheick, D. (2002). Mastering group leadership. *Psychological Nursing and Mental Health Services, 40*(9), 35-36.

KEY POINTS

- Middle adulthood is the period after the early adult reproductive years and before retirement. It includes the period between 40 and 60 years of age.
- Erikson's developmental task of middle adulthood is Generativity versus Stagnation.
- Other developmental tasks of middle adulthood include managing finances and a career, nurturing marriage and family relationships, managing a household, and maintaining a positive self-image.
- Middle adulthood is a time of self-reflection, reevaluation, and prioritization.
- Gradual hormonal changes occur before menopause; these changes may begin as early as age 35.
- The climacteric is when hormonal changes result in cessation of menstruation in women and decreased muscle mass and sex drive in men.
- Concerns of middle-aged men are typically related to role changes, work-related stress, decreased physical fitness, and performance anxiety.
- Preventive health care for men includes testicular self-evaluation, annual dental examinations, blood pressure and blood lipid levels, and prostate and colorectal cancer screenings.
- Middle age is referred to as a sandwich generation, where responsibilities include the care of children and older parents.

CRITICAL THINKING

Gender-appropriate health education is important in middle adulthood. Outline two health education plans, one for men and one for women. Include information about preventing illness, recognizing midlife mental health issues, and managing the approach of the climacteric.

MULTIPLE-CHOICE REVIEW QUESTIONS

1 Middle adulthood includes the period between the ages of:
   1 20 to 29 years
   2 30 to 39 years
   3 40 to 60 years
   4 60 to 80 years
2 The main task or crises of middle adulthood is:
   1 Intimacy versus isolation
   2 Generativity versus stagnation
   3 Identity versus role confusion
   4 Dependence versus independence

3 Menopause includes:
  1 Cessation of sexual activity
  2 Loss of sexual ability
  3 Cessation of menstrual period
  4 The beginning of a midlife crisis
4 Preventative health care for men in middle adulthood should include:
  1 Annual chest X-rays
  2 Testicular self-examination
  3 Annual pap tests
  4 Daily recording of pulse rate
5 The *sandwich generation* refers to:
  1 People who do not have time to cook
  2 People who care for children and grandchildren
  3 People who prefer sandwiches to hot meals
  4 People who care for elderly parents in addition to young children

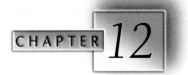

CHAPTER *12*

Late Adulthood

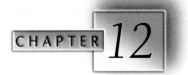
OBJECTIVES

Upon completion of this chapter, the student will be able to:

1 Discuss the major goals of Healthy People 2010 related to late adulthood.
2 Identify common health concerns of late adulthood.
3 Describe challenges and developmental tasks of late adulthood.
4 Discuss lifestyle changes that may be necessary for late adulthood.
5 Define elder abuse and state one way it can be prevented.
6 Discuss the ways menopause may affect women in the late adulthood phase of the life cycle.
7 List the learning needs of later adulthood.
8 Select appropriate teaching techniques to promote effective learning and coping for late adulthood.

KEY TERMS

Assistive devices
Autonomy
Competence
Disengagement
Elder abuse
Polypharmacy
Relatedness

GOALS OF *HEALTHY PEOPLE 2010* FOR LATE ADULTHOOD
Definition

The U.S. government defines old age as over age 65, when full social security benefits become available, retirement usually occurs, and a leisurely lifestyle is assumed. Late adulthood is considered to encompass the ages between 65 and 74 years. Increased technology and improved health care practices have enabled people to live longer and remain active and productive. Today many people in the late adulthood phase of the life cycle postpone retirement and remain active in the workforce as senior employees or part-time consultants.

> One of the major goals of *Healthy People 2010* for older adults is to increase the lifespan and the quality of life by focusing on wellness, prevention of illness, and treatment of disease.

Maximizing health as much as possible promotes mobility and independence. The older adult can develop meaning and enjoyment in life despite physical limitations.

> The most common health risks and leading causes of death in the older adult include cancer, heart disease, stroke, pneumonia, and influenza. These risks can decrease through preventative measures, medical treatment, social support, and healthy behaviors.

Some health concerns of the older adult include the following:
- Development of osteoporosis
- Risks for falls and fractures
- Poor awareness of healthy behavior options
- Increased risk of influenza and pneumonia

- Development of cataracts
- Compensation for developing hearing deficits

Statistics

According to the Department of Health and Human Services (USDHHS), in the year 2000 the number of people age 65 and older was three times higher than that in 1900 and increased 12% between 1990 and 2000 (DHHS, 2000). It is estimated that by 2030 the older adult population will number 70 million, or double the year 2000 figures, because the baby boom generation will have reached age 65.

Income

The income sources for older persons in the United States include social security, pensions, personal assets, and earnings. Approximately 23% of persons over age 65 reported an annual income of more than $25,000 in the year 2000. Approximately 10% of persons over 65 were considered below poverty level, with another 6.7% at near poverty level. Those persons living alone were at greatest risk for financial crisis. Approximately 12% of persons over age 65 continue to work. Table 12-1 shows the elderly population of each state in the United States and the percent below poverty level.

Education Level

As of 2001, approximately 46% of African Americans, 63% of Asians or Pacific Islanders, and 74% of Caucasians in the over-65 age group had a high school education. Approximately 16% of the over-65 age group had a bachelor's degree or higher. Approximately 28% of persons 65 or older have Internet access, with 12% using computers at home (USDHHS, 2000). Understanding these statistics enables the health care worker to plan for the needs and limitations of the elderly population they serve in the twenty-first century. The living arrangement, support systems, income, and educational level all influence the plan of care for the older person. The nurse or health care worker can refer to the Administration on Aging section of the DHHS Web site to locate nationwide elder care resources and obtain other information concerning the geriatric population. The World Health Organization (WHO) has urged governments around the world to consider the health needs of the older adult in the general health programs of their countries (Kumar, 1999).

CHALLENGES

Several factors influence the health and well-being of older adults:

- *Access to Health Care*—Access to health care to maintain optimum physical and mental health is often blocked by lack of health insurance coverage. When access to health care is blocked, preventive care is neglected and health care is only obtained after an illness or disease develops.
- *Reduced Income*—Reduced income is a problem for many older adults. Social security and pension incomes may not cover daily living and health care expenses. Working past retirement age is a potential solution for some older adults. In 1986

TABLE 12-1

THE 65+ POPULATION BY STATE FOR YEAR 2000

	Number of Persons	Percent of All Ages	Percent Increase 1990-2000	Percent Below Poverty 1999-2001*
U.S. Total	34,991,753	12.4	12.0	9.9
Alabama	579,798	13.0	10.9	14.8
Alaska	35,699	5.7	59.6	5.9
Arizona	667,839	13.0	39.5	7.7
Arkansas	374,019	14.0	6.8	14.2
California	3,595,658	10.6	14.7	8.0
Colorado	416,073	9.7	26.3	6.3
Connecticut	470,183	13.8	5.4	8.4
Delaware	101,726	13.0	26.0	6.9
District of Columbia	69,898	12.2	−10.2	16.7
Florida	2,807,597	17.6	18.5	9.0
Georgia	785,275	9.6	20.0	12.4
Hawaii	160,601	13.3	28.5	7.4
Idaho	145,916	11.3	20.3	7.9
Illinois	1,500,025	12.1	4.4	8.3
Indiana	752,831	12.4	8.1	7.8
Iowa	436,213	14.9	2.4	6.3
Kansas	356,229	13.3	4.0	6.8
Kentucky	504,793	12.5	8.1	12.4
Louisiana	516,929	11.6	10.2	14.5
Maine	183,402	14.4	12.3	9.7
Maryland	599,307	11.3	15.8	11.4
Massachusetts	860,162	13.5	5.0	10.3
Michigan	1,219,018	12.3	10.0	8.0
Minnesota	594,266	12.1	8.7	10.3
Mississippi	343,523	12.1	6.9	17.7
Missouri	755,379	13.5	5.3	8.4
Montana	120,949	13.4	13.6	8.3
Nebraska	232,195	13.6	4.1	9.9
Nevada	218,929	11.0	71.5	8.1
New Hampshire	147,970	12.0	18.3	7.8
New Jersey	1,113,136	13.2	7.9	7.9
New Mexico	212,225	11.7	30.1	13.6
New York	2,448,352	12.9	3.6	11.8
North Carolina	969,048	12.0	20.5	15.2
North Dakota	94,478	14.7	3.8	11.4
Ohio	1,507,757	13.3	7.2	7.3
Oklahoma	455,950	13.2	7.5	11.7
Oregon	438,177	12.8	12.0	6.9
Pennsylvania	1,919,165	15.6	4.9	8.3

(Continued)

TABLE 12-1

THE 65+ POPULATION BY STATE FOR YEAR 2000—cont'd

	Number of Persons	Percent of All Ages	Percent Increase 1990-2000	Percent Below Poverty 1999-2001*
Rhode Island	152,402	14.5	1.2	10.6
South Carolina	485,333	12.1	22.3	13.1
South Dakota	108,131	14.3	5.7	8.3
Tennessee	703,311	12.4	13.7	13.0
Texas	2,072,532	9.9	20.7	12.6
Utah	190,222	8.5	26.9	7.8
Vermont	77,510	12.7	17.2	11.5
Virginia	792,333	11.2	19.2	10.4
Washington	662,148	11.2	15.1	8.5
West Virginia	276,895	15.3	3.0	11.6
Wisconsin	702,553	13.1	7.9	7.9
Wyoming	57,693	11.7	22.2	10.0

Data from the Administration on aging, profile of general demographic characteristics for the United States, 2000; poverty data is from the 2002 current population surveys, aoa.gov/ada/stats/profile/6.html
*Calculated on the basis of the official poverty definitions for the years 1999 to 2001.

age-based mandatory retirement was abolished, but age-discrimination remains a problem for those seeking new jobs.

- *Changes in Living Arrangements*—Adjusting to changes in living arrangements can also influence the physical and mental well-being of the older adult. Evidence suggests that living as extended family, or near family members, is optimum. As another option, assisted living communities help the older adult maintain independence, social interaction, and a positive self-concept. Some older adults may live in inadequate housing, whereas others may be institutionalized in nursing homes and may lose independence and control over their lives.

- *Cost of Health Care*—Private insurance and Medicare cover some of the clinic or office care, but the focus is often on treatment and recovery rather than preventive care. According to the Centers for Disease Control and Prevention (CDC), the most common activities of daily living that require assistance by home health care aides include body hygiene, bed-to-chair transfer, toileting, shopping, meal preparation, and light housework. Ambulatory care clinics and home care organizations can be helpful to the older adult in accessing health care.

- *Altered Nutritional Needs*—Dental problems, inability to cook, dislike of eating alone, pain or malaise due to a medical condition, or lack of accommodation for special needs related to cultural or religious food traditions may be the cause of altered eating habits. Attention to diet and nutrition improves and maintains good health in the older adult. Caloric needs may decrease with age, but a balanced nutritional intake remains essential. Assessment of the nutritional needs of the older adult is essential, and community resources such as Meals on Wheels can be utilized.

- *Assistive Devices*—**Assistive devices** may be needed by the older adult to help maintain independent living. Assistive devices include such items as walkers, canes, respiratory equipment, hearing aids, and electronic emergency response devices.
- *Preventing Falls*—Preventing falls becomes more important as the older adult develops vision or hearing problems and slower response times. The use of certain medications can cause dizziness or imbalance that can also increase the vulnerability of the older adult to falling. The nurse or health care worker can assess the older adults environment and help with securing loose rugs, improving tracking on slippery floors, clearing general clutter, and improving lighting, especially near stairways. Installing handgrips in showers or tubs can also be instrumental in preventing accidents. Reaching for items on high shelves, changing light bulbs, going up and down stairs, and opening simple medicine bottles are some activities that may require assistance or improved safety strategies.
- *Polypharmacy*—The problem of polypharmacy arises with the use of medications by older adults. **Polypharmacy** is the ingestion of multiple medications in one day. Medications may be prescribed for various medical conditions or purchased over the counter. Drug-drug interactions, drug-food interactions, and drug-environment interactions (such as increased sensitivity to sun exposure) can occur. Optimum or average drug dosages are determined by research on young adults, and little research is available concerning modifications in dosages required by older adults. In older adults the decreased ability of the liver and kidneys to excrete drugs from the body can result in an accumulation of the drugs to toxic levels. The older adult may forget to take a dose of medication or may accidentally take an extra dose and therefore may be undermedicated or overmedicated and prone to undesirable side effects. Patient monitoring and education is essential. The use of memory aids such as notebooks or labeled pill boxes may be helpful.

There are many developmental tasks of the older adult and related challenges (Box 12-1). Older adults with healthy attitudes and coping skills typically do not mourn their lost youth but are able to find fulfillment and meaning in their life despite health limitations. However, weight gain, dental problems, diminished eyesight and hearing, decreased mobility, and changes in body image are some issues

---

BOX 12-1   Tasks and Challenges of the Older Adult

Older adults must adjust to the following:
- Menopause
- Retirement and redirection of goals and energy
- Decreased income
- Grandparenting
- Reentry into the job market
- Maintaining access to health care

that create difficulty. Older adults may show a readiness for learning if they recognize old age is near and that physical health and life circumstance may change. Developing a healthy lifestyle with access to preventative care is a primary goal in the education and care of the older adult.

GRANDPARENTING

When healthy older adults assume the role of grandparents, they often do more for their children than their children do for them. The grandparenting role can be quite satisfying for the older adult because it enhances self-image, increases activity level, creates feelings of self-worth and usefulness, and contributes to the meaning and quality of life. Many older adults may enjoy their grandchildren more because they know the children's parents will take over when they tire. Some older adults serve as volunteer adoptive grandparents to children in need or seek useful volunteer activities in the community. The role of the grandparent in the home can be a positive experience for grandchildren when healthy relationships between all generations are maintained.

It is when grandparents become ill or disabled that the roles can reverse and the older adult needs more assistance. This role reversal can result in family stress and financial strain. Many families are not aware of community programs available for assistance with older adults and for caregiver support. Family education concerning the older adult's limitations and abilities can increase compassion and motivation to assist and improve verbal communication and the quality of the relationship. Nurses and health care workers can educate and guide families concerning resources available to them before emotional stress, financial strain, caregiver burnout, and older adult alienation occur.

ELDER OR DEPENDENT ABUSE

Elder abuse affects more than 2 million older adults each year. **Elder abuse** is defined as infliction of harm or neglect through actions or acts of omission. Abuse can be physical, emotional, or financial and can include neglect or obstruction of personal rights (Berliner, 1999).

The family or health care worker can observe interactions between older adults and the caregivers and alert other family members to potentially abusive situations. Referral of the caregiver to community agencies for respite care may decrease stress that can lead to abuse.

POSTMENOPAUSAL CARE

There are more than 14 million women between the ages of 50 and 60 in the United States. Eighty-five percent are high school graduates and 20% have some college education (Census Bureau, 1998). In 2001, 16 million women between the ages of 40 and 60 were single (widowed, divorced, or never married), and they may face this transition to menopause with varying levels of support. Adjusting to the postmenopausal phase of life is an important developmental task of the older woman. Menopause is defined as the absence of menstruation for a period of at least 1 year (due to decline or cessation of hormonal production and function).

Menopause is not a disease or illness; it is a natural occurrence in the life cycle. However, there are discomforts and risks associated with the postmenopausal phase that can be averted with healthy lifestyles and access to preventative medical care. Some discomforts associated with postmenopause include genital atrophy, vasomotor instability, heart disease, breast cancer, or osteoporosis. Hormone replacement therapy (HRT) was designed to relieve some of these discomforts, but controversy exists concerning the safety and advisability of routine HRT. Complementary and alternative medical therapies (CAM) are also available when HRT is not recommended. Complementary therapy refers to nontraditional therapies, such as relaxation or biofeedback, that are used *with* traditional therapy. Alternative therapy refers to nontraditional therapy, such as herbs and oils, that are used *instead of* traditional therapy. A healthy lifestyle is essential because habits such as smoking can reduce the beneficial effects of estrogen therapy (Porter et al, 2001). See Appendix B for cultural aspects of aging.

LIFESTYLE CHANGES
Simple Lifestyle Changes

Simple lifestyle changes for women experiencing menopausal and postmenopausal symptoms include dressing in layers to deal with hot flashes, using a portable fan, adjusting heat and air conditioning in the room, limiting alcohol and caffeine intake, and drinking more fluids. Vaginal dryness can be overcome by the use of water-based gels or lubricants. Mood swings can be recognized and managed by increasing self-awareness and reframing thoughts and interpretations of situations. Understanding partners can also be supportive. The use of CAM therapy such as herbal supplements to prevent the development of depression requires close evaluation for possible interaction with prescribed medicines or other treatments. Soy, soy nuts, or tofu have been successful in relieving some symptoms of menopause without deleterious effects (Lobo, 2000).

Decreases in estrogen often cause vaginal wall thinning and urine leakage when sneezing or laughing. Panty liners, pads, and adult diapers can be of help in dealing with these embarrassing problems that can cause the woman to otherwise want to stay at home.

Driving Safety

Many adults over age 65 are driving on the roads of the United States. Some may have early undetected impairments that can affect their safety on the road. Occupational and physical therapy can help maintain driving safety and delay loss of their driver's license, but when driving is no longer safe, the license must be taken away. Counseling concerning other methods of transportation is essential. Isolation, loneliness, stagnation, or depression may occur if alternative transportation options are not offered.

HEALTH SCREENINGS

Health screenings can identify developing health issues in early stages and can lead to early interventions and prevention of greater difficulties. Screenings should include dental and eye checkups and a physical evaluation that includes weight, blood pressure, thyroid, and blood glucose and lipid levels. It is useful to assess for substance abuse, overmedication, sexual dysfunction, urinary incontinence, and other indications for necessary lifestyle changes. Papanicolaou (Pap) smears for cervical cancer are recommended at 1- to 3-year intervals in healthy older women. Mammography screening for breast lesions and screening for colorectal cancer and prostate cancer in men are also recommended. Routine cardiovascular screening should be done for patients who present with two or more risk factors, such as increased lipid levels, hypertension, or smoking. Postmenopausal bone loss and osteoporosis should be assessed regularly, and preventive measures such as increased calcium intake, vitamin D, and daily weight-bearing exercise can be emphasized during routine office visits. A nutritional health assessment is essential. Referral for dental care or community services such as Meals on Wheels may be an option to assist in the maintenance of nutrition if transportation is an obstacle.

In late adulthood, decreased organ size and function can cause increased toxic effects related to alcohol use. Assessing for alcohol abuse is therefore also an important aspect of health screening.

Two affirmative answers to the CAGE questions indicate a need for further evaluation or follow-up (Box 12-2).

SEXUALITY

As people age, specific changes in sexual responses occur. However, the notion that the older adult is sexually inactive is untrue. Some older adults may feel guilty or abnormal because they continue to have sexual feelings. The most common cause of sexual dissatisfaction is the lack of a partner. In this age group, divorces, widowhood, or ill or disabled spouses are common problems. Men may develop erectile dysfunction, which is now treatable with a high rate of success. Painful intercourse (dyspareunia) for women may be the result of atrophy of the vaginal tissues and a decrease in natural lubrications. Both problems can be easily overcome.

HRT or CAM therapy can alleviate menopausal symptoms that interfere with sexual pleasure. A health care provider must evaluate the suitability of HRT for individual patients before determining the appropriate approach to care. Sex therapy is available and can be helpful. The main obstacle in maintaining a healthy sexual lifestyle is the tendency to avoid talking about it due to embarrassment. Therefore it is the nurse or health care worker's responsibility to assess sexual functioning in older adults, both men and women.

BOX 12-2   **CAGE Assessment Questions**

- Have you ever felt the need to "**C**ut down" on alcohol intake?
- Have you ever felt "**A**nnoyed" by criticism of your drinking?
- Have you ever felt "**G**uilty" about drinking?
- Have you ever had to take a morning drink as an "**E**ye opener"?

Modified from Ewing, J. (1984). Detecting alcoholism: the CAGE questionnaire. *JAMA, 252*, 1905.

MEMORY

The older adult experiences memory changes, particularly in remembering names and faces of people. Normal memory loss can be associated with aging, and temporary memory loss can be due to depression or anxiety (Zelinski et al, 1997). Preclinical manifestations of Alzheimer's disease are a common worry when normal memory loss becomes noticeable (Boxes 12-3 and 12-4).

Active lifestyles that routinely exercise memory skills are thought to help maintain memory function. Perhaps this is another "use it or lose it" phenomenon (Morrow et al, 1994). However, studies have shown that older adults need more time to process thoughts and perform tasks than younger adults (Salthouse, 1999). Knowledge or information that is deeply processed rather than superficially memorized will be remembered longer. See Table 12-2 for memory decline due to normal aging, depression, or dementia.

BOX 12-3   **Warning Signs of Problematic Memory Decline**

- Memory loss affecting job functioning
- Difficulty remembering steps in familiar tasks
- Disorientation
- Lack of awareness of time, place, or date
- Decrease in abstract thinking (increased need for concreteness)
- Associated problems with mood, language, or personality changes

---

BOX 12-4   **Preventable Causes of Memory Problems**

- Drug toxicity
- Depression
- Metabolic problems (kidney or liver dysfunction, hypoglycemia)
- Sensory problems (difficulty hearing, seeing, or sensing information)
- Nutritional deficiencies (dehydration, B_{12}, iron deficiency)
- Illness (pneumonia and other infections)

TABLE 12-2

MEMORY DECLINE DUE TO NORMAL AGING, DEPRESSION, OR DEMENTIA

Normal Age-Related Memory Decline	Depression-Related Memory Problems	Dementia-Related Memory Problems
Onset age specifically identifiable.	Onset with depression.	Hard to establish onset.
Slow progression of symptoms.	Rapid or sudden progression of symptoms.	Slow or stepwise progression.
History of depression less common.	History of depression less common.	History of depression less common.
Complains about memory loss.	Complains about memory loss.	Usually unaware of memory loss.
May emphasize disability.	May emphasize disability.	Conceals disability.
May decrease or increase efforts to perform.	Decreases effort to perform.	Struggles to perform.
Uses notes and other memory aids.	May not try to keep up.	Needs instruction to use memory aids.
No lasting mood change associated.	Consistent depressive mood.	Emotional lability and shallowness.
Behavior may or may not change.	Behavior change is greater than impairment.	Behavior change may be appropriate.
Nocturnal drop in performance unusual.	Nocturnal drop in performance unusual.	Nocturnal drop in performance common.
"Don't know" answers common.	"Don't know" answers common.	Guesses or "near miss" answers common.
Recent and remote memory losses are equal.	Recent and remote memory losses are equal.	Recent memory impaired, remote is intact.
	Memory gaps for specific events common.	Memory gaps for specific events unusual.

EMOTIONS IN THE OLDER ADULT

Emotions and emotional control develop during the growth and development process, as a person copes with the challenges in each phase of the life cycle. Earlier theorists believed **disengagement** was a task of the older adult. This implies that removing emotional attachments to people, places, and objects is part of the natural aging process. This may be true of the depressed older adult but is likely not a natural or healthy process. Newer studies (Carstensen et al, 1998) found that aging healthy adults do not naturally disengage. Instead they continue emotional learning and emotional competencies. Past experiences from the long lives of older adults may influence their expression of emotional responses. Culture and expectations play a role in the emotional status of the older adult. In cultures with close families, more respect and inclusion in the lives of their families or maintenance of communication and relationships with their families will encourage and maintain emotional competencies and enhance quality of life for older adults.

PSYCHOSOCIAL ISSUES FOR THE OLDER ADULT

The social network of friends usually narrows for the older adult due to the death of peers. This may result in fewer peer social experiences unless older adults live in a retirement community or are connected with organized social activities for their specific age group. Remaining an integral part of an extended family provides valuable social activity and relationships, but they may be different than peer relationships.

Basic needs for **autonomy** (self-direction), **competence** (effective interactions), and **relatedness** (a sense of belonging) motivate social activities that enhance general well-being (Baumeister et al, 1995). An environment that helps meet these basic needs enables the older adult to maintain positive social interactions (Figure 12-1).

Complete dependency often does not support autonomy, social competence, or relatedness in satisfying ways unless the situation is specifically designed to provide assistance in achieving these goals. Many assisted living facilities for older adults are designed to offer assistance with living without taking away these three basic needs.

CLINICAL DISEASE IN THE OLDER ADULT

Good health in older people is often defined as absence of disease or disability. However, normal body changes due to aging, such as ovarian failure or menopause, place a risk on the cardiovascular, bone, and metabolic systems. This occurs at a time when emotional stress may increase due to other life changes.

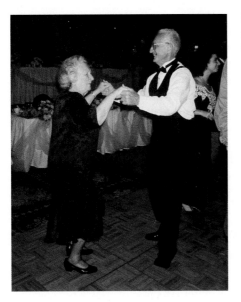

FIGURE 12–1 Social activities and positive social interactions enhance a feeling of well-being in the older adult.

The combination of subclinical cardiovascular changes associated with aging and response to stressful life events can affect the risk factors for the development of a clinical disease. Individuals who characteristically hid or suppressed their emotions in young adulthood and held a pessimistic view toward life events may be at a higher risk for clinical disease as they age (Menkes, 1989). This may indicate that prevention of disease in the older adult lies partially in the development of attitudes and coping skills.

DEPRESSION IN THE OLDER ADULT

Depression should not be automatically expected in the older adult. In some older adults, depression occurs as a continuation of a negative attitude from young adulthood. A young person who looks at life's events in a pessimistic way may be vulnerable to developing depression as an older adult. However, late-onset depression (or a change in personality) may be attributed to changes in the brain itself (Leuchter, 1994). The traditional symptoms of depression as listed in the *Diagnostic and Statistical Manual of Mental Disorders,* fourth edition, text revision (DSM-IV-TR) criteria for diagnosis of major depression may not be completely accurate for older adults (Koenig et al, 1995). Older adults may be taking medications for various medical conditions that have side effects that mimic depression. Therefore depression can be overdiagnosed or underdiagnosed (AAGP, 2002). Several factors increase the vulnerability of the older adult to depression. Chronic poor health can lead to stress, decreased activity, and social interactions, which can trigger depression. Prescribed treatment of the medical conditions can induce changes that result in a deepened depression. Depression itself can in turn also trigger physical illness.

Helping the older adult deal with stressful life events, strengthening coping strategies, and providing social support can help avoid the development of depression for many older adults. Any person who first develops depression as an older adult usually has experiences and coping styles that can be utilized by a professional therapist in individual or group sessions to help treat the depressive symptoms (Terri et al, 1996). Providing access to mental health care and early screening for the presence of risk and depressive symptoms can empower older adults to be in control of their own emotions.

Some of the challenges to early mental health screening and intervention are limited by managed care. Although managed care plans provide benefits to a large segment of the population across the nation, a limited number of psychotherapy sessions per year are available. The sessions focus primarily on crisis intervention or short-term problems with obvious symptoms. Referrals from a primary care physician may be needed to access mental health care, and this may delay access to the care needed. The ratio of drug therapy to psychotherapy for treatment of mental health problems is 4:1 (AAGP, 2003), and the use of drugs may not be the optimum approach for the older adult. The new mental health parity law requires unlimited doctors visits for conditions such as major depression. However, the managed health care systems have been overwhelmed and referrals for short-term care still delay treatment.

The American Psychiatric Association (APA) Division of Clinical Psychology and the American Association of Geriatric Psychiatry (2003) have developed evidence-based practice guidelines that recommend specific treatments for a variety of psychological problems. However, there is little research concerning the application of these guidelines to the older adult population.

Obstacles in accessing mental health care have led to the emergence of self-help techniques that are available to all at low cost. Self-help resources can be useful for those who need some guidance (Kurtzweil et al, 1996). Self-help resources include books and support groups led by clergy, peer counselors, and others who advertise their success stories. Many psychologists prescribe self-help resources to supplement their therapy (Norcross et al, 2000). The combination of various types of interventions has been embraced by the interdisciplinary Society for the Exploration of Psychotherapy Integration (SEPI). This and other professional networks, such as the American Association of Behavior Therapist (AABT) and Anxiety Disorder Association of America (ADAA), offer conferences and newsletters on effective mental health care. The American Association of Retired Persons (AARP) is also an advocate for the older adult regarding education for healthy living.

TEACHING TECHNIQUES AND GOALS FOR THE OLDER ADULT

Human growth and development occurs in a sequential pattern and developmental tasks are often related to the phases or stages within these patterns. Therefore within any stage or phase of development there can be a wide variation in abilities that are mastered. A person's ability and readiness to learn depends on his or her stage of development; physical, psychological, and social health; support systems and environmental stress; and personal motivation. It must be noted, however, that chronological age is not a specific indicator of a stage of development.

A *teaching moment* has been defined as the point at which the learner is most receptive to a situation (Havighurst, 1974). The learner must be motivated to learn and the teaching must be relevant to the learner and appropriate to the developmental stage and abilities of the learner.

For the older adult, learning is enhanced if mutual respect exists between teacher and learner. The teacher should recognize the lifelong accomplishments of the older adult, be nonjudgmental, and foster an environment conducive to learning. Visual aids should have large print in a bright color. Vision decline in the older adult often causes color distortions, so medication or pills should not be referred to by color.

Hearing loss in the older adult usually affects perception of high-pitched sound or rapid speech. Therefore shouting or raising volume is not helpful. Speaking clearly and slowly, making eye contact while speaking, wearing lipstick or lip gloss (to assist visual perception), and using an interactive style to obtain feedback from the older adult will confirm that information was understood.

Scheduling short teaching sessions enables the older adult to concentrate and absorb all the information throughout the session without losing concentration due to fatigue or other interference, such as having to leave the room to go to the bathroom. The teacher can counteract avoidance or denial of the need to change lifestyle practices during educational sessions by validating the older adults experiences and needs and by keeping topics related to the here and now. Relating learning topics to autonomy, social acceptability, and strong coping skills can boost effectiveness of learning. Repetition of information helps encode information into long-term memory, especially if memory skills are in decline. Presenting information in different ways, visually, verbally, and experientially (hands-on), can also be an important aid to learning. However, repetition of material already known by the older adult is a turn-off to learning.

Important goals in managing the aging process include preventing illness and disability, maintaining cognitive functioning, and maintaining an active and healthy lifestyle. Assessment for cardiovascular risks, nutritional needs, bone density, visual, hearing and memory loss, depression, and specific concerns of the individual are helpful in developing a meaningful teaching plan for the individual.

The *Physician's Desk Reference for Herbal Medicines* can be used as a guide in helping the older patient evaluate complementary therapy that they may choose to use.

Decreasing stress and maintaining a positive attitude are essential to successful living.

KEY POINTS

- A *Healthy People 2010* goal for the older adult is to increase the lifespan and quality of life by focusing on wellness and preventive care.
- Some health challenges for the older adult include maintaining access to health care, managing on a reduced income, adjusting to a changes in living arrangements, accessing preventive health care, maintaining nutrition, and preventing accidents.
- Elder abuse is the infliction of harm or neglect through actions or acts of omission.
- Menopause is not a disease; it is a natural occurrence in the life cycle.
- Hormone replacement therapy or CAM therapy may be helpful in relieving menopausal discomfort.
- Health screenings for the older adult may include dental and vision check-ups; screening for breast, cervical and prostate cancer; checking blood glucose and lipid levels; weight and blood pressure monitoring, and alcohol and depression screening.

- The most common cause of sexual inactivity in the older adult is loss of a partner.
- Keeping an active mind and lifestyle can enhance memory performance in the older adult.
- An older adult can benefit from the use of memory aids such as lists or calendar notes.
- Basic needs for autonomy, social competence, and relatedness in the older adult motivate continued social interactions and prevent isolation and disengagement.
- Several factors make older adults vulnerable to developing depression.
- Providing access to mental health care, early screening, and a combination of social and psychological interventions can help avoid development of depression in the older adult.
- Specific teaching techniques can enhance the learning process for the older adult.

CRITICAL THINKING

Health care teaching is important for older adults. What teaching techniques might be helpful for effectively teaching a group of older adults?

MULTIPLE-CHOICE REVIEW QUESTIONS

1 Old age is defined by the U.S. government as the time when full Social Security benefits become available, which is when one reaches the age of:
   1 55
   2 65
   3 75
   4 85
2 The problem of polypharmacy involves:
   1 Inaccessible drugstores
   2 Ingestion of multiple medications
   3 Online drug availability
   4 Use of prescription medications
3 Complementary and alternative medicine involves:
   1 Use of herbs, biofeedback, or soy products
   2 Use of hormones to treat menopause
   3 Use of antibiotics to treat infections
   4 Use of contraceptive pills
4 One method that will help prevent osteoporosis includes:
   1 Sedentary activities
   2 Weight-bearing exercises
   3 A diet high in potassium
   4 Bone density study
5 A teaching moment occurs when the learner:
   1 Is motivated and receptive
   2 Is quietly listening
   3 Is momentarily distracted
   4 Answers a question

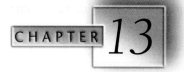

Geriatrics: Advanced Old Age

O B J E C T I V E S

Upon completion of this chapter, the student will be able to:

1 Explain the concept of geriatrics.
2 Discuss the anticipated future increase in the advanced old age population as related to the development of geriatrics as a specialty.
3 State four normal physiological changes that occur in the geriatric adult.
4 List the major developmental tasks of the geriatric adult.
5 Name three psychological changes or challenges that occur in the geriatric adult.
6 Discuss three specific psychosocial problems associated with aging.
7 List four specific health-promoting activities for the geriatric adult.
8 Discuss the sexuality needs of the geriatric adult.
9 Discuss six health maintenance requirements for adults who are in advanced old age.
10 Discuss various modifications of the environment necessary to the geriatric adult.
11 State four factors to consider when helping to select a nursing home for placement.
12 Discuss alternatives to nursing home care.
13 Define *activities of daily living.*
14 Discuss principles of elder care and the role of the health care worker.
15 Discuss the teaching needs of the geriatric adult.

K E Y   T E R M S

Activities of daily living
Ageism
Alzheimer's disease
Apoptosis
Atrophy
Biological clock
Free radicals
Geriatrics
Immune theory
Osteoporosis
Senescence
Wear-and-tear theory

GERIATRICS: WHAT IS IT?

There are many ways to define geriatrics, such as the study of the aged, of advanced old age, or of old-old adults. Some define old age according to physiological decline, such as the occurrence of menopause and skin or hair changes. Others define old age as one in which psychological changes occur.

Senescence is referred to as a period in an adult's life in which the body begins to age and weaken. Senescence is a gradual process, and people age in different ways and rates. The health needs of advanced old age may differ slightly from those of late adulthood. For example, the incidence of chronic disease increases markedly after age 80. As a result, senescence is now categorized as follows (Ebersole et al, 1998):

- Young-old—65 to 75
- Old—76 to 84
- Old-old—85 to 99
- Elite-old—100 years and older

Geriatrics is an age group that is rapidly expanding and has become a specialty in the health care field. There is a growing need for health care workers and providers to care specifically for this age group.

Geriatrics is defined as the study of old-age and includes the biological, psychological, physiological, and sociological aspects of aging. The goal in the care of an advanced old age adult is to maximize the ability to function and live independently and shorten the period of illness and disability. *Healthy People 2010* goals for the aged adult are listed in Box 13-1.

THEORIES OF THE AGING PROCESS

The process of aging is due to multiple factors, including the genetic lifespan of cells. The past lifestyle, level of activity, dietary practices, and social support all play a role in the process of aging. Selected theories concerning the aging process follow.

Cellular Changes
Free Radicals

Ions travel in pairs within cells and are stable. For example, sodium and chloride are paired in the cell as sodium chloride (salt). When one ion breaks off and is no longer paired, it becomes a **free radical.** Free radicals are unstable. They attack other molecules in the body and result in cell damage that cannot be repaired. The numbers of free radicals increase in people as they age.

Biological Clock (Programmed Cell Death)

Also known as **apoptosis,** the membrane surrounding a cell starts breaking down. As this process continues, the debris is phagocytized (eaten) by surrounding cellular mate-

---

BOX 13-1 *Healthy People 2010:* **Goals for the Aged**
• Reduce osteoporosis
• Reduce fractures
• Increase access for colon screening
• Encourage health promotion activities
• Reduce pneumococcal infections and influenza
• Increase hearing and vision screening and care
These goals are designed to increase the number of healthy aged people in the population who continue to enjoy life and contribute to society.

Adopted from USDHHS (2000). *Healthy People 2010.* Washington, DC: U.S. Government Printing Office.

rials. This **biological clock** process dictates the occurrence of menopause in women and contributes to the body changes that ultimately result in death. Interestingly, the ovary is the only organ that appears to have a "programmed senescence in adult life that leads to predictable complete loss of function during aging in all human populations" (Finch et al, 2000).

Wear-and-Tear Theory

Wear-and-tear theory can be equated with a machine. Just as the parts in a machine begin to wear out or break down, so too does the human body. With humans, not all parts are so easily replaced or repaired. An example would be the ease and frequency of hip or knee replacement surgery versus heart transplantation.

Immune Theory

As one ages, the body finds it more difficult to tell the difference between healthy and defective cells. Therefore the body responds by destroying both types of cells. **Immune theory** states that the end result is that the body's immune response is impaired. This causes the aging person to be more susceptible to a variety of illnesses or infections. Decreased immune function of the thymus gland, lymph nodes, spleen, and possibly bone marrow are thought to also be contributing factors.

Cellular damage or decline over a number of years results in the activation of the stress responses in the body in an attempt to try to repair what it can. When the body is unable to repair itself as efficiently, changes occur in the various body systems.

PHYSIOLOGICAL CHANGES
Bones and Cartilage

The loss of body water and bone mass and degeneration of spinal disks result in a decrease in height during the aging process. A decrease in body mass and a loss of body water occur after age 65. Collagen in the body becomes rigid, and elastin in the body becomes brittle. These substances transport material between cells, and the changes that occur during the aging process results in decreased function of the cells.

The loss of estrogen decreases the ability of the body to utilize calcium to maintain bone density. Loss of bone mass can result in **osteoporosis**, which is a thinning of the bone. This predisposes the geriatric adult to fractures. Posture and balance may change, and falls become a common problem.

Blood Vessels

Arterial walls thicken with fatty deposits and connective tissue that result in a narrowing of the arteries. As a result, coronary arteries provide less oxygenated blood to the heart muscle. The heart muscles become less elastic. Oxygen exchange slows, and so blood pressure may rise to compensate for the lowered oxygen supply. These processes predispose the geriatric adult to developing high blood pressure, which can result in a stroke. It takes longer for the heart to beat faster in response to activity or stress, and therefore the observable response to pain, stress, or anxiety may be delayed. This means that the nurse or health care worker cannot rely on observing changes in the vital signs to determine the presence of pain, stress, or anxiety.

Lungs

The ribs and cartilage become more rigid, and thus the respiratory muscles have to work harder. Lung tissue loses elasticity, so geriatric adults may not breathe as deeply or cough as effectively, making them more vulnerable to respiratory infections.

Kidneys and Bladder

The rate that the kidneys filter the blood slows, so medications and other substances take longer to leave the body. This can result in an accumulation of medication in the blood and subsequent overdose reaction. Bladder capacity decreases, with urinary frequency a common result. In men an enlarged prostate may block the urethra, resulting in urinary frequency or complete obstruction of urinary flow. This obstruction of urinary flow is known as urinary retention and requires prompt medical intervention.

Metabolism

A slowed metabolism can cause retention of glucose (sugars) and lipids (fats). Therefore the geriatric adult is at risk for developing elevated serum lipids. In the geriatric person, a fasting blood glucose level will be more accurate than a glucose level taken 2 hours after a meal has been consumed (Kane et al, 1999).

Digestion

The decreased motility of the gastrointestinal system results in slower emptying of the stomach. Digestive enzymes also decrease, which can result in poor appetite and digestive disturbances. A slowed gag reflex increases the risk of choking, so the geriatric adult should eat slowly while sitting upright. A decrease in *peristalsis* (a wavelike motion that causes intestinal contents to be moved through the gastrointestinal tract) can cause constipation and gas discomfort. This often results in the older person using laxatives and antacids, which may decrease nutrient absorption and cause other health problems.

Teeth

Tooth loss is common, and the remaining teeth often do not provide optimum cutting or chewing abilities. This influences nutritional intake and may also have a negative impact on self-image. Over time, receding gums can lead to ill-fitting dentures and gum lesions (sores). Regular follow-up with a dentist is essential. Providing nutritious foods that are attractively prepared and easy to chew will help meet the nutritional needs of the geriatric adult.

Skin

With aging, the body takes longer to repair and replace skin cells. Due to the loss of subcutaneous fat and collagen, the skin becomes thinner and *turgor* (elasticity) is poor. This makes the geriatric person more vulnerable to skin injury, and healing of skin wounds is slower. The thin, dry skin develops wrinkles and spotty pigmentation. The ability to perceive cold and hot sensations also decreases and therefore geriatric adults are at an increased risk for burns. A decrease in the number and function of sweat glands in the skin results in difficulty adjusting to changes in environmental temperature. Chilling (hypothermia) and heat exhaustion occur more easily.

Eyes

A loss of cells in the optic nerve makes it more difficult to see details. Eyesight declines. The pupil of the eye opens and closes more slowly, so when moving from light to dark areas, more time is needed to adapt to the surroundings. Cataracts develop in the lens of the eye, which further decreases vision in advanced old age. Fifty percent of persons older than 75 may develop cataracts due to the natural aging process. Advancing age and diabetes are two of the risk factors for the development of glaucoma. Glaucoma is an atrophy of the optic nerve and increased intraocular pressure. It is the leading cause of blindness and occurs in 15% of people over age 80. All adults should be periodically screened for the development of glaucoma. Age-related macular degeneration (AMD) is a retinal degeneration that causes loss of central vision in the geriatric adult. Some peripheral vision may be retained and total blindness is rare.

Ears

Degenerative changes in the bones of the middle ear result in a decrease in hearing ability. Certain frequencies of sound become difficult to distinguish, and the older person finds it difficult to locate the sound. Communication with geriatric persons is often a problem because they might not hear all the words in the sentence and possibly misinterpret what is said. Therefore when teaching geriatric patients, it is wise to ask them to repeat what was said to ensure clear communication.

Nervous System

Neurons **atrophy** (decrease in size) during the aging process, and transmission of impulses to the brain becomes sluggish. Because of the fatty deposits within the walls of the blood vessels, blood flow to the brain slows. Motor responses and reaction time to stimulus is delayed, and maintaining environmental safety is a challenge.

SEXUALITY IN THE GOLDEN YEARS

As people age, specific changes in sexual responses occur. However, the notion that the aged person is sexless is a myth. Part of the reason for this myth is that the concept of love and romance, as portrayed in the media, focuses more on the young adult and the relationship of sex to having children. People of advanced old age may even feel guilty or abnormal because they recognize that they continue to have sexual feelings. Some older women may believe they are less sexually attractive than younger women and often choose to dress in what they think is a more appropriate style for their age. The media advertises surgery for facelifts, and cosmetic surgery is becoming more popular. Older men are also having more cosmetic surgery in an effort to maintain attractiveness to potential partners. Some men attempt to take a partner decades younger for a variety of reasons. Aging without protest is becoming more popular today, with the older woman taking pride in maintaining her physical and mental competencies while allowing her face and body to show the natural consequences of age and experience.

Medications are often prescribed to the geriatric patient without considering or educating the geriatric person regarding the effects on sexual performance. Many medications prescribed for conditiqons common to the aged have an inhibitory effect on sexual interest, arousal, and performance. To ensure compliance with the medication regimen, appropriate education about these effects must be an integral part of the overall provision of health care in the aging population. It is also important to instruct the aging adult on prevention of sexually transmitted diseases (STDs), including human immunodeficiency syndrome/acquired immunodeficiency syndrome (HIV/AIDS), because this age group is just as likely as their younger cohorts to receive or transmit a communicable disease (Catania, 1989). Because pregnancy prevention is not a concern of the geriatric population, condoms may not be considered as necessary, and therefore the rate of STDs in this age group continues to increase.

Personality and behavior are important dimensions in sexuality. According to the World Health Organization (WHO, 1986), there are three key elements to consider within the concept of sexuality: (1) the capacity to enhance and control sexual and reproductive behavior in accordance with a social and personal ethic; (2) freedom from fear, shame, guilt, false beliefs, and other psychological factors inhibiting sexual responses; and (3) freedom from organic disorder, disease, and deficiencies that interfere with sexual or reproductive function. When working with the geriatric adult, one must take into consideration these three primary elements of sexuality. Box 13-2 reviews details concerning the aging process and its effects on sexuality.

BOX 13-2 **Factors That Influence Sexuality in the Geriatric Adult**

Attitude/Interest
- Prior life experiences
- Body image perception
- Mental function
- Self-expectations and image promotion
- Social contact/isolation
- Environment/privacy

Sexual Health
- Incontinence, urinary/fecal devices
- Reduction in mobility
- Impotence and menopause
- Chronic or terminal illness
- Medications and their side effects

Sexual Responses in the Aging Woman

Menopause, or climacteric, in women does not decrease sexual response, because androgens are no longer inhibited by estrogens. Due to the varying levels of hormones, the woman will notice dryness in the vaginal mucosa, hot flashes, and other assorted hormone-related body changes. Frequent sexual activity, use of creams and water-soluble lubricants in the vagina, exercise, proper nutrition, and soy supplements can be alternatives to hormone replacement therapy (HRT), which may be contraindicated in some women. Although the erotic responses of the nipple and clitoris do not decrease, the intensity of vaginal lubrication and tissue expansion during sexual arousal does decrease with age and can make sexual activity uncomfortable. This is primarily due to decreased levels of estrogen. The ability to achieve multiple orgasms continues, although the intensity is decreased. As part of a health maintenance plan, women should continue regular health screenings, which include regular Papanicolaou (Pap) smears and mammography.

Sexual Responses in the Aging Man

Testosterone production decreases between the ages of 40 and 60 but remains stable thereafter. This leads to a decrease in the size and firmness of the penis and reduced production, motility, and lifespan of sperm. Men are often able to retain fertility into their eighth decade of life, despite the decline in actual sperm count and activity by up to 30% (Christiansen et al, 1993).

The ability to attain and maintain an erection may be delayed and requires increased physiological stimulation as men age. Anxiety may also contribute to increased delay or sexual dysfunction. However, men soon realize that once the erection is achieved it can be maintained for a longer period compared with earlier years. The intensity of orgasm may be decreased, but the pleasurable response is usually retained.

A decrease in men's sexual function is similar to that in women and is referred to as the male climacteric. Some men experience similar symptoms of hot flashes, feelings of suffocation, and depression. These symptoms can usually be treated with hormonal replacement, such as testosterone, synthetic androgens, and in some cases estrogen (Guyton, 2001). A consequence of decreased sexual activity is the increased risk of inflammation and enlargement of the prostate gland.

The Impact of Illness on Sexuality

Cancer of the prostate is a risk, and preventive screening via yearly examinations, which include prostate-specific antigen (PSA) blood levels and professional guidance, are essential in this age group. Hormone treatments for cancer of the prostate can interfere with achieving and maintaining penile erection. Some men who have had surgery of the prostate gland experience retrograde ejaculation into the urinary bladder rather than out through the urethra.

After a heart attack, the aged man is given extensive information about dietary changes he needs to follow. Rarely is he or his partner educated about possible alternatives that can be used to fulfill sexual needs. Hospitals and nursing homes are often insensitive to the sexual needs of the aged. Sexual opportunity, privacy, and programs having to do with sexuality are often absent from the care plan of the aged population in nursing homes, hospitals, and community settings. Postoperative instructions concerning surgery that involve reproductive organs should include an understanding of the effects on sexuality and options available to deal with them.

Health care workers, such as nurses, have the opportunity to discuss discomforts or problems with sexual functioning in the aging patient, in the postoperative patient, and in the perimenopausal and postmenopausal woman. Patients should be taught that maintaining physical activity can help them enjoy erotic activity. Studies by Masters and Johnson (1976) reveal that regular sexual activity with a partner, or through masturbation, also contribute to maintaining the capacity for sexual pleasure. Overeating, drinking alcohol, and a sedentary lifestyle all negatively affect sexual vigor. The normal alterations of aging may decrease but do not eliminate the ability to have a satisfactory sex life.

The nurse should help the aged understand the normal changes and responses in their bodies to avoid misinterpretations. Intimacy is a lifelong need. For some, cuddling and caressing is all that is needed, whereas others prefer to form an increased intellectual and emotional closeness with friends and develop interests that will meet their intimacy needs. Sexual concerns in the geriatric adult can be discussed with the health care provider for assessment and interventions.

PSYCHOLOGICAL CHANGES IN THE AGING PROCESS

Throughout the life cycle the attractiveness of personal appearance has high value. The media and the marketplace offer makeup and clothes that value appearing eternally young. A person's negative self-image may affect his or her ability to function. Fortunately the aging process is a gradual one that provides time for coping and adaptation to the physical changes that are evident in the aging process. Roles may change. The dependent wife may become the caregiver and decision maker if the husband becomes disabled. An older man may take on homemaking duties if the younger wife continues to work. These various role adjustments require adaptation or acceptance.

Culture also affects the aging process. In cultures where people of advanced old age are valued and respected, the feeling of self-worth contributes to general health. In cultures where people of advanced old age are avoided (**ageism**), a feeling of usefulness declines and depression can set in. Geriatric persons usually fear loss of independence and disability that will make them a burden to their family.

The loss of peers, siblings, and even a spouse can result in loneliness. **Disengagement** is the process in which an older adult withdraws from social contacts and relinquishes independence and control to others. A decline in income may require relocation, and a new environment may intensify the feeling of loneliness. Some guidance may be needed to help the older person seek new relationships and activities that are enjoyable. Grandparenting can be a source of satisfaction if the children and grandchildren live nearby (Figure 13-1). People of advanced old age often are afraid to try new things and may be slow to learn as concentration and memory decline with advancing age.

DEVELOPMENTAL TASKS OF THE AGED

Mastering the crisis of Ego-Integrity versus Despair is the challenge of the older adult. Mastering the crisis of Immortality versus Extinction is the major task of advanced old age. Reflecting on their own accomplishments and the legacy of their life brings ego integrity and satisfaction to geriatric adults. Achieving ego integrity and immortality from their legacy implies successful mastery of the developmental tasks from previous stages of the life cycle. Reminiscing about past experiences is therapeutic. If reflection about life's experiences brings feelings of unresolved conflicts and failures, then a feeling of despair will overcome the person. This will result in anxiety, bitterness, and perhaps even stress and illness.

Ego integrity is achieved when reminiscing reveals satisfaction with past achievements and a sense of leaving a positive legacy or memory behind. If geriatric adults can focus on prioritizing activities that bring them pleasure, they can enjoy daily life.

A major developmental task of old age is adjusting to retirement. The work setting is no longer the center for maintaining a feeling of self-worth. Having a hobby or interest to pursue that offers a sense of fulfillment and satisfaction is essential in maintaining good mental health (Figure 13-2). Another developmental task for this age group is adjusting to and accepting the frailties of aging and the changes in physical appearance and lifestyles.

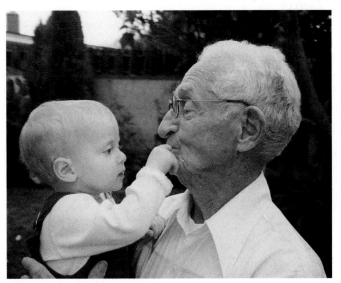

FIGURE 13–1 Grandparenting can be a source of satisfaction to the geriatric adult. The interactions benefit both the child and the grandparent.

FIGURE 13–2 Older adults can engage in hobbies or activities that bring them pleasure and help maintain an active mind and body.

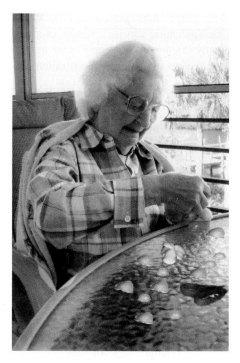

HEALTH MAINTENANCE FOR ADVANCED OLD AGE

Physical Exercise

"Use it or lose it" is an old adage, and it is true. The losses in physiological functioning may be related to activity (Waillant, 2002). Regular exercise promotes mental and physical health. In accordance with *Healthy People 2010* goals, regular exercise should be maintained as long as possible. Natural activities such as walking, jogging, running, or swimming are appropriate and can provide pleasure.

Occupational Activities

Adjusting to retirement from the life's work and finding fulfillment and self-worth from volunteer activities, hobbies, or travel can help maintain an active mind and body. This is often referred to as the *activity theory* and is related to a positive transition in the phase of aging adult.

Nutrition

Maintaining an adequate nutrition intake is important for health maintenance. There are challenges to overcome, such as dental loss, adaptation to dentures, slowed digestion, constipation, and a decline in ability to buy or prepare nutritious meals. Many communities offer a Meals on Wheels service that delivers one meal a day to geriatric residents. Senior centers within the community often serve one meal a day, with the added advantage of socialization.

Prevention of Illness

Providing regular health checkups and follow-up for abnormal symptoms is essential for health maintenance. Annual immunizations recommended by the health department or the Centers for Disease Control and Prevention (CDC), such as the pneumococcal vaccine (pneumonia) and flu shots, are also advisable (see Appendix A). Close monitoring of chronic illnesses such as heart disease, high blood pressure, arthritis, and visual disturbances is important. Providing access to regular medical care is often a challenge. The geriatric adult should be screened periodically for colon cancer, breast cancer, prostate cancer, and lipid disorders.

Mental Health

Depression is the most common mental health problem in the geriatric age group. It is typically brought on by isolation from social contacts, change in environment, low self-esteem, and loss of loved ones. Suicide is also common in this age group. Psychological counseling, establishment of social contact and support, and engaging in pleasurable activities on a daily basis help avoid the development of depression. To maintain mental health, the person of advanced old age must be realistic, use strengths and coping strategies to deal with physiological changes, and set new goals that are positive and attainable.

Environmental Controls

Reducing the risks of falls and fractures can be achieved by providing a safe home environment. Avoiding the use of slippery area rugs, using handrails in the bathroom to assist with changes in body position, and maintaining effective lighting are easy to achieve environmental modifications.

Elder Abuse

Elder abuse is the intentional infliction of mental, emotional, or physical pain or failure to provide care necessary for survival. In some cases the abuse may be economic, depriving geriatric adults of their life savings. Physical abuse is common. Dependency, frailty, illness, and metal disability may make the geriatric adult more vulnerable to abuse. When the caregiver is a family member, the combined effect of fatigue and overwhelming responsibilities to spouse, children, and job, as well as the care of the geriatric adult, may cause caregiver strain that results in some type of elder abuse. The nurse or health care worker can intervene by offering resources for caregiver support, such as respite care, support groups, education, and stress management. Signs of abuse may include depression, social isolation, clusters of bruises, unexplained burns, contractures, undernutrition, dehydration, and missed follow-up health care appointments. All caregivers should be alert to elder abuse because it may go unreported by the geriatric adult, whose self-esteem may have been destroyed. Referral to adult protective services may be necessary, or placement in another environment may be advisable.

Polypharmacy

Polypharmacy is the use of many medications prescribed for different chronic illnesses. The medications taken may interact with each other and produce unwanted side effects. The geriatric person may forget to take one dose or accidentally take a double dose, which can result in toxicity and illness. Monitoring of medications should be a priority in elder care. The decreased organ function found in advanced old age contributes to a delay in excretion of the drug from the body, and toxicity can also develop. Drug dosages and effects need to be carefully monitored and explained to patients and their caregivers.

Placement Alternatives

Sometimes geriatric adults suffer from multiple chronic illnesses. They also may have cognitive impairments such as **Alzheimer's disease**, which involves loss of memory, disorientation, and loss of ability to communicate and function in social situations. The complete dependence on others for **activities of daily living** (ADLs) such as bathing, tooth-brushing, dressing, and eating may lead to the need for placement in a nursing home or long-term care facility (Box 13-3).

Some nursing homes offer basic nursing care; others offer physical and recreational activities as well. Entering a nursing home often requires giving up independence and control over one's life, and many geriatric patients decline rapidly in this type of impersonal environment. Selection of a nursing home should include such factors as cost, insurance coverage, accessibility to medical services, philosophy of care, staffing, availability of occupational, physical and speech therapy, and social services. Some facilities offer *pet therapy,* which is the use of pets as friends and dependents. Providing a clean homelike setting with open visiting hours, spiritual care, and pleasant visual surroundings is important (Box 13-4).

There are alternatives to nursing home care for the adult in advanced old age. Long-term care insurance, if purchased before it is needed, can provide in-home care and assistance. Some apartment rentals offer assisted living in a residential setting for the geriatric adult who needs minimal or moderate supervision and care. Some families build additions to their home for geriatric parents, so that their independence is maintained yet they are close by. In some communities, visiting nurses can visit the homebound geriatric person and provide supervision, care, and education.

BOX 13-3   Activities of Daily Living

- Eating
- Toileting, bathing, and grooming
- Cooking
- Shopping
- Taking medication

The ability to manage these activities of daily living (ADLs) is essential for independent living. Assisted living facilities can help with cleaning, laundry, meals, and recreational activities.

ROLE OF THE NURSE AND HEALTH CARE WORKER

Most geriatric adults develop coping strategies to deal with the gradual aging process. Often, minor changes in the environment can enhance their ability to function. For example, the geriatric person with decreased lung capacity and high blood pressure may manage well in a ground floor apartment but may have difficulty if walking up steps is a required daily activity.

It is important to observe family interaction. An overprotective family that insists on restraining the geriatric person in a wheelchair or bed for fear of their falling will foster dependency that can result in dysfunction and psychological decline. Changes in aging include physiological, psychological, social, economic, and cultural factors that influence the way one ages and the rate of the aging process.

There are many positive aspects of aging. Geriatric adults offer a wealth of experience, expertise, and wisdom. They provide a grandchild with a relationship that cannot be equaled and one that contributes to the development of the child and the well-being of the geriatric adult (Figure 13-3). Understanding the developmental tasks of advanced old age, knowing the physiological and psychological changes and challenges geriatric persons face, and empowering those in advanced old age to maintain autonomy or control over their lives is the focus in geriatric care (Box 13-5).

BOX 13-4   Concerns Related to Placement

- Access to health care and assessment
- Individual perception of move as "dumping" or as assistance
- Control of patient's finances
- Personal space allowed
- Accommodation of special needs
- Privacy or sharing room
- Providing pet care, allowing plants in room
- Peer group activity
- Rehabilitation and therapies available

FIGURE 13–3 Adults in the geriatric age group can benefit from assisted living facilities that enable them to maintain personal independence. Friends, family, and visitors to their home are offered the benefits of experience, wisdom, and expertise of geriatric adults.

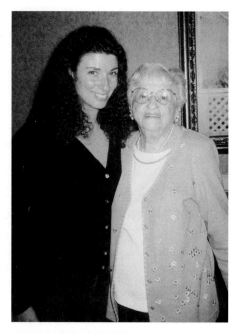

BOX 13-5   **Principles of Elder Care**

- Encourage confidence
- Raise self-image
- Provide empowerment
- Demonstrate kind, caring manner
- Identify and include family and social support systems
- Actively listen
- Integrate spirituality, hope, and faith
- Assist in setting personal goals
- Monitor exercise and nutrition
- Follow-up on health concerns

KEY POINTS

- Senescence is categorized as including the young-old, old, old-old, and elite-old.
- The physiological changes in advanced old age affect all body systems, but the degree is dependent on genetics, lifestyle, dietary practices, and social support.
- Immortality versus distinction is the major task or challenge that the advanced old age population must face.
- Some health promotion activities the geriatric adult can participate in are physical exercise, balanced nutrition, preventive health maintenance (such as getting the flu vaccine), and controlling the safety of their environment.
- The need for a sense of being loved and valued continues throughout the lifespan and includes fulfilling the sexual needs of the geriatric adult.

- Elder abuse is the physical, mental, social, or financial neglect or mistreatment of the geriatric adult.
- A variety of living options are available to geriatric adults, including living in their own homes, with other family members, in assisted living apartments, or in skilled/long-term care facilities.
- Activities of daily living involve the ability to independently feed, dress, wash, toilet, and communicate.
- The health care worker can provide education and guidance in meeting the life tasks of the geriatric adult.

CRITICAL THINKING

Discuss some advantages and disadvantages of three different living arrangements available for geriatric patients. What factors should be considered when helping a geriatric patient select a living arrangement?

MULTIPLE-CHOICE REVIEW QUESTIONS

1 Osteoporosis is:
   1 The loss of bone mass
   2 The occurrence of bone fractures
   3 The development of mental confusion
   4 An inevitable part of the aging process
2 Senescence is a period in an adult's life when:
   1 The body begins to age and weaken
   2 Sexual desires disappear
   3 Mental confusion occurs
   4 Death is imminent
3 In men, fertility may be retained until:
   1 The age of 65
   2 The age of 70
   3 The age of 80
   4 The midlife crisis occurs
4 Preventative screening for the presence of early cancer of the prostate includes:
   1 Prostate-specific antigen (PSA) test
   2 Radiograph of the prostate
   3 Annual magnetic resonance imaging exam
   4 Annual Pap test
5 The major task of the advanced old age adult includes:
   1 Immortality versus Extinction
   2 Identity versus Role Confusion
   3 Intimacy versus Isolation
   4 Ego-Integrity versus Despair

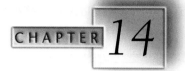

CHAPTER *14*

Planning for the End of a Generation

OUTLINE

DEATH AS PART OF THE LIFE CYCLE
SIGNS AND SYMPTOMS OF DEATH
THE PROCESS OF DYING
    Psychological Responses of the Dying Patient
    Family Behaviors Related to the Dying Process
CULTURE AND DYING
OPTIONS FOR END-OF-LIFE CARE
    Acute Care of the Dying Patient
    Hospice Care
ETHICAL AND LEGAL ISSUES
    Advance Directive
    Durable Power of Attorney for Health Care
    Living Will
    Do Not Resuscitate Order
    Assisted Suicide and Euthanasia
ROLE OF THE NURSE OR HEALTH CARE WORKER IN END-OF-LIFE
    CARE
DEATH OF A CHILD
    Developmental Concepts of Death and Dying
NURSING RESPONSIBILITIES WHEN DEATH OCCURS

OBJECTIVES

Upon completion of this chapter, the student will be able to:

1 Describe the grieving process of the patient facing death.
2 List the stages of the dying process.
3 Discuss behaviors related to the dying process.
4 Describe the philosophy of hospice and palliative care.
5 Define quality of life from a child's-eye view.
6 List the dying person's bill of rights.
7 Discuss the response and needs of the family of the dying patient.
8 Review ethical and legal issues involved in end-of-life care.
9 State the role of the nurse or health care worker in end-of-life
    care.
10 State three cultural practices related to end-of-life care.

11 Describe the development of the concept of death and dying in young children.
12 Discuss similarities and differences in end-of-life care for adults and children.
13 List signs of impending death.

KEY TERMS

Advance directives
Assisted suicide
Culturally competent
Durable power of attorney for health care
Euthanasia
Hospice
Informed consent
Palliative care
Therapeutic communication
Therapeutic presence

DEATH AS PART OF THE LIFE CYCLE

Death is a normal part of the life cycle. Most people who think about death associate it with the elderly. Many older people prepare for death by writing a last will and testament or advance directives for health care or by making advance funeral arrangements, including the purchase of a burial plot. Few people are really prepared for the actual event.

Death is not unique to the aged. The sudden, unexpected death of a young person causes different emotions and behaviors in the survivors. The process of death can occur in the acute care hospital amid the surroundings of whirring machines, twisted tubes, and medical and nursing staff who are strangers, or it can occur in the peaceful home or hospice environment of a room surrounded by family and familiar caregivers.

The care of a dying person, called *end-of-life care* (EOL), involves ethical and legal issues and religious and cultural responsibilities that need to be addressed by the nurse or health care team.

Surveys have shown that the two most common fears associated with death are the fear of pain and the fear of being a burden to the family (NHPCO, 1996). The biggest barrier to accessing hospice or palliative care facilities is the fear of letting go of all hope for survival.

No specific technique or procedure can describe for a nurse or health care worker what to do for a patient who is dying or the family who is in anguish. A flexible approach is needed to meet the needs of the patient and family. Often the mere presence of a nurse or health care worker provides the caring and support that is needed. Remaining near the patient and family, or simply holding a hand, provides strength while facilitating expressions of emotions and grief. This is known as **therapeutic presence.**

Understanding the patient's and the family's wishes, religious and cultural needs, and legal and ethical protocols are essential for the nurse or health care worker. (See Appendix B for cultural aspects related to death.) The physical, psychological, spiritual, and social needs of the family as a unit are part of the care of a dying patient. Most care plans focus on a positive outcome of care provided, and few see any positive outcome when death occurs. However, providing death with dignity is a quality process in the closure of a life. Decreasing pain, promoting comfort, and reducing stress are considered positive outcomes in the care of dying patients and their families.

SIGNS AND SYMPTOMS OF DEATH

The family should be prepared for symptoms that accompany death (Box 14-1), and the information should be communicated with sensitivity. Even when the death of a person is expected, the finality of the actual death still will come as a shock to most family members.

THE PROCESS OF DYING

The process of dying is psychological and physiological. Psychological dying starts when a person is told he or she has a terminal illness. Sometimes the death of a spouse or peer causes persons to believe their own death is near. Physiological death starts when the body processes decline in function.

BOX 14-1   **Common Signs of Impending Death**

- Increasing weakness, immobility
- Weight loss
- Decreased appetite
- Loss of bowel and bladder control
- Decreased awareness of surroundings
- Diaphoresis (sweating)
- Lung congestion (loose gurgling sound, referred to as the death rattle)
- Altered breathing patterns (periods of apnea)
- Decreased urine output
- Slowed pulse
- Cold and mottled extremities
- Relaxed and open jaw

NOTE: Even though the patient may appear to be asleep or in a coma, hearing is the last sense to be lost. Family and caregivers should continue to talk to the patient.

Psychological Responses of the Dying Patient

Death, as part of the life cycle, is accompanied by tasks and responses. Most people who realize they are facing death go through a grieving process. (See Table 14-1 for stages of dying as described by Kübler-Ross.) The process may start with disbelief: "This can't be happening to me." It is often accompanied by periods of crying and sadness concerning what will be left behind and future events that will be missed. Patients may mourn missed opportunities in relationships and activities. This grief process may or may not proceed to clinical depression. The normal sadness of grieving the end of life may occur in spurts, as the person realizes he or she needs increasing assistance in activities of daily living (ADLs) and the sense of deterioration of a condition becomes real. This kind of decrease in independence may trigger a period of sadness.

Disability and increasing dependence on others may cause the patient to lose self-esteem and be concerned with body image. The normal grief process can be interrupted by visits from close family or friends. Periods of pleasure can occur during the grief process if the patient is not clinically depressed. A glimmer of hope is often seen during the grief process. There is always the thought that some last minute reprieve or mistake in diagnosis will occur. This glimmer of hope is typically not seen if the patient is clinically depressed. A good social support system can assist the dying patient through the preparatory grief process. The nurse or health care worker can help the person prepare for death by understanding and accepting the stages of grieving, mobilizing support systems, and utilizing coping strategies. Therapeutic presence is just being there, providing support and comfort. **Therapeutic communication** involves accepting the patient's emotional outbursts and expressions of anger and encouraging venting and verbalization. The nurse or health care worker should maintain communication with the family and explain the stages of grief and the related behaviors. Talking with the patient about family, past achievements, and legacies can also be helpful. Clinical depression can often be avoided by identifying common fears of patients facing death and making efforts to alleviate these fears, such as fear of abandonment. Therapeutic presence of family and staff can alleviate this stress. Fear of the unknown can be avoided by education of the family and patient and by offering support. Complementary or alternative therapy, using simple relaxation techniques, is often

TABLE 14-1

BEHAVIORS AND STAGES OF DYING

Stages	Behaviors
Denial: "This can't be real"	Shock, numbness
Anger: "Why me?"	Disruptive behaviors, turmoil
Bargaining: Making deals with a god	Anxiety, conflict, confusion
Depression: Feeling of loss	Withdrawal, guilt, grief
Acceptance: "My time has come"	Vulnerability

Modified from Kübler-Ross, E. (1969). *On death and dying*. New York: Macmillan; and Kinney, M., et al. (Eds.) (1996). *AACN's Clinical reference for critical care nursing*, (4th ed.). St. Louis: Mosby.

helpful. A spiritual history obtained as part of the care plan can enable assessment of spiritual or cultural needs and practices that would be helpful to use when providing individualized care. The health care team, working closely with the patient and family, can help provide a death with peace and dignity. The stages and typical behaviors of the dying patient are outlined in Table 14-1.

Some patients do not progress through the stages as outlined by Kübler-Ross and may never pass beyond the stage of denial. Some people regress to previous stages such as anger from time to time during their journey toward death. Hope need not be abandoned during any stage. It has long been understood that a terminally ill patient can prolong his or her life by the desire to be present at an important family event, such as a birth or a wedding, and then die soon afterward. Some people faced with the diagnosis of a terminal illness lose the will to live, whereas others decide to live life to the fullest as long as they are able. There is no norm for the process of dying.

Family Behaviors Related to the Dying Process

Family members may show a variety of responses when a loved one is dying. In many ways these behaviors are similar to the dying person's responses. All these behaviors, regardless of who is exhibiting them, need to be recognized and acknowledged. The nurse or health care worker is able to help the family most by assessing their needs and informing them about what they may see on entering the patient's room. Preparation and education are the keys to helping the family to cope with what lies ahead.

Two specific behaviors should be quickly recognized, so that appropriate interventions can be implemented as soon as possible. These behaviors are *helplessness* and *guilt*. To minimize the sense of helplessness, the health care worker needs to educate and inform family members of what is happening and allow the family to assist in providing care, such as washing the patient's face, adjusting a pillow, or just sitting at the bedside so they may hold hands with their loved one.

Guilt is a much more difficult behavior for the nurse or health care worker to manage. The setting often determines the level of guilt a family member may experience. For example, if in an intensive care unit, the family may feel not only overwhelmed with all the machinery but also additional guilt secondary to the different types of invasive procedures that may be required to keep the patient alive. If the guilt of one family member is related to an interpersonal conflict with the patient that occurred before the dying or death of the patient, this family member may be in direct conflict with the rest of the family regarding what type or extent of interventions they want performed. In many cases the guilt experience may cause the family member to insist on everything being done regardless of the outcome or level of suffering the dying person may have to endure. Therefore it is imperative to help the family member to resolve feelings of guilt, so that a more individualized approach can be taken in the treatment and plan of care for the dying patient.

Pain appears to be a common fear that most people have related to dying. Many state that they "hope it's quick and painless." The nurse can now use a variety of pain-relieving techniques to help make the dying person as comfortable as possible. These techniques range from back rubs, position changes, scented oils or candles, acupressure, acupunc-

TABLE 14-2

THERAPEUTIC COMMUNICATION

Therapeutic Comments (What to Say)	Nontherapeutic Comments (What Not to Say)
"Tell me how you are feeling"	"You need to be strong for your family"
"It's okay to cry"	"Don't cry"
"It sounds like you are dealing with painful memories"	"It was God's will"
"I'm here if you want to talk"	"He/she is out of pain now"
"He/she was very special"	"It could have been worse"

ture, herbs, and nonnarcotic pain relievers or opioid pain relievers. The nurse attempts to find a balance to ensure that the pain is relieved as much as possible while still allowing the dying person time to complete any tasks he or she may want to finish.

Family, friends, and sometimes even health care workers seek advice concerning what to say to a person who is dying. This fear of saying the wrong thing often keeps people away from the bedside of a person who is dying, and therefore their needs and the needs of the patient remain unmet. Table 14-2 offers some suggestions for what to say and what not to say. This is often referred to as therapeutic communication.

 Culture and Dying

The behaviors of the family related to the care of a terminally ill relative may be influenced in part by their cultural beliefs and practices. Nurses and health care workers must be **culturally competent**; that is, they must be aware of the cultural practices of others and accept the practices in a nonjudgmental way. Cultural competence is developed through cultural awareness, knowledge of various cultural practices, skill in incorporating cultural beliefs into a patient care plan, and experience with persons from diverse cultures. Part of nursing education includes encounters with patients and coworkers from diverse settings. Understanding that culture influences thought; language; symbolic artifacts (such as bracelets or amulets); and actions that reflect specific traditions, customs, and rituals helps the nurse or health care worker understand behaviors and practices common to specific cultural groups. Culture and health care are interrelated. Culture influences an individual's attitude toward illness, nutrition, health care, and health care providers. A cultural assessment and history are important parts of a patient's care plan. A family care plan facilitates a more comprehensive cultural assessment, especially when related to end-of-life care. Interpreters should be provided whenever necessary to ensure accurate communication. Table 14-3 describes the dying rituals of selected cultures.

TABLE 14-3

DYING RITUALS OF VARIOUS CULTURES

	Preparation	Home vs. hospital	Special Needs
American Indians	May avoid contact with the dying person. Grieving is usually done in private, away from the person who is dying.	Concern for comfort and naturalness of the dying process.	May request shaman or healers to address spiritual health of the dying.
Arab Americans	Head of family to be informed privately of pending death. He will then determine how the rest of the family is to be informed.	Generally, prefer hospital to home setting in the hope that Western medicine may be able to hold off death.	Muslims do not need Imam in attendance until the process of dying begins or the patient has died. Have a private room available for the family, so that they may grieve together.
Cambodian (Khmer)	Parents or older children are to be notified, so that religious leader and other family members may be contacted.	Comfortable with death occurring in home or hospital environment.	Incense is used. Family grieves quietly and wears white while mourning.
East Indian	Believes only the body dies and that the soul lives on. Hindus and Sikhs believe in the concept of reincarnation. Dying person is typically not told of impending death.	Prefer death to occur in the privacy of their own home, so family and friends can visit. Religious ceremonies can also be conducted at home without interruption from hospital staff.	Family must be notified if death is imminent and be allowed to remain at bedside until death has occurred. Those of Hindu faith will mourn for 40 days.
Filipino	Prefer that the family tell the patient he or she is dying.	Prefer to die at home if terminal because they want to die with dignity intact as much as possible.	Family prays at bedside. Patient usually has religious medallion of some kind on body or in hand. Will want a chaplain/priest at bedside to receive the Sacrament of the Sick or to have Last Rites performed.

(Continued)

TABLE 14-3

DYING RITUALS OF VARIOUS CULTURES—cont'd

	Preparation	Home vs. hospital	Special Needs
Hispanic	May wish to protect ill person from knowledge of impending death. Family prefers to inform patient. Family may want time alone with person to say good-bye. May call clergy.	Prefer death at home to preserve dignity and location of spirit. Privacy is important to the family. Family usually stays with patient. Do not resuscitate (DNR) orders usually not acceptable.	Pregnant women and children may be prohibited from contact with dying patient. Amulets, prayer beads at bedside are common. Document that eldest child may be responsible for health care decisions.
West Indian	Prefer to see the body immediately after death. Remaining spouse is to be notified of death with children present.	Terminally ill usually taken home to be cared for as a sign of respect, loyalty, and obligation.	As death approaches, family and friends will want to be at the bedside to witness the death and pray for the person's passing on.

Modified from Smith, S.F., Duell, D.J., & Martin, B.C. (2000). *Clinical nursing skills: basic to advanced skills.* New York: Prentice-Hall; Leifer, G. (2003). *Introduction to maternity and pediatric nursing.* (4th ed.) Philadelphia: W.B. Saunders; Lipson, J.G., Dibble, S.L., & Minarik, P.A. (1996). *Culture & nursing care: a pocket guide.* San Francisco: UCSF Nursing Press.

OPTIONS FOR END-OF-LIFE CARE
Acute Care of the Dying Patient

Over the past several decades, medicine has seen a number of positive changes in the ability to care for the sick, injured, or dying. With the advent of new technology in the hospital environment, nurses and health care workers are now able to resuscitate premature infants and help them survive with the aid of machines until their own small bodies are able to take over the task. A gravely ill patient may be kept alive for an indefinite amount of time. This extended time may allow the family to gather at the bedside to say their final good-byes.

However, there are times when modern technology cannot keep someone alive. For whatever reason, the person's body has taken all it can and is unable to fight to survive. It is usually at this time when the physician speaks to the family to discuss the options and possible outcomes. These options can include continuation of full life support, such as a ventilator (breathing machine), intravenous medications to keep the heart beating and the blood pressure high enough to circulate blood throughout the body, and full cardiopulmonary resuscitation (CPR). They can also include removing all life support or sustaining equipment and stopping all drugs except those that can provide sedation and relief of pain. The dying person's bill of rights is outlined in Box 14-2.

BOX 14-2 **The Dying Person's Bill of Rights**
• I have the right to be treated as a living human being until I die.
• I have the right to maintain a sense of hopefulness, however its focus may change.
• I have the right to be cared for by those who can maintain a sense of hopefulness, however its focus may change.
• I have the right to express my feelings and emotions about my approaching death in my own way.
• I have the right to participate in decisions concerning my care.
• I have the right to expect continuing medical and nursing attention even if "cure" goals must be changed to "comfort" goals.
• I have the right not to die alone.
• I have the right to be free from pain.
• I have the right to have my questions answered honestly.
• I have the right not to be deceived.
• I have the right to have help from and for my family in accepting my death.
• I have the right to die in peace and with dignity.
• I have the right to retain my individuality and not to be judged for my decisions, which may be contrary to the beliefs of others.
• I have the right to discuss and enlarge my religious and spiritual experiences, regardless of what they may mean to others.
• I have the right to expect that the sanctity of the human body will be respected after death.
• I have the right to be cared for by caring, sensitive, knowledgeable people who will try to understand my needs and will be able to gain some satisfaction in helping me face my death.

Created at the workshop "The terminally ill patient and the helping person," sponsored by the Southwestern Michigan In-service Education Council and conducted by Amelia J. Barbus, associate professor of Nursing, Wayne State University, 1975. From Barbus, A. (1975). The dying patient's bill of rights. *Am J Nurs, 75,* 99.

Hospice Care

Hospice care is a program that supports the patient and family through the dying process and the survivors through the period of bereavement. The program originated in England as a response to the growing awareness of the unmet needs of the dying patient. The hospice plan is based on the philosophy that death is a part of the normal life cycle. The physical, psychological, spiritual, and social needs of the dying patient are addressed. The hospice program of care started in the eastern United States in 1974 and became a recognized Medicare benefit in 1982. The hospice plan involves **palliative care.** Palliative care is defined by the World Health Organization as the "active total care of patients whose disease is not responsive to curative therapy" (WHO, 1990). The goal is the best possible quality of life for patients and their families. Aggressive curative efforts are not part of hospice care. The varied settings for hospice care can include the home, nursing facilities, or long-term care facilities. Medication is prescribed for relief of pain and discomfort rather than for curative reasons. The hospice palliative care program provides comprehensive patient-centered care with a physician and nurse as the key links of a multidisciplinary team. Financing sources for hospice care are insurance companies, veteran's benefit services, Medicare/Medicaid, and private payments. The eligibility requirements for hospice care may be restricted by the rules of the funding source used.

ETHICAL AND LEGAL ISSUES

Ethical issues concerning death are influenced by values, culture, and religion, whereas legal issues are rooted in the law. The responsibilities of nurses and health care workers are to be familiar with the laws, recognize the cultural needs of the patient and family, and make the family aware of options available and the consequences of each option. Informed consent is based on respect for the dignity and rights of individuals and their right to make decisions about themselves and their health care.

In 1971 the Kennedy Institute of Ethics was established in Washington, D.C. This group deals with laws (formal rules), ethics (informal rules), and bioethics (health care regulations and research). In 1978 the President's Commission for the Study of Ethical Problems in Medicine and Research was established and reported on issues in the health care system. Decisions concerning end-of-life care, such as terminating life support, consenting to organ donation, and protecting the rights of incompetent patients, were researched. As a result of the research findings, policies were developed that addressed **informed consent, advance directives**, and **durable power of attorney for health care.**

Advance Directive

The advance directive (ADR) is used to inform health care providers and family members of the wishes of the patient concerning the level of lifesaving measures or heroics to be used when patients are near death and unable to express their own wishes. In 1990 the U.S. Congress passed, as part of the Omnibus Budget Reconciliation Act of 1990, the Patient Self-Determination Act. It became law in December 1991 (U.S. Public Law 101-508). This law mandates that, at the time of admission to an acute care or long-term care facility, all patients must be asked if they have executed an advance directive. If they have not, they are to be given information defining ADRs and informed that they have the right to state such directives at the time of admission. However, there is a significant drawback to waiting until they are ill or hospitalized to draw up an ADR. Many times, patients are admitted to hospital with an acute illness or in a crisis. These types of situations typically involve a great deal of stress, both physically and emotionally. Medication may be given that dulls the senses and prevents rational, clear thinking. Patients must also be informed of their rights to accept or refuse any medical treatment. Ultimately, advanced directives help lessen the burden of decisions that must be made by the family members.

Durable Power of Attorney for Health Care

The durable power of attorney is a type of advance directive that gives the decision-making power concerning health care choices to a person designated by the patient.

It is used when the patient cannot speak for himself or herself. This designation must be set up and signed before the person becomes incapacitated.

Living Will

A living will is usually drawn up before a patient is terminally ill or incapacitated. It describes the wishes of the person concerning end-of-life care that is respected by the courts. State laws vary concerning recognition of living wills but such a document is more valid as an expression of a person's wishes than casual statements made during family discussions.

Do Not Resuscitate Order

A do not resuscitate (DNR) order can only be written by a physician and can be based on the patient's living will or durable power of attorney for health care. DNR means that if a patient stops breathing or the heartbeat is incompatible with life (e.g., asystole or "flat line"), aggressive methods of resuscitation such as CPR will not be attempted.

Assisted Suicide and Euthanasia

Suicide is the taking of one's own life. **Assisted suicide** is the action of a person other than the patient to facilitate suicide. The word **euthanasia** comes from the Greek *eu* ("good") and *thanatos* ("death"). It is an intentional act such as the lethal injection of a drug that causes death. Both assisted suicide and euthanasia involve legal, moral, and ethical issues that have been tested in the courts through the years and remain controversial.

Health care professionals are often asked by the patient or family to participate in hastening the end of life. Oregon was the first state to legalize physician-assisted suicide (Oregon Death with Dignity Act of 1997). The core of the debate against assisted suicide and euthanasia is the premise that providing effective palliative, pain-free, end-of-life care will eliminate the need for people to request such action.

ROLE OF THE NURSE OR HEALTH CARE WORKER IN END-OF-LIFE CARE

The nurse or health care worker must understand the process of dying, offer support and empathy to the patient and family, and assist the family to recognize and manage options and supportive resources. Standards of professional practice in nursing have been developed jointly by the Hospice and Palliative Nurses Association, the American Nurses Association, and the National Hospice and Palliative Care Organization. The role of the nurse in end-of-life care is to perform the following:

- Ensure education of the patient and family concerning the diagnosis
- Ensure informed consent is provided with a clear offer of all available options of care
- Ensure that the patient's and family's cultural and personal wishes are respected
- Communicate with the multidisciplinary health care team when death is imminent or has occurred

DEATH OF A CHILD

An understanding of death is first taught to children as they learn about the life cycle of plants and animals in school. Sociology classes discuss cultural and religious customs of funerals and burials. The media reviews the life and death of celebrities. High school classes may be assigned an opinion paper concerning the right to die or the final destiny of death.

Nurses and other health care workers often help parents guide children in developing a positive attitude toward and an understanding of death. Discussion of experiences with loss in everyday life, using a flower, pet, or movie character, creates opportunities to discuss death in a nonthreatening manner. Many children's books are available to introduce the concept of death at an age-appropriate level. Discussion of life and death should be a normal part of the growth and development experience to prepare a child to understand and deal with death whenever it occurs. The concept of death is often influenced by exposure and discussion in school, although the understanding of death is closely related to Piaget's stages of cognitive development (see Chapter 4). A child's first experience with death usually occurs when a pet dies. Telling a child that a pet is being put to sleep does not add to the understanding of death and in fact may make the child afraid to go to sleep. Often the child's first experience with the death of a person may occur when a grandparent dies. The occurrence of death should not be hidden but should be openly discussed to enable effective coping strategies to be developed.

Children who have a terminal illness typically progress through specific stages as they prepare for death and are often more aware of their condition than parents may realize. Children as young as age 2 respond to their parents' emotions and nonverbal behavior. Therefore truthfulness, explained in age-appropriate terms in a supportive, nonthreatening manner, is the optimum approach in the care of a terminally ill child. Efforts at covering up or hiding the terminal nature of the condition merely obstruct vital communication between the parent and child, and communication could be more useful than false cheer. The initial stage of awareness (Bluebond-Langner, 1996) involves the child adapting to an identity or niche in the family as the sick child. Special privileges or attention may be given to the child, and siblings often do not understand the favored status. The dying child soon learns there is a relationship among medications, treatments, and recovery and adapts to the need for daily medication. Eventually, as the child's condition deteriorates, the child begins to realize he or she is different from peers. As the illness progresses, the child sees the illness as a lifelong challenge and feels he or she will always be sick. In the final stage the child develops an awareness of the terminal nature of the illness, often asks direct questions about death, and may express inner fears and fantasies. The focus of care may initially be on educating the child and family about the disease. Later, specific fears expressed by the child or family are an appropriate focus of care. Siblings should be included in the plan of care, so they do not feel abandoned or punished or do not develop an overwhelming sense of sibling rivalry and, later, guilt feelings.

The role of the nurse or health care worker is to provide support to and for the patient, parents, siblings, family, and school contacts. The death of a child is not part of the natural life cycle, and so the emotional impact on the family is often devastating. The dying child should be provided with age-appropriate routines and activities for as long as possible. Contact with all family members should be encouraged. Questions should be answered truthfully, and the nurse or health care worker should try to empower the child as much as possible. The adolescent is most aware of the loss of expected life experiences when facing death. Outbursts of anger are common and should be accepted and understood. Nurses and other caregivers also need a support system of peers to cope with the death of a child. Parents will need help with coping strategies and assistance with care of other children and family members during the grief process. Community resources should be used to help the family through the difficult time.

Developmental Concepts of Death and Dying

Death and dying are understood in different ways by children of different ages and developmental stages. It is important to recognize the ability of the child to understand what is happening and to help the family communicate with the dying child.

Toddler

The toddler views separation as temporary because he or she is just learning to separate from parent and to understand object permanence. The toddler's behavior may reflect a response to changes in caregivers and routines.

Preschooler

The thinking of a preschooler is not logical. The preschool-age child thinks of death as reversible. The preschooler employs magical thinking and may believe his or her own negative thoughts caused the sibling to go away. He or she may also fear abandonment.

School-Age Child

Concrete thinking enables the school-age child to realize death is permanent and the deceased sibling will miss family activities. The school-age child should attend the funeral or memorial service. The school-age child does not yet understand his or her own mortality.

Adolescent

Adolescents can think abstractly. The adolescent mourns and understands the effect of death on others in the family and community. A dying teen resents his or her dependence on others. Comfort and pain relief are very important, and the adolescent should be involved in decision making. Adolescents may have difficulty dealing with their own death and will often deny their own mortality by engaging in risk-taking activities.

It is important to understand that quality of life for a child means participating in age-appropriate activities as normal, healthy children do. Visits from friends and attending school, even part time, help the child and the family cope with what is happening.

NURSING RESPONSIBILITIES WHEN DEATH OCCURS

The physical care of the patient is carried out according to the protocols of the institution. The nurse should communicate with the family concerning policies and routines related to care and transport of the body because cultural or religious practices may require flexibility in the procedure. The time of death may be the last opportunity for some family members to see or touch their loved one, so they may appreciate some private time with the deceased to help with closure. Often when a child dies the parents may wish to hold the child snugly wrapped in a blanket for a time.

Family may need assistance in notifying extended family and friends; therefore facilitating phone calls is helpful. Talking about the death is part of the healing process. Providing referral for funeral and memorial service planning may also be helpful to the family. Utilizing community resources for bereavement support groups helps survivors realize they are not alone. See Chapter 15 concerning the bereavement process.

KEY POINTS

- The grieving process of a patient facing death includes the stages of denial, anger, bargaining, depression, and acceptance.
- Hospice care is based on the philosophy that death is a normal part of the life cycle. The physical, psychological, spiritual, and social needs of the dying person are addressed in hospice care.
- Palliative care is the total care of patients without the use of aggressive curative efforts. Comfort is the core of care.
- Quality of life for children involves inclusion in age-appropriate routines and activities for as long as possible.
- Some ethical and legal issues involved in end-of-life care include understanding of advanced directives, living wills, and DNR orders.
- Cultural practices of the family should be respected during end-of-life care.
- Family and friends should continue talking to the dying patient because hearing is the last sense to be lost.
- An understanding of death is taught to children as they study the life cycle of plants and animals in school. Sociology classes discuss customs and cultures. The death of a family pet may be a common experience children share concerning death.
- Death and dying are understood in different ways by children of different ages and developmental stages. Communication with children at their level of understanding is important.
- Some signs of impending death include weakness, immobility, altered breathing patterns, cold and mottled extremities, and decreased awareness of surroundings.
- The role of the nurse in end-of-life care is to educate the family and patient concerning options and resources, provide support, and maintain communication with the health care team. The nurse or health care worker can provide the family with strategies and resources to cope with end-of-life care.

CRITICAL THINKING

An 84-year-old man states that he is afraid he may be dying. He further states that he does not want to be alone or experience the pain of a slow death and asks the nurse to help him die now with dignity. What ethical issues, legal issues, and alternative options should be discussed with this person?

MULTIPLE-CHOICE
REVIEW QUESTIONS

1 The biggest barrier to accessing hospice care is the:
    1 Cost of care provided
    2 Required referral by health care provider
    3 Loss of hope for a cure
    4 Lack of insurance coverage
2 Hospice care involves:
    1 Palliative measures
    2 Curative therapy
    3 Custodial measures
    4 CAM therapy
3 Advance directives are used to:
    1 Determine end-of-life care measures
    2 Determine who will inherit property
    3 Provide consent for surgery
    4 Determine visitors allowed for the patient
4 A durable power of attorney for health care is set up:
    1 When illness strikes
    2 Before illness strikes
    3 When death is imminent
    4 After death occurs
5 The preschool-age child views death as:
    1 A permanent loss
    2 A temporary separation
    3 Abandonment of care
    4 Relief from pain

CHAPTER *15*

Bereavement

OBJECTIVES

Upon completion of this chapter, the student will be able to:

1 List the normal losses that occur during the stages of the life cycle.
2 State how the response to normal losses influences responses to loss of life.
3 Explain the difference between grief, mourning, and bereavement.
4 List the stages and tasks of the grieving process.
5 Describe an emotional, cognitive, and behavioral response to grief.
6 State two religious and two cultural practices related to death.
7 List two components from the DSM-IV-TR that define an abnormal grief response.
8 State the response to loss and grief at different development stages within the lifespan.

9 Discuss the achievement of the letting-go phase of the grief process.

10 State four ways condolences can be expressed.

KEY TERMS

Anticipatory grief
Bereavement
Condolence
Culture
Grief
Legacy
Mourning

THE CONCEPT OF LOSS

Loss is a part of life. Loss is often painful and requires an adjustment that may be difficult. However, the experience of loss occurs at almost every stage of life, not just at life's end.

NORMAL LOSSES DURING THE LIFE CYCLE

Perhaps the first experience of loss is the newborn's loss of the security of the womb. When the newborn later develops an attachment to the mother, the goal of the newborn is to prevent the loss of the mother, who is needed for survival. The very act of attachment of the infant to his or her mother or the husband to his wife makes the person vulnerable to the experience of loss.

The toddler endures the loss of being the exclusive focus of his or her parents when a rival sibling arrives who must share the love of the parents. Puberty involves the loss of the perceived body image of adulthood. The boy who does not attain 6 foot height or the girl who never develops a 36C breast size both deal with the loss of what they thought was to be.

When the teen leaves home for college, the teen loses the securities of home and family and the parents lose the control over their child. We lose our dreams of what might be when we settle for more realistic life goals. We lose our youth and beauty, our energy, our sight and health. We learn to cope with all these losses.

The normal losses of each stage of the life cycle involve some form of letting go and adapting. How a person responds to the various losses during life contributes to the development of that person's personality and how bereavement is managed when loss of life occurs.

Community Disasters

Families across the nation suffered a loss of national security when Pearl Harbor was bombed on December 7, 1941. Confidence in the safety and security of our country was again lost when the World Trade Center towers were attacked on September 11, 2001. Families in the United States had felt protected by their isolation from war-torn countries by the moatlike surroundings of the oceans that seemed impenetrable. The loss of that feeling of security affected everyone in the country.

RESPONSES TO LOSS

To adapt to the various normal losses in life, the individual must learn how to cope with disappointments. The ability to deal with disappointments and move on results in maturity and personality growth. The response to normal losses during each phase of the life cycle determines how loss in old age is perceived and managed. Those who deny aging may turn to techniques such as plastic surgery to restore youthful looks. Others seemingly dance through old age gracefully. The attitude toward loss often determines the quality of life. When past losses are not resolved, the losses involved in retirement may reactivate old, unresolved sorrows. Passing successfully through Erikson's stages of the life cycle determines whether the older person will enjoy life to its end with new strengths and goals or just spend time waiting in the corner to be claimed by death.

TASKS OF DEATH

Death is the ultimate loss—the loss of life. It is important to establish communication with those who are dying, but many people avoid discussing death. The experience of death is a stage in life with its own tasks. Some people wish not to be present when death occurs. They opt for sedation; they yearn for death during sleep. The hospice movement has enabled the terminally ill to experience the task of dying with dignity. Being satisfied with the legacy one leaves to the world or the family may give the person a feeling of immortality. The **legacy** can be a grandchild, property, a culture, an organization, or writings. A spiritual connection and belief that there is an afterlife, a final reunion of all, also can be a meaningful task of death.

GRIEF

Understanding the dynamics of loss, dying, and grief is essential to help the patient and family go through the process of bereavement. Verbal and nonverbal communication, therapeutic presence, and collaboration with the multidisciplinary health care team are the core responsibilities of the health care professional.

Grief Process

Grief is the emotional response to a loss and is a process through which a survivor accepts the loss. The grief process involves a series of stages, but travel through these stages is not always orderly. Grief can occur before the actual loss, when a terminal illness is diagnosed, or it may be initiated upon the actual death of the loved one. Grief that occurs before the loss is known as **anticipatory grief** (Lindeman, 1944). **Mourning** is the outward expression of grief. Mourning is often based on cultural practices and traditions. For example, in Jewish tradition, mirrors in the home are covered and the immediate family sits on hard surfaces for a prescribed period after a loved one dies. **Bereavement** involves grief and mourning. It involves the time survivors first react to the reality of the loss, the adjustment to the loss, and the entering of a period where they can move on and continue a fabric of life (Figure 15-1).

Culture, Religion, and Death

How individuals grieve is often directed by cultural and religious traditions and practices. **Culture** is a pattern of behavior, language, and practices that are transmitted through the generations. Within each culture, these practices may vary. Table 15-1 reviews the death rituals and practices of selected cultures, and Table 15-2 reviews common religious practices related to death. Understanding common religious and cultural practices enables health care workers to individualize their approach to the grieving survivor and family following the death of a loved one.

Normal Grief Responses

Normal grief reactions often involve *physical* symptoms, such as lack of energy, weight gain or loss, or insomnia; *emotional* symptoms, such as anger, anxiety, relief, or despair; *cognitive* reactions, such as disbelief, confusion, or inability to concentrate; and *behavioral* symptoms, such as crying, impaired functioning, withdrawal, or changing of relationships.

Schulz (1978) and Bowlby (1980) outlined three stages of grief that involve (1) initial shock and disbelief; (2) numbness and overwhelming sadness, with yearning and protest; and (3) reflection in search of meaning. Elisabeth Kübler-Ross suggested three stages or tasks of the grieving process. See Table 15-3 for a description of the tasks of the grieving process and suggested interventions.

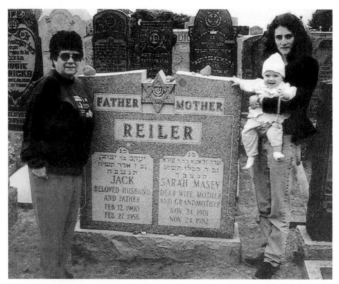

FIGURE 15–1 Most cultures include a ritual of memorializing family members who have died. Periodic visits to the cemetery to reflect, offer respect, and say prayers are healthy adaptations in the grief process.

TABLE 15-1

DEATH RITUALS OF VARIOUS CULTURES

	Preparation	Special Needs	Care of the Body	Organ Donations and Autopsy
Native American Indian	Portrays obvious signs of grief, such as crying, singing, or hugging of the deceased.		An open window with special position of the body may be preferred to allow for the spirit to leave the body.	Generally not desired.
Arab American	Family should be allowed to grieve together in privacy.	Grief tends to be open, loud, and unrestrained. Once death has occurred, an Imam will read passages from the Koran over the body.	Special bathing of the body is required after death, and the body is turned toward Mecca.	Believe presenting the intact body to Allah preserves integrity.
Cambodian (Khmer)	Immediate family is responsible for notifying clergy and extended family.	Incense is used. Family grieves quietly and wears white while mourning.	Family members or monk cleanse the body. On night of death, prayers by monk are important.	Prefer body to be intact, even though it will be cremated. Believe in rebirth or reincarnation.
East Indian	Believe it is only the body that dies; the soul lives on. Hindus and Sikhs believe in the concept of reincarnation. Dying person is typically not told of impending death.	Family must be allowed to remain at bedside until death has occurred. Hindus will mourn for 40 days.	Body is washed and prepared by immediate family members, placed in new clothing, and prepared for the cremation ceremony. Ashes are typically saved until they can be taken and placed in the Ganges River in India.	Not allowed.

(Continued)

TABLE 15-1

DEATH RITUALS OF VARIOUS CULTURES—cont'd

	Preparation	Special Needs	Care of the Body	Organ Donations and Autopsy
Filipino	Will want a chaplain or priest at bedside to receive the Sacrament of the Sick or Last Rites.	Family prays at bedside. Patient usually has religious medallion of some kind on body or in hand. Family tends to be somewhat vocal at time of death. Allow for privacy as much as possible.	Family will take part in washing/ cleansing the body before it is taken away. Death is handled with dignity because it is a highly spiritual event in this culture.	Cremation not the norm. May allow organ donation in some cases.
Hispanic	Will have multiple family members at bedside. Prefer priest to provide Last Rites and pray over patient/ body, usually with family present.	Pregnant women may not be present at bedside or at funeral.	No special treatment or ritualistic cleansing or preparation of the body is done.	Typically not permitted.
West Indian	Prefer to see the body immediately after death has occurred. Remaining spouse is to be notified of death with children present.	As death approaches, family and friends want to be at bedside to witness the death and pray for the loved one's passing.	Prefer hospital personnel to prepare the body for transfer to the morgue.	Preserving the integrity of the body is very important; therefore organ donation unlikely.

Modified from Smith, S.F., Duell, D.J., & Martin, B.C., (2000). *Clinical nursing skills: basic to advanced skills.* New York: Prentice-Hall; Leifer, G. (2003). *Introduction to maternity and pediatric nursing* (4th ed.). Philadelphia: W.B. Saunders; Lipson, J.G., Dibble, S.L., & Minarik, P.A. (1996). *Culture & nursing care: a pocket guide.* San Francisco: UCSF Nursing Press.

TABLE 15-2

COMMON RELIGIOUS PRACTICES RELATED TO DEATH

Religion	Common Practices
Christian	Anointing by a priest. Funerals held within 2 to 3 days. Mass held on annual anniversary of death. A memorial service may be held at 40-day anniversary. Adventist, Christian Scientist, Jehovah's Witness, and Methodist religions do not require Last Rites. Roman Catholic and Eastern Orthodox religions require last rites.
Muslim	Male cousins or uncles take leadership roles. The head is elevated above the body and faces Mecca. Rarely express fear of death because of belief in Allah. Ritual hitting of the body may be common.
Jewish	The body is ritually washed after death and must not be moved on a Saturday. The body should not be left alone. Casket is made of wood with no metal parts. Funeral is held within 24-hours. Family sits Shiva for 7 days with mirrors covered. Mourning continues for 30 days, with wearing of a cut black ribbon on the lapel.
Hindu	May tie a thread around the wrist of the dying or place a basil leaf on the tongue. These should not be removed after death.
Mormon	Baptism can be done by proxy if not done in early life.

The nurse and health care worker should maintain a pleasant nonjudgmental attitude while providing therapeutic presence and help the survivor identify and mobilize a strong support system. Referral to support groups or bereavement counselors for needed guidance is important. Hospice agencies can assist with accessing these resources.

TABLE 15-3

TASKS OF THE GRIEF PROCESS

Stage	Task	Interventions
Notification of death	Share event with extended family and friends	Assist with initial coping or refer to community resources needed Assess support system
Recognition of reality of death	Share the response by expressing grief	Understand anger may be directed at health care professional Survivor may need help with feelings of guilt
Adjustment or reintegration	Reorganize family structure and life goals	Survivor may need help setting up memory book and also planning for future and reintegrating into society

Adapted from Kübler-Ross, E. (1969). *On death and dying.* New York: Macmillan

Abnormal Grieving: DSM-IV-TR

The *Diagnostic and Statistical Manual of Mental Disorders,* fourth edition, text revision (DSM-IV-TR, 2000) lists a specific set of criteria required for the diagnosis of a mental illness or behavior disorder. The DSM-IV-TR also discusses certain signs and symptoms that would be seen in both the healthy and unhealthy phases of bereavement. In some instances the signs and symptoms appear to be similar to a major depressive episode. These signs and symptoms include insomnia, emotional lability, changes in appetite, and withdrawal from friends or social support systems (Box 15-1).

It is important to note that some of the signs and symptoms may be normal for the first few months after the death of a loved one. Typically the bereaved slowly begin to resume normal activities of daily living (ADLs) and maintain contact with family, friends, and other forms of support. It is not normal, however, to continue to remain isolated or removed from the real world for prolonged periods. Some form of intervention, whether medical, psychological, or both, may be necessary if the bereavement process is prolonged. The death of a loved one by suicide affects the grief process. Box 15-2 describes the typical grief response following a death by suicide.

Role of the Nurse or Health Care Worker

The responsibility of the nurse or health care worker does not end at the death of the patient. Preparing the family for the grief process and utilizing community resources to refer family for counseling and other assistance are important. The focus of care is on the patient and family unit, as described in Chapter 3. Cultural competence is the key to successful communication and support. Cultural competence is described in Chapter 14. See Table 15-4 for some suggestions of what to say and not say. See also Appendix B.

Tasks of the Family

Family tasks related to loss of a family member may include the reorganization of roles. Decisions need to be made regarding who will do the laundry, cook, and care for the young or disabled or earn money to pay the bills. Often children are required to fill the adult roles. Parents who suffer a loss of a loved one may not be able to respond to the needs of young children. The resources of the family need to be assessed and utilized. In the first days after

---

BOX 15-1 **Signs and Symptoms of Dysfunctional Bereavement**

- Guilt at things other than actions taken or not taken by the survivor at the time of death
- Thoughts of death or suicide
- Morbid preoccupation with worthlessness
- Marked psychomotor retardation
- Prolonged or marked functional impairment
- Excessive and uncontrolled crying
- Inability to accept the reality of the death

Modified from American Psychological Association (2000). Diagnostic and statistical manual of mental disorders (4th ed.), text rev. (DSM-IVTR). Washington D.C.: APA.

BOX 15-2   **Special Aspects of Grief Following a Suicide**

- Event involves social stigma
- Blaming often occurs
- Police investigation increases guilt
- Survivors feel death could have been prevented
- Survivors may feel decreased self-esteem
- Survivors feel rejected and deserted
- Family may worry about inherited predisposition

---

a death, families usually gather together to make funeral arrangements. There is opportunity to talk with survivors, express feelings, and offer support. In the weeks, months, and years after the death, however, overt support wanes, especially if family members live many miles apart. Professional help may be needed if financial issues spark animosity among survivors. Survivors who have had the opportunity to anticipate the death of a loved one may be better prepared for the changes and challenges they will face. However, the actual event usually sets in motion the typical stages of the grief process.

GRIEF EARLY IN THE LIFE CYCLE
Pregnancy

Because women who are pregnant experience movement of the fetus by the second trimester of pregnancy, a close relationship or attachment between the mother and fetus begins to evolve. Typically the mother and father join together in planning their future and the future of their unborn infant. When a stillbirth occurs, both parents respond, but often the mother suffers a more intense grief reaction, which may spark some interpersonal problems. The health care team must take the time to provide much needed support during this difficult time. Acknowledging the existence of the baby as a sepa-

TABLE 15-4

COMMUNICATING WITH THE BEREAVED*

What to Say	What Not to Say
"I am sorry for your loss."	"I know how you feel."
"It is okay to be angry with God and everyone else."	"You must not blame God. You should not feel like that."
"Grieving takes time. Take your time. Don't feel pushed to do anything."	"You will be okay in a week or so."
"It is not easy for you. Tell me about the person you lost."	"He lived a long and full life."
"Would you like to talk? I will listen."	"Tell me what happened."
"You did the best you could. It is okay to cry."	"Do not feel guilty. Do not cry."

*The most important thing to do is to *listen*.

rate person is important and may include taking careful pictures or footprints or snipping (cutting) and preserving a curl of hair as a memento (Figure 15-2).

Some parents wish to hold their infants to say good-bye. Parents should be taught about the grieving process, so each will understand what behaviors to expect. Options for funeral arrangements should be offered and parents should be referred to support groups that may be beneficial in the weeks and months following their loss. Providing empathetic listening, therapeutic touch, and nonverbal support to the parents are most helpful. Attention to siblings and extended family is also important because they may not verbalize their feelings as readily as the parents.

Clear information should be given about the cause of death and any implications for future pregnancies. Anxieties relating to the outcome of future pregnancies need to be addressed. Women who become pregnant after experiencing a loss in a previous pregnancy need to be taught the positive milestones of the subsequent pregnancy to promote a positive attitude and anticipate a positive outcome.

If the mother experiencing a pregnancy loss is an adolescent, the responses may be complicated by the thinking process of that level of development and the attitude of the adults around her. Often the unmarried adolescent who experiences a miscarriage is not given permission to grieve because some may feel the pregnancy was unwanted and would have complicated the adolescent's life. Therefore adolescents have a greater risk for developing depression, anger, or feelings of guilt that will affect their own growth and development process. Nurses or health care workers need to offer the adolescent information about the grief process, referral for counseling, and general empathy and support.

Infant

By the age of 10 months, when they have established an attachment, infants are capable of responding to loss. This response to loss may resurface in adulthood and may

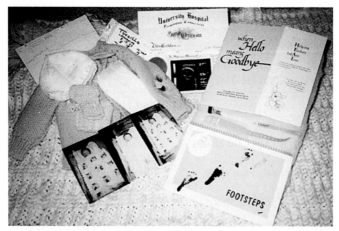

FIGURE 15–2 After pregnancy loss, the mother may take home a memory kit. This kit can include pictures of the infant, the death certificate, footprints, identification bands, an ultrasound picture, and the first set of clothing. (From Lowdermilk, D.L., Perry, E., & Bobak, I.M. [2000]. *Maternity and women's health care,* [7th ed.]. St. Louis: Mosby.)

manifest as an inability to form attachments or as a more intense response to normal loss experiences.

Child

Young children may react to death in a manner reflecting their developmental stage. By age 6, children realize death is not reversible. Children may show *anger* at the person who left them, *guilt* because they blame themselves for the loved one leaving, and *fear* that they will not be cared for and loved. Their immaturity prevents them from coping with these feelings and often prevents them from expressing these feelings. Young children need the support and guidance of understanding adults to help them through this stressful experience (Box 15-3).

Adolescent

Adolescents who lose a parent are usually at the point of moving into the adult role and may mourn the adult-to-adult relationship they had anticipated. The adolescent is establishing a sense of identity and may mourn the loss of sharing accomplishments with the parent who died. Adolescents may feel the need to take on the role of the deceased parent to help the surviving parent or they may slip back into a complete dependency role.

Young Adult

Young adults who are in a newly established marriage or family and are separated by death from the spouse may respond with rage at lost opportunities.

Communicating with a grieving survivor is the responsibility of the nurse, because contact is often continued in the community setting. Helping the survivor through the grief process toward reintegration and adjustment is both challenging and rewarding.

THE HEALING PROCESS
Reintegration and Adjustment

Many people remain in emotional pain years after the loss of a loved one. Grief is considered to be a private emotion, and others may be glad not to intrude because they

---

| BOX 15-3 | Children Coping with Loss |

- Don't overload children with too much information because they are concrete thinkers.
- Answers should be given in a simple and honest manner.
- Play activities are a way children express grief.
- Take the time to listen to children verbalize fears of the future and their own mortality.
- Allow children to remember and talk about the deceased.

Modified *Helping children cope with loss,* from National Mental Health Association, 2001, Alexandria, VA.

really do not know what to say or do. Some people say, "Don't feel bad" or "Don't cry." This type of response implies that the person who is grieving should not show the grief.

When a child loses a pet dog, parents may avoid having the child cope with grief by saying, "Don't worry—we will get you another dog." This implies that the loss can be replaced. Not showing the grief that is felt and trying to replace what is lost are not appropriate responses to grief because they do not allow recovery to occur. There is no process or task to be mastered. The loss is covered up by burying and replacing it, leaving the child to grieve all alone.

Encouraging the cover-up of grief forces the person to act as if he or she has successfully managed the loss in order to be comfortably accepted back into his or her social group. These unresolved feelings may be buried, but they are never buried very deep because their effects can last a lifetime. However, burying or hiding the grief may appear to be the better choice for the grieving person rather than being isolated from social contacts who may feel uncomfortable when he or she shows grief. Social isolation adds to emotional pain, and sleeplessness, confusion, and changes in behavior can result. Unresolved issues in the grieving process can lead to physical and mental illness. The nurse or health care worker should try to help the grieving survivor master tasks toward healthy grief healing.

Mastering Tasks Toward Grief Healing

The nurse or health care worker can help survivors in the task of grief healing by offering the following suggestions:

1. Find others who have experienced grief with whom feelings can be openly expressed. This can be a close friend, fellow widower, or grief recovery group. Meet with these people on a regular basis.
2. Recognize that change has occurred and what has changed. Recognize that things cannot be the same as they were before the loss.
3. Accept change. Because nothing will be the same after a great loss, one must accept that change will occur. Change is beyond the person's control, so acceptance of change makes the task easier.
4. Make changes slowly. Most psychologists advise not to make drastic changes in the first year following the loss. Disposing of possessions or selling the house, for example, are decisions that need to be carefully thought out to avoid regrets.
5. Become aware of what was and recognize the good, the bad, the intense, and all other aspects of the relationship that were lost. This prevents placing the lost one on a pedestal and creating a shrine, which may really be a distortion of the reality. Selecting the memories that will become permanent is important. Recognize that you did the best you could in the relationship and what could have or should have been done was just not possible at that time.
6. Avoid thinking of "what could have been," "should have been," "might have been," "if only." Avoid blame—especially blaming God, which may result in losing the spiritual side of life.
7. Let go of the past. This does not mean forgetting, it just means to letting go. Letting go and saying good-bye to a loved one need not mean saying good-bye to the loving memories. Letting go is saying good-bye to the pain, to the feeling of isolation,

and to the physical nearness of the loved one. This type of letting go will enable moving on. The nurse or health care worker can assess the successful achievement of the letting-go stage, which is manifested by the ability of the survivor to express positive and negative memories of the deceased without feeling deep anguish.

8. Financial decisions will need inventory and review. New goals will have to be established and new strategies designed. Updating the last will and testament and other legal documents should reflect the changes incurred by the loss of a loved one.

HELPING GRIEVING SURVIVORS
Condolence

The word **condolence** means to express sympathy or grieve together. To offer condolence to a survivor, one must elect to confront the grieving person. As one offers comfort and understanding to the survivor, profound perceptions about life and loss are sparked. Disturbing questions arise, such as "What would I do if this were me?" Often the one offering condolence does not know what to say and is concerned about saying the wrong thing. A feeling of helplessness follows, and the challenge of offering condolence may become overwhelming.

The nurse or health care worker may offer condolences to the family after the death of a patient by sending a letter to the survivor or family. Friends of the deceased patient often look to the health care worker for advice on how to offer condolences to the grieving survivors. The grief experience is a life-changing experience. The goal is to move into a new life that has many changes and is not clouded by the unknown. The nurse or health care worker is often called on to help support the bereaved. Supporting the bereaved means helping them preserve their dignity and understand the process they must journey through. The outcome of condolence is not meant to cure grieving persons of their feelings of loss. It is not meant to cheer them up. However, condolence may ease the emotional pain and help facilitate a healthy passage through the grieving process. A person providing condolence may receive the reward of strengthening his or her own coping strategies. Some ways to offer condolence include:

1. **Writing a letter.** Perhaps include a poem or a quotation that would be appropriate. The letter should not diminish the intensity of the grieving person's feelings and so should not say "I know exactly how you feel." It should not offer advice to bury the feelings by saying "Don't cry." It should basically be a letter of compassion and support, reminiscence of a memory, and offer of assistance.

2. **Visiting the survivor.** A spoken word of comfort, a supporting hand on the shoulder, and face-to-face encounters are very meaningful to the grieving person. Touch breaks through the numbness stage of grief and may bring the grieving person out of isolation.

3. **Helping with phone calls and arrangements for the funeral and receptions.** Try to help with hotel accommodations for family who must travel to attend the funeral.

4. **Selecting a gift or service to provide,** such as cooking a meal, babysitting for the younger children, or any other activity that will relieve the responsibilities of the grieving survivor.

5. **Helping the adjustment of the household** by offering to assist with disposition of clothes or helping to list the legal responsibilities and set a list of priorities.

6. **Including the survivor in occasional positive activities**, especially during holiday times.
7. **Remembering the anniversary of the death**, offering support, and reinforcing coping strategies during any remembrance services.
8. **Offering resources for coping**, such as a book, an Internet source, or a community support group that will help the grieving survivor move through the grieving process.

The nurse or health care worker has an important role in helping the grieving survivors through the bereavement process. The end of a life is part of the life cycle. Coping with loss is a developmental task in any stage of the life cycle.

KEY POINTS

- Loss is a part of life. Normal loss occurs in every stage of life, and coping strategies are developed in response to these losses.
- When past losses are not resolved, dealing with the losses involved in retirement, aging, and the loss of a spouse may be dysfunctional.
- Understanding common religious and cultural rituals related to death (cultural competence) enables the health care worker to meet the individual needs of the grieving survivor and family.
- Grief is the emotional response to loss.
- Anticipatory grief occurs before the death of a loved one, when death appears imminent. Some preparation for the grief process may occur, but the stages of the grief process remain the same.
- Mourning is the outward experience of grief.
- Bereavement involves grief and mourning.
- Stages of grieving generally involve shock, disbelief, and numbness; overwhelming sadness with yearning and protest; and reflection and search for meaning.
- The tasks of the grieving process include sharing the event, recognition of the reality of the loss, sharing the expression of grief, and reorganizing and reintegrating life goals.
- Alterations of the grieving process may occur in the case of sudden deaths, in unanticipated deaths, and in deaths involving children.
- Hiding the expression of grief or attempting to replace what is lost does not allow for healthy adaptation and recovery.
- Expressing grief, accepting changes, and establishing positive and negative memories help a person progress through the grieving process.
- The ability to express positive and negative memories of the deceased without suffering severe anguish may indicate that the survivor has successfully achieved the letting-go phase of the grieving process.
- Condolence is the sharing of grief with the survivors. There are many ways condolences can be expressed.

CRITICAL THINKING

Plan a condolence visit to a neighbor whose husband died a week ago. Discuss how you would determine whether her grieving was normal or dysfunctional. How would you offer comfort to this person? What might you plan to say during the visit?

MULTIPLE-CHOICE REVIEW QUESTIONS

1 Normal losses that occur during the life cycle most often involve:
   1 Death of a loved one
   2 Any experience of letting go
   3 Wartime deaths
   4 Loss of property
2 Anticipatory grief is:
   1 Grief that occurs before a loss
   2 Grief that occurs after a person dies
   3 Mourning a loved one who dies
   4 A fear of death
3 Normal grief responses may include:
   1 Inability to concentrate
   2 Rage
   3 Violence
   4 Inability to communicate
4 According to the DSM-IV-TR, a sign of dysfunctional grief may include:
   1 Prolonged functional impairment
   2 Initial denial that death occurred
   3 Temporary social withdrawal
   4 Crying
5 The role of the nurse or health care worker after the patient's death involves:
   1 Terminating professional responsibilities
   2 Preparing the family for the grieving process
   3 Referring the family to a psychiatrist
   4 Notifying the priest

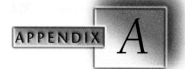

Child and Adult
Immunization Schedules

Recommended Childhood and Adolescent Immunization Schedule – United States, 2003

Age▶ Vaccine▼	Birth	1 mo	2 mos	4 mos	6 mos	12 mos	15 mos	18 mos	24 mo	4-6 yrs	11-12 yrs	13-18 yrs
	range of recommended ages				catch-up vaccination				preadolescent assessment			
Hepatitis B[1]	HepB #1	only if mother HBsAg (-)								HepB series		
		HepB #2				HepB #3						
Diphtheria, Tetanus, Pertussis[2]			DTaP	DTaP	DTaP		DTaP			DTaP	Td	
Haemophilus influenzae Type b[3]			Hib	Hib	Hib	Hib						
Inactivated Polio			IPV	IPV		IPV				IPV		
Measles, Mumps, Rubella[4]						MMR #1				MMR #2	MMR #2	
Varicella[5]						Varicella				Varicella		
Pneumococcal[6]			PCV	PCV	PCV	PCV				PCV	PPV	
Hepatitis A[7]										Hepatitis A series		
Influenza[8]						Influenza (yearly)						

Vaccines below this line are for selected populations

This schedule indicates the recommended ages for routine administration of currently licensed childhood vaccines, as of December 1, 2002, for children through age 18 years. Any dose not given at the recommended age should be given at any subsequent visit when indicated and feasible. ▢ Indicates age groups that warrant special effort to administer those vaccines not previously given. Additional vaccines may be licensed and recommended during the year. Licensed combination vaccines may be used whenever any components of the combination are indicated and the vaccineÕs other components are not contraindicated. Providers should consult the manufacturers' package inserts for detailed recommendations.

1. Hepatitis B vaccine (HepB). All infants should receive the first dose of hepatitis B vaccine soon after birth and before hospital discharge; the first dose may also be given by age 2 months if the infantÕs mother is HBsAg-negative. Only monovalent HepB can be used for the birth dose. Monovalent or combination vaccine containing HepB may be used to complete the series. Four doses of vaccine may be administered when a birth dose is given. The second dose should be given at least 4 weeks after the first dose, except for combination vaccines which cannot be administered before age 6 weeks. The third dose should be given at least 16 weeks after the first dose and at least 8 weeks after the second dose. The last dose in the vaccination series (third or fourth dose) should not be administered before age 6 months.

Infants born to HBsAg-positive mothers should receive HepB and 0.5 mL Hepatitis B Immune Globulin (HBIG) within 12 hours of birth at separate sites. The second dose is recommended at age 1-2 months. The last dose in the vaccination series should not be administered before age 6 months. These infants should be tested for HBsAg and anti-HBs at 9-15 months of age.

Infants born to mothers whose HBsAg status is unknown should receive the first dose of the HepB series within 12 hours of birth. Maternal blood should be drawn as soon as possible to determine the mother's HBsAg status; if the HBsAg test is positive, the infant should receive HBIG as soon as possible (no later than age 1 week). The second dose is recommended at age 1-2 months. The last dose in the vaccination series should not be administered before age 6 months.

2. Diphtheria and tetanus toxoids and acellular pertussis vaccine (DTaP). The fourth dose of DTaP may be administered as early as age 12 months, provided 6 months have elapsed since the third dose and the child is unlikely to return at age 15-18 months. **Tetanus and diphtheria toxoids (Td)** is recommended at age 11-12 years if at least 5 years have elapsed since the last dose of tetanus and diphtheria toxoid-containing vaccine. Subsequent routine Td boosters are recommended every 10 years.

3. Haemophilus influenzae type b (Hib) conjugate vaccine. Three Hib conjugate vaccines are licensed for infant use. If PRP-OMP (PedvaxHIB or ComVax [Merck]) is administered at ages 2 and 4 months, a dose at age 6 months is not required. DTaP/Hib combination products should not be used for primary immunization in infants at ages 2, 4 or 6 months, but can be used as boosters following any Hib vaccine.

4. Measles, mumps, and rubella vaccine (MMR). The second dose of MMR is recommended routinely at age 4-6 years but may be administered during any visit, provided at least 4 weeks have elapsed since the first dose and that both doses are administered beginning at or after age 12 months. Those who have not previously received the second dose should complete the schedule by the 11-12 year old visit.

5. Varicella vaccine. Varicella vaccine is recommended at any visit at or after age 12 months for susceptible children, i.e. those who lack a reliable history of chickenpox. Susceptible persons aged ³13 years should receive two doses, given at least 4 weeks apart.

6. Pneumococcal vaccine. The heptavalent **pneumococcal conjugate vaccine (PCV)** is recommended for all children age 2-23 months. It is also recommended for certain children age 24-59 months. **Pneumococcal polysaccharide vaccine (PPV)** is recommended in addition to PCV for certain high-risk groups. See *MMWR* 2000;49(RR-9);1-38.

7. Hepatitis A vaccine. Hepatitis A vaccine is recommended for children and adolescents in selected states and regions, and for certain high-risk groups; consult your local public health authority. Children and adolescents in these states, regions, and high risk groups who have not been immunized against hepatitis A can begin the hepatitis A vaccination series during any visit. The two doses in the series should be administered at least 6 months apart. See *MMWR*1999;48(RR-12);1-37.

8. Influenza vaccine. Influenza vaccine is recommended annually for children age ³6 months with certain risk factors (including but not limited to asthma, cardiac disease, sickle cell disease, HIV, diabetes, and household members of persons in groups at high risk; see *MMWR* 2002;51(RR-3);1-31), and can be administered to all others wishing to obtain immunity. In addition, healthy children age 6-23 months are encouraged to receive influenza vaccine if feasible because children in this age group are at substantially increased risk for influenza-related hospitalizations. Children aged ²12 years should receive vaccine in a dosage appropriate for their age (0.25 mL if age 6-35 months or 0.5 mL if aged ³3 years). Children aged ²8 years who are receiving influenza vaccine for the first time should receive two doses separated by at least 4 weeks.

For additional information about vaccines, including precautions and contraindications for immunization and vaccine shortages, please visit the National Immunization Program Website at www.cdc.gov/nip or call the National Immunization Information Hotline at 800-232-2522 (English) or 800-232-0233 (Spanish).

Approved by the Advisory Committee on Immunization Practices (www.cdc.gov/nip/acip), the American Academy of Pediatrics (www.aap.org), and the American Academy of Family Physicians (www.aafp.org).

Recommended Adult Immunization Schedule, United States, 2002-2003

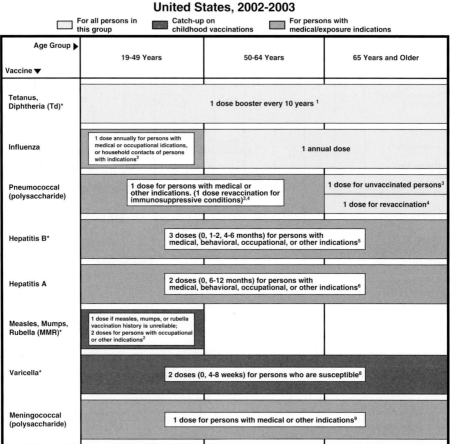

☐ For all persons in this group	▨ Catch-up on childhood vaccinations	☐ For persons with medical/exposure indications

Age Group ▶ Vaccine ▼	19-49 Years	50-64 Years	65 Years and Older
Tetanus, Diphtheria (Td)*	1 dose booster every 10 years [1]		
Influenza	1 dose annually for persons with medical or occupational idications, or household contacts of persons with indications[2]	1 annual dose	
Pneumococcal (polysaccharide)	1 dose for persons with medical or other indications. (1 dose revaccination for immunosuppressive conditions)[3,4]		1 dose for unvaccinated persons[3] 1 dose for revaccination[4]
Hepatitis B*	3 doses (0, 1-2, 4-6 months) for persons with medical, behavioral, occupational, or other indications[5]		
Hepatitis A	2 doses (0, 6-12 months) for persons with medical, behavioral, occupational, or other indications[6]		
Measles, Mumps, Rubella (MMR)*	1 dose if measles, mumps, or rubella vaccination history is unreliable; 2 doses for persons with occupational or other indications[2]		
Varicella*	2 doses (0, 4-8 weeks) for persons who are susceptible[8]		
Meningococcal (polysaccharide)	1 dose for persons with medical or other indications[9]		

See Footnotes for Recommended Adult Immunization Schedule, United States, 2002-2003 on back cover.

*Covered by the Vaccine Injury Compensation Program. For information on how to file a claim call 800-338-2382. Please also visit www.hrsa.gov/osp/vicp. To file a claim for vaccine injury write: U.S. Court of Federal Claims, 717 Madison Place, N.W., Washington D.C. 20005.202.219-9657.

This schedule indicates the recommended age groups for routine administration of currently licensed vaccines for persons 19 yeras of age and older. Licensed combination vaccines may be used whenever any components of the combination are indicated and the vaccine's other components are not contraindicated. Providers should consult the manufacturers' package inserts for detailed recommendations.

Report all clinically significant post-vaccination reactions to the Vaccine Adverse Event Reporting System (VAERS). Reporting forms and instructions on filing a VAERS report are available by calling 800-822-7987 or from the VAERS website at www.vaers.org.

For additional information about the vaccines listed above and contraindications for immunization, visit the National Immunization Program Website at www.odc.gov/nip/ or call the National Immunization Hotline at 800-232-2522 (English) or 800-232-0233 (Spanish).

Approved by the Advisory Committee on Immunization Practices (AOP), and accepted by the American College of Obstetricians and Gynecologists (ACOG) and the American Academy of Family Physicians (AAFP)

Recommended Immunizations for Adults with Medical Conditions, United States, 2002-2003

| | For all persons in this group | Catch-up on childhood vaccinations | | For persons with medical/exposure indications | | Contraindicated |

Medical Conditions ▼ / Vaccine ▶	Tetanus-Diphtheria (Td)*	Influenza	Pneumococcal (polysaccharide)	Hepatitis B*	Hepatitis A	Measles, Mumps, Rubella, (MMR)*	Varicella*
Pregnancy		A					
Diabetes, heart disease, chronic pulmonary disease, chronic liver disease, including chronic alcoholism		B	C		D		
Congenital immunodeficiency, leukemia, lymphoma, generalized malignancy, therapy with alkylating agents, antimetabolites, radiation or large amounts of corticosteroids			E				F
Renal failure/end stage renal disease, recipients of hemodialysis or clotting factor concentrates			E	G			
Asplenia including elective splenectomy and terminal complement component deficiencies			E, H, I				
HIV infection			E, J			K	

A. If pregnancy is at 2nd or 3rd trimester during influenza season.

B. Although chronic liver disease and alcoholism are not indicator conditions for influenza vaccination, give 1 dose annually if the patient is ³ 50 years, has other indications for influenza vaccine, or if the patient requests vaccination.

C. Asthma is an indicator condition for influenza but not for pneumococcal vaccination.

D. For all persons with chronic liver disease.

E. Revaccinate once after 5 years or more have elapsed since initial vaccination.

F. Persons with impaired humoral but not cellular immunity may be vaccinated. MMWR 1999;48(RR-06):1-5.

G. Hemodialysis patients: Use special formulation of vaccine (40 ug/mL) or two 1.0 mL 20 ug doses given at one site. Vaccinate early in the course of renal failure disease. Assess antibody titers to hep B surface antigen (anti-HBs) levels annually. Administer additional doses if anti-HBs levels decline to < 10 milliinternational units (mIU)/mL.

H. Also administer meningococcal vaccine.

I. Elective splenectomy: vaccinate at least 2 weeks before surgery.

J. Vaccinate as close to diagnosis as possible when CD4 cell counts are highest.

K. Withhold MMR or other measles containing vaccines from HIV-infected persons with evidence of severe immunosuppression. MMWR 1996;45:603-606, MMWR 1992;41(RR-17):1-19.

Footnotes for
Recommended Adult Immunization Schedule, United States, 2002-2003

1. **Tetanus and diphtheria (Td)**—A primary series for adults is 3 doses: the first 2 doses given at least 4 weeks apart and the 3rd dose, 6-12 months after the second. Administer 1 dose if the person had received the primary series and the last vaccination was 10 years ago or longer. *MMWR* 1991;40 (RR-10):1-21. The ACP Task Force an Adult Immunization supports a second option: a single Td booster at age 50 years for persons who have completed the full pediatric series, including the teenage/young adult booster. *Guide for Adult Immunization.* 3rd ed. ACP 1994:20.

2. **Influenza vaccination**—Medical indications: chronic disorders of the cardiovascular or pulmonary systems including asthma; chronic metabolic diseases including diabetes mellitus, renal dysfunction, hemoglobinopathies, immunosuppression (including immunosuppression caused by medications or by human immunodeficiency virus [HIV]), requiring regular medical follow-up or hospitalization during the preceding year; women who will be in the second or third trimester of pregnancy during the influenza season. Occupational indications: health-care workers. Other indications: residents of nursing homes and other long-term care facilities; persons likely to transmit influenza to persons at high-risk (in-home caregivers to persons with medical indications, household contacts and out-of-home care givers of children birth to 23 months of age, or children with asthma or other indicator conditions for influenza vaccination, household members and caregivers of elderly and adults with high-risk conditions); and anyone who wishes to be vaccinated. *MMWR* 2002;51(RR-3):1-31.

3. **Pneumococcal polysaccharide vaccination**—Medical indications: chronic disorders of the pulmonary system (excluding asthma), cardiovascular diseases, diabetes mellitus, chronic liver diseases including liver disease as a result of alcohol abuse (e.g., cirrhosis), chronic renal failure or nephrotic syndrome, functional or anatomic asplenia (e.g., sickle cell disease or splenectomy), immunosuppressive conditions (e.g., congenital immunodeficiency, HIV infection, leukemia, lymphoma, multiple myeloma, Hodgkins disease, generalized malignancy, organ or bone marrow transplantation), chemotherapy with alkylating agents, anti-metabolites, or long-term systemic corticosteroids. Geographic/other indications: Alaskan Natives and certain American Indian populations. Other indications: residents of nursing homes and other long-term care facilities. *MMWR* 1997;47(RR-8):1-24.

4. **Revaccination with pneumococcal polysaccharide vaccine**—One time revaccination after 5 years for persons with chronic renal failure or nephrotic syndrome, functional or anatomic asplenia (e.g., sickle cell disease or splenectomy), immunosuppressive conditions (e.g., congenital immunodeficiency, HIV infection, leukemia, lymphoma, multiple myeloma, Hodgkins disease, generalized malignancy, organ or bone marrow transplantation), chemotherapy with alkylating agents, anti-metabolites, or long-term systemic corticosteroids. For persons 65 and older, one-time revaccination if they were vaccinated 5 or more years previously and were aged less than 65 years at the time of primary vaccination. *MMWR* 1997;47(RR-8):1-24.

5. **Hepatitis B vaccination**—Medical indications: hemodialysis patients, patients who receive clotting-factor concentrates. Occupational indications: health-care workers and public-safety workers who have exposure to blood in the workplace, persons in training in schools of medicine, dentistry, nursing, laboratory technology, and other allied health professions. Behavioral indications: injecting drug users, persons with more than one sex partner in the previous 6 months, persons with a recently acquired sexually-transmitted disease (STD), all clients in STD clinics, men who have sex with men. Other indications: household contacts and sex partners of persons with chronic HBV infection, clients and staff of institutions for the developmentally disabled international travelers who will be in countries with high or intermediate prevalence of chronic HBV infection for more than 6 months, inmates of correctional facilites. *MMWR* 1991:40(RR-13):1-25. (www.cdc.gov/travel/diseases/hbv.htm)

6. Hepatitis A vaccination—For the combined HepA-HepB vaccine use 3 doses at 0, 1, 6 months). Medical indications: persons with clotting-factor disorders or chronic liver disease. Behavioral indications: men who have sex with men, users of injecting and noninjecting illegal drugs. Occupational indications: persons working with HAV-infected primates or with HAV in a research laboratory setting. Other indications: persons traveling to or working in countries that have high or intermediate endemicity of hepatitis A. *MMWR* 1999;48(RR-12):1-37. (www.cdc.gov/travel/diseases/hav.htm)

7. Measles, Mumps, Rubella vaccination (MMR)—Measles component: Adults born before 1957 may be considered immune to measles. Adults born in or after 1957 should receive at least one dose of MMR unless they have a medical contraindication, documentation of at least one dose or other acceptable evidence of immunity. A second dose of MMR is recommended for adults who:

- are recently exposed to measles or in an outbreak setting
- were previously vaccinated with killed measles vaccine
- were vaccinated with an unknown vaccine between 1963 and 1967
- are students in post-secondary educational institutions
- work in health care facilities
- plan to travel internationally

Mumps component: 1 dose of MMR should be adequate for protection. Rubella component: Give 1 dose of MMR to women whose rubella vaccination history is unreliable and counsel women to avoid becoming pregnant for 4 weeks after vaccination. For women of child-bearing age, regardless of birth year, routinely determine rubella immunity and counsel women regarding congenital rubella syndrome. Do not vaccinate pregnant women or those planning to become pregnant in the next 4 weeks. If pregnant and susceptible, vaccinate as early in postpartum period as possible. *MMWR* 1998:47(RR-8):1-57.

8. Varicella vaccination—Recommended for all persons who do not have reliable clinical history of varicella infection, or serological evidence of varicella zoster virus (VZV) infection; health-care workers and family contacts of immunocompromised persons, those who live or work in environments where transmission is likely (e.g., teachers of young children, day care employees, and residents and staff members in institutional settings), persons who live or work in environments where VZV transmission can occur (e.g., college students, inmates and staff members of correctional institutions, and military personnel), adolescents and adults living in households with children, women who are not pregnant but who may become pregnant in the future, international travelers who are not immune to infection. Note: Greater than 90% of U.S. born adults are immune to VZV. Do not vaccinate pregnant women or those planning to become pregnant in the next 4 weeks. If pregnant and susceptible, vaccinate as early in postpartum period as possible. *MMWR* 1996;45(RR-11):1-36, *MMWR* 1999;48(RR-6):1-5.

9. Meningococcal vaccine (quadrivalent polysaccharide for serogroups A, C, Y, and W-135)—Consider vaccination for persons with medical indications: adults with terminal complement component deficiencies, with anatomic or functional asplenia. Other indications: travelers to countries in which disease is hyperendemic or epidemic ("meningitis belt" of sub-Saharan Africa, Mecca, Saudi Arabia for Hajj). Revaccination at 3-5 years may be indicated for persons at high risk for infection (e.g., persons residing in areas in which disease is epidemic). Counsel college freshmen, especially those who live in dormitories, regarding meningococcal disease and the vaccine so that they can make an educated decision about receiving the vaccination. *MMWR* 2000;49(RR-7):1-20.
Note: The AAFP recommends that colleges should take the lead on providing education on meningococcal infection and vaccination and offer it to those who are interested. Physicians need not initiate discussion of the meningococcal quadravalent polysaccharide vaccine as part of routine medical care.

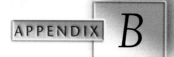

APPENDIX B

Paradigms of Cultural Influences Across the Lifespan

Cultural aspects of growth and development across the lifespan are integrated throughout the text chapters. The following table is designed to provide some specific illustrations of some differences in cultural or religious traditions that the nurse or health care worker should be aware of when planning culturally competent care.

Culture is defined as a set of learned values, beliefs, customs, and behaviors that is shared by a common social group and passed down through generations of family. Culture can influence food choices, parenting styles, and preferences for treatment measures. A nurse or health care worker can demonstrate *cultural sensitivity* by observing, using, and showing knowledge of culturally appropriate verbal language, body language, use of personal space, and gestures of respect toward family members while providing health care or teaching. Religion is closely related to culture, and a nurse may also include religiously appropriate interventions to sensitively meet the spiritual needs of patients and their families.

Cultural competence is the awareness of, acceptance of, and respect for beliefs, values, traditions, and practice that are different from one's own. The ability to adapt health care so that it does not violate the culture or religion of the patient is at the core of cultural competence. Achieving cultural competence is aided by knowledge, skills, and encounters with others of different cultures.

Nurses and health care workers must remember that there are always individual differences among people in cultural groups. People from specific cultures or religions should not be stereotyped. Individual members of a culture group may not each strictly adhere to all traditions of the culture (see Chapter 3). The assumption that all the people of one culture behave the same way and believe the same thing is called *cultural stereotyping* and can be offensive. It is particularly important to be sensitive to individual differences when working with a diverse population.

Often, some of the patient's traditional practices can be incorporated into the care plan. For example, an Asian woman who refuses to eat or take oral medication after giving birth may not have been offered the appropriate hot foods and may have been expected to drink ice water with her oral medication. In this example the care provided conflicted with the woman's cultural practices. However, offering hot soup to eat and room temperature water without ice with medications easily solves the problem.

Following are two important factors to consider when providing culturally competent care:

1. **Communication**—Obtain interpreters to aid in data collection and when providing information to patients who primarily speak other languages. Gestures and body language are important. Some cultures value eye-to-eye contact, whereas others tend to avoid direct eye contact.
2. **Personal space**—In the American culture an intimate zone is considered to be up to 1.5 feet, personal distance is 1.5 to 4 feet, social distance is 4 to 12 feet, and public distance is 12 feet away (Hall, 1963). Comfortable personal space may differ among individuals and cultures.

Further information concerning culture can be found in Chapters 3 and 5 and throughout the text and in the sources listed in the Bibliography.

CULTURE AND PREGNANCY

The cultural background of the family may strongly influence   their view of the birth experience.

An appropriate approach is to ask the pregnant patient what she considers normal practice:

1. Is pregnancy viewed as a healthy time, a vulnerable time, or an illness?
2. Is the birth process viewed as dangerous?
3. Is the birth a public or private experience?
4. What type of help is needed/accepted?
5. What is the expected role of the family?

Some cultures restrict the behavior of the husband during the perinatal phase. In *American Indian* culture the husband avoids eating meat while the woman is in labor and delivery. In *Arabic, Chinese, Cuban,* and *Ethiopian* cultures, the husband remains in control of the care but does not participate. In the *Orthodox Jewish* religion the husband may not participate in prenatal classes or during labor and may not view the newborn as it is born. Only verbal encouragement is usually allowed. In *South American, Vietnamese,* and *West Indian* cultures the husband is expected to be nearby. Most other cultures allow the husband to be present and participate during the birth process.

Many non-Western cultures expect the woman to have at least 20 to 40 days of bedrest after giving birth. *Southeast Asian, Hispanic, African American,* and *Chinese* cultural practices usually avoid full washing of the hair or body until lochia has ceased. Because pregnancy, labor, and delivery are considered "cold" conditions, air-conditioned rooms and cold fluids are avoided.

Cambodian women often discard colostrum and do not eat vegetables during the first week after delivery. Traditional Japanese cultural practices dictate bathing the newborn twice a day for a week with loud noise and playing music to ward off evil spirits. In the United States the baby is the focus of gift-giving following birth, whereas in many non-Western cultures the mother is the focus of attention. A cross-cultural maternal health information catalogue may be obtained from www.alpha.org/pp/red/index.htm.

CULTURE AND THE CHILD

Cultural practices can influence the timing of developmental stages. For example, the development of initiative may be later for children in families that practice an authoritarian style of parenting, because these families put a great value on obedience and conformity in children.

CULTURE AND THE ADOLESCENT

Independence in adolescents is not valued equally by all cultures. The *Chinese* culture does not recognize adolescence as a period of development. There is no word for it in their language. Adolescents understand abstract thinking, and the religious practices and symbols that are traditional at this stage help stabilize the adolescent's developing identity. Many cultures have specific rituals that recognize passage of the individual from childhood to adulthood. These practices can be symbolic rituals or celebrations, such as a bar mitzvah in the Jewish religion, or can be an actual test that demonstrates mastery of specific survival skills to determine that the adolescent is ready to take on adult responsibilities.

CULTURE AND THE ADULT

In *Jewish* religious culture, women are considered to be in a state of impurity during menstruation and after giving birth. Very religious husbands may not touch their wives during these periods. Health care workers or nurses can inquire about and be sensitive to this cultural practice and provide physical assistance when needed, such as after a cesarean section.

In many religions, birth control is not encouraged. The *Roman Catholic Church* and *the Mormon Church (Latter-Day Saints)* allow only natural family planning, using abstinence as the technique of choice. The *Christian Science* religion approaches health care with a spiritual framework and may decline preventive medicines, although some required vaccinations or personal birth control drugs may be accepted. The *Unitarian Universalist Association* advocates birth control practices and supports women's rights related to abortions.

The *Islamic* culture permits contraception but forbids abortion.

CULTURE AND THE OLDER ADULT

A positive attitude toward life and health is encouraged for older adults in most cultures. Most cultures look to elders as a source of wisdom, and often elders play a major role in raising or disciplining grandchildren. In many cultures, elders are also welcomed as the preferred babysitters and parenting consultants. Many geriatric patients who are confined to a wheelchair or nursing home may have limited contact with family but may place a high value on any available assistance in accessing family contact.

Women from different cultures have different experiences of menopause. In cultures where age is revered, menopause may be a nonevent. In the United States, where sometimes a high value is placed on youth, sex appeal, and physical beauty, menopause and related body changes may challenge feelings of self-worth.

CULTURE AND HEALTH BELIEFS

Many non-Western cultures believe that balances between hot and cold affect health and illness. This belief is known as the humoral theory. *Latin American, African, Hispanic, Haitian,* and *Chinese* cultures have traditional cold remedies to treat hot diseases and hot remedies to treat cold diseases. Cold illnesses or conditions include pregnancy, earache, chest pain, paralysis, gastrointestinal diseases, rheumatism, and tuberculosis. Hot illnesses include dental problems, sore throat, rashes, and kidney disorders. In *Asian* cultures the forces of yang (light heat or dryness) and yin (darkness, cold, or wetness) influence the balance and harmony of a person's state of health. Yin (cold foods) includes fruits, vegetables, cold liquid, and beer. Yang (hot foods) includes meat, eggs, hot soup, cantaloupe, and fried foods. Foods are classified as hot or cold according to their effects on the body when metabolized rather than their thermal temperature.

The *American Indian* culture defines wellness as harmony in body, mind, and spirit. A holistic approach to healing is valued.

CULTURE AND ILLNESS

Specific holidays may involve some restriction of activity. *Orthodox Jews* do not turn electricity, such as lights or television, on or off or use the telephone from sunset on Friday night to sunset on Saturday. During times of culturally restricted behavior, medical appointments or procedures should be postponed if it is possible without endangering the patient. Shaving can be done with an electric razor if a beard must be removed, but a razor blade must not touch the skin.

In the *Roman Catholic* and many other Christian faiths, a sacrament is offered to the seriously ill person. To enable this practice, the nurse should notify the priest before the patient loses consciousness if possible. Abstinence from solid food is required for at least 15 minutes before clergy offers the consecrated host in people receiving communion. Rosary beads or religious medallions may be pinned to the gown or bed of the ill person. *Mennonite* women may wear head coverings during hospitalization. Persons of the *Christian Science* faith often decline medications or psychotherapy. For *Jehovah's Witnesses,* receiving blood transfusions or medications containing blood products violates religious guidelines. However, today there are some alternatives to blood transfusions, such as plasma expanders and autologous transfusions.

Religious *Mormons* wear a sacred undergarment that should not be removed unless an emergency occurs. Patients of the *Islamic* faith may request that the Koran be kept at the bedside and that nothing be placed on top of it. Religious jewelry or prayer strings should not be removed from the body unless medically necessary.

Buddhist and *Hindu* cultural beliefs suggest that illness is the result of sins committed in a previous life or abuse of the body. Time for concentrated meditation (yoga) may be requested or viewed as required for healing.

Social behavior consistent with the sick person role may vary from demanding to silent passivity depending on the cultural background and other personal variables of the patient.

CULTURE AND DEATH

The Self-Determination Act of 1991 granted patients in the United States the legal right to full disclosure of medical information, to allow individuals to participate in their own care.

In some non-Western cultures, information is released to the patient at the discretion of family members. In most Western cultures a high value is placed on individual life. In many non-Western cultures the welfare of the family is primary and life and death decisions are made by group approval.

Judaism and some other cultures believe that dying persons must have someone with them as their soul leaves the body. Traditionally the body is not left alone until burial, which must occur within 24 hours (or as soon as possible) after death. The body is dressed in a shroud and no metal objects, including nails, may be in the coffin. No flowers are permitted during the funeral or for the 7 days of mourning immediately following. Mirrors are covered and immediate family may sit on low, hard benches during the mourning period.

Last rites are obligatory for many *Christian* cultures. The *Unitarian Universalist* faith prefers cremation to burial. The *Islamic* culture requires the body be placed in a position facing Mecca. According to the Islamic culture, persons do not own their body, and so cremation, autopsy, and organ donation are prohibited.

A *Hindu* priest may place a thread around the neck or waist of the deceased as a blessing before cremation, which is preferred over burial. *Buddhist* culture teaches acceptance of the inevitability of death and believes the person's state of mind at the moment of death influences rebirth. Suicide, violent death, or the death of a child may require special rituals because the state of mind at death may not have been optimum. Buddhist culture also considers it bad luck for a pregnant woman to attend a funeral.

In *American Indian* cultures a dying person may be surrounded by a positive celebratory atmosphere of family and children. Some *African Americans* believe that dying in the home brings bad luck to the house. They prefer that death occur in the hospital and may prefer that professionals prepare the body for burial.

In *Central American* cultures, death with dignity in the home setting is preferred over a hospital setting because death is considered a spiritual event.

The *Hmong* culture suggests a person must be well dressed at the time of death. A nurse may inform the family if the patient's death is imminent, so that the family can bring the desired clothing to the hospital. Internal metal objects such as plates, bullets, or medical devices must be removed from the body before burial, and metal objects such as zippers or buttons touching the body after death are prohibited.

CULTURE AND TEACHING

People from cultures that place a high value on pleasing others may answer questions with information they think you want to hear to maintain a harmonious relationship. To collect accurate data, questions should be phrased in a neutral fashion. *Asian, Native American Indian,* and *Muslim* patients consider direct eye contact impolite and may stare at the floor as a symbol of respect during contact with the nurse. The nurse should avoid misinterpreting this behavior as not paying attention. *Hispanic* patients may view extended eye contact as related to the evil eye, which will bring bad luck. Many *Asians* believe the head is sacred and therefore must not be touched or patted. Palpating the fontanel of an infant may be interpreted as a disrespectful action unless the medical procedure is properly explained to and accepted by the parents. *Native American Indian, Chinese, and Japanese* cultures suggest that silence indicates respect for another person, whereas *Russians, French,* and *Spanish* cultures may interpret silence as agreement with the speaker. Yet other cultures make every effort to fill silent moments with conversation. These factors should be considered and interpreters used when appropriate. Whenever possible, family members should not be used as interpreters when embarrassing or confidential issues are discussed.

CULTURE AND FOOD

Many cultures and religions include specific foods as an integral part of holiday celebrations and may restrict consumption of specific foods. For example, *Mormons* do not consume alcohol or any beverage containing caffeine and many fast on the first Sunday of each month. The *Hindu* culture prohibits consumption of all meats, whereas *Islamic* culture specifically prohibits pork. The nurse should be aware that some gelatin preparations might contain a pork product. Mixing dairy and meat products at the same meal is prohibited in the *Jewish* religion. Pork is also avoided, all meats must be specially prepared or koshered, and only fish with scales are permitted. The *Seventh Day Adventist* religion encourages a vegetarian diet. *Hispanic* diets incorporate the concept of cold foods, such as vegetables, fruit, and dairy, and hot foods, such as garlic, grains, and selected cuts of meat.

Bibliography

Dreher, H., & MacNaughton, N. (2002). Cultural competence in nursing: foundation or fallacy? *Nursing Outlook*, 50(5), 181.

Giger, J., & Davidhizar, R. (1999). *Transcultural nursing: assessment and intervention* (3rd ed.). St. Louis: Mosby.

Hall, E. (1963). Proxemics: the study of man's spatial relations. In I. Galdston (Ed.), *Man's image in medicine and anthropology*. New York: International Universities Press [classic].

Harkreader, H. (2000). *Fundamentals of nursing: caring and clinical judgment*. Philadelphia: WB Saunders.

Kim-Godwin, Y. (2003). Postpartum beliefs and practices among non-western cultures, *MCN: The American Journal of Maternal Child Nursing*, 28(2), 75.

Lipson, J. G., Dibble, S. L., & Minarik, P. A. (1996). *Culture and nursing care: a pocket guide*. San Francisco: UCSF Nursing Press.

Lipson, J. G., & Steiger, N, J. (1996). *Self-care nursing in a multicultural context*. Thousand Oaks, CA: Sage.

Luckmann, J. (Ed.). (1997). *Saunders manual of nursing care*. Philadelphia: WB Saunders.

Mazanec, P., & Tyler, M. (2003). Cultural considerations in end-of-life care. *American Journal of Nursing*, 103(3), 51.

Nies, M. A., & McEwen, M. (2001). *Community health nursing: promoting the health of populations* (3rd ed.). Philadelphia: WB Saunders.

Internet Resources

www.cns.org

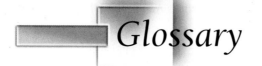

Glossary

Abstinence: A voluntary refrain from indulging in intercourse.

Activities of daily living: Tasks that enable a person to meet basic needs, such as toileting, eating, and dressing.

Adolescence: The period between childhood and adulthood, between ages 10 and 21.

Advance directive: A legal document that guides health care personnel concerning a patient's wishes when that patient is no longer capable of making decisions.

Age-appropriate toys: Toys that are safe and promote the cognitive and motor development of the specific age group.

Ageism: Discrimination against an aged person.

Allele: A pairing of genes that contain specific inheritable characteristics.

Apgar score: A scoring system to evaluate the physical condition of the newborn at birth.

Apoptosis: The programmed death of cells. Referred to as the biological clock, it leads to menopause and senescence.

Assisted suicide: An action of a person other than the patient to facilitate suicide.

Assistive devices: Items such as canes, walkers, and hearing aids that help a person maintain independent living.

Asynchronous: When different parts of the body mature at different times, causing an awkward appearance, usually during adolescence.

Atrophy: A decrease in the size of an organ or tissue.

Attachment: An affectionate tie that occurs over time as a result of interaction.

Autonomy: Functioning independently.

Behaviorist theory: A theory that describes how and why behavioral learning changes behavior.

Bereavement: A period of sadness after the loss of a loved one.

Biological clock: A programmed cell death that leads to menopause and deterioration associated with senescence.

Blended family: A family consisting of a mother or father, a stepparent, and children. Both parents may bring children from a previous marriage to form a new, blended family.

Bonding: The development of a strong emotional attachment between individuals, such as a mother and her infant.

Cephalocaudal: The progression of the growth pattern that proceeds from head to toe.

Chromosome: A thread of protein and DNA contained in the nucleus of every cell.

Classical conditioning: Relates a positive or negative event to a specific behavior to promote or prevent that behavior from recurring.

Climacteric: The change of life in which hormonal shifts result in cessation of the reproductive ability in women and a corresponding decrease in sexual drive in men.

Clique: A social group with a fixed exclusive membership, sharing similar interests, values, and tastes.

Cognitive style: A pattern of thought and reasoning.

Coitus: Sexual intercourse.

Competence: Effective interactions; ability.

Conception: The union of the male sperm and female ovum; fertilization.

Condolence: To express sympathy or grieve together.

Cooperative play: A group of children cooperate by playing together with each other.

Coping skill: A behavior that helps an individual adapt to or manage a stressful situation.

Corporal punishment: Spanking; focuses on the pain of the punishment, role models aggression, and rarely accomplishes the true goal of discipline.

Cultural assimilation: A process by which members of a specific cultural group lose the characteristics of that group and adapt practices of another group.

Cultural competence: Involves cultural awareness, acceptance, and respect toward behaviors and practices that are different from one's own.

Cultural relativism: The concept that normalcy comes from the standard social practices of a specific culture.

Cultural sensitivity: Observing, using, and showing knowledge of culturally appropriate verbal language, body language, use of personal space, and gestures of respect toward family members while providing health care or teaching.

Culture: A set of learned values, beliefs, customs, and behaviors that is shared by interacting individuals, such as a family.

Culture shock: The effect of a sudden, drastic change in the cultural environment of an individual or family.

Defense mechanism: A reaction that is protective to the individual or helps conceal conflicts or anxieties.

Dental caries: Tooth decay.

Determinants of health: Genetic makeup, lifestyle behaviors, social and physical environment, and general policies and interventions that affect the health of the population.

Developmental stage: Patterns of development related to perception and response to environment.

Discipline: A technique used to guide, teach, or correct behavior; it is not punishment.

Disengagement: Implies removing of emotional attachments to people, places, and objects.

Dizygotic: A type of twin that occurs when two ova are released at ovulation and each ovum is fertilized by a separate sperm.

Dominant gene: A gene that overpowers other genes, so that its characteristics will be inherited.

Durable power of attorney for health care: A type of advance directive that gives decision-making power concerning health care to a person designated by the patient, to be used when the patient cannot speak for himself or herself.

Dysfunctional family: A family unit that does not offer consistency of members or rules, may exhibit poor interpersonal relationships among its members, deals poorly with conflicts and problems, and often cannot reach out to the community for help.

Early childhood: A period that includes children between age 1 to 6. Early childhood is typically separated into two phases; ages 1 to 2 is the *toddler phase* and ages 2 to 6 is the *preschool phase*.

Ectopic pregnancy: A pregnancy that occurs outside the uterus, usually in the fallopian tube.

Ejaculation: Release of sperm during orgasm.

Elder abuse: The infliction of harm or neglect through actions or acts of omission on an older person. The abuse can be physical, emotional, or financial and can include neglect or obstruction of personal rights.

Electra anxiety: Occurs when little girls compete with their mothers for the love and attention from their fathers.

Empowerment: Providing tools and knowledge to the family to enable informed participation in decision making.

Empty nest syndrome: Occurs when grown children start to leave home for the first time, causing parents to feel lonely or isolated.

En face: Face to face.

Engrossment: When fathers or significant others develop an intense focus on the newborn.

Ethnocentrism: The belief that one's own culture is the standard of behavior and is better than other cultures.

Euthanasia: An intentional act, such as the lethal injection of a drug, that causes death.

Expressive language: The ability to express thoughts in the words of a language.

Extrovert: An outgoing person who focuses on others in the environment.

Family systems theory: Theories that explain interconnected family functions and responses.

Federal Register: Federal legislation concerning health care is recorded and published in this document.

Fetal alcohol syndrome: A group of symptoms present in a newborn infant resulting from maternal ingestion of alcohol during pregnancy.

Fetus: An unborn infant from the ninth week of conception to birth.

Free radicals: When one ion of a molecule breaks off and is no longer paired. Free radicals produce a harmful effect on body tissues.

Gene therapy: Involves placing a therapeutic gene on the back of a virus vector, which will then carry the new gene into the cell that has a missing or defective gene.

Generativity: Contributing in a positive way to family or community. This contribution improves self-image and promotes subjective well-being.

Genetic code: The code contained in the genes of living cells that will determine what characteristics will be inherited.

Genetic counseling: The communication between a geneticist (a specialist in inherited conditions) and the parents to discuss the risk of their infant inheriting genes that can result in an abnormality.

Genome: A complete set of chromosomes and DNA that contain all the genetic information in the human cell.

Geriatrics: The study of old age; includes the biological, psychological, physiological, and sociological aspects of aging.

Gestation: The length of time from conception to birth.

Gonads: A term used to refer to ovaries in females and testicles in males.

Health indicators: The public health issues and concerns linked to the objectives of *Healthy People 2010.*

Health maintenance organization (HMO): A group medical practice that offers prepaid care for members.

Health status: Details concerning illness and other factors that affect health; measured by factors such as birth and death rates, life expectancy, and accessibility to health care.

Homeopathy: The use of minute portions of chemicals for their healing power.

Hospice: A plan of terminal care that is based on the philosophy that death is a part of the normal life cycle; involves palliative care that meets the physical, psychological, spiritual, and social needs of the dying patient.

Hot flashes: A sensation caused by blood rushing to the surface of the skin as a result of dilation of capillaries.

Identity accommodation: Changing the concept of one's own identity to fit what is real, rather than what was dreamed.

Immune theory: A theory of aging that involves the concept that as one ages, the body finds it more difficult to tell the difference between healthy and defective cells.

Immunity: The body's resistance to disease-causing organisms.

Infant: The period between ages 4 weeks and 1 year.

Infant mortality rate: The number of deaths that occur before age 1 per 1000 live births.

Information processing: The inputting of information followed by a thought mechanism that results in an output of judgment or decision making.

Informed consent: Providing the patient with information regarding risks, advantages, and alternatives available to a procedure in a language that can be understood by the patient.

Initiative: The ability to take the first step or leading movement.

Intimate partner violence: A new term related to domestic violence, which can include psychological, physical, sexual, financial, and social abuses between intimate partners.

Introvert: A quiet person who focuses inwardly on himself or herself.

Latchkey children: Children who are left unsupervised after school because both parents work and extended family are not available to care for them.

Late adulthood: The ages between 65 and 74 years.

Life expectancy: The average number of years a person born in that year is expected to live.

Looking-glass self: The development of a self-image by combining how we portray ourselves to others and how others evaluate us.

Managed care organization: An organization that standardizes medical practice guidelines to maintain quality of care provided while at the same time controlling costs of health care.

Medicaid: A type of federal welfare program in which benefits are provided on a basis of need or level of poverty.

Medicare: A type of a government-provided insurance program in which benefits are received after contributions are made through payroll deductions.

Menarche: The very first menstrual period.

Menopause: The cessation of the menstrual period as a result of hormonal changes in the body.

Menstrual cycle: Consists of (1) maturing of the egg in the ovary, (2) formation of blood and mucus in the lining of the uterus, (3) ovulation, (4) and expulsion of the unfertilized egg with the blood and mucous lining from the uterus. This cycle lasts approximately 28 days and repeats until menopause.

Middle adulthood: The ages between 40 and 60 years.

Middle childhood: Children between ages 6 and 12 years.

Midlife crisis: A stressful period when an adult tries to make up for lost opportunities of the past or challenge the inevitability of the future.

Mnemonic technique: The use of rhymes for remembering certain things, such as the number of days in each month.

Monozygotic: A type of twin that develops when one single fertilized ovum separates into two separate embryos.

Moral behavior: Actions based on moral reasoning.

Moral reasoning: Occurs as the child learns to understand rules and determine if an action is right or wrong.

Mourning: The outward expression of grief.

Multifetal: More than one fetus—that is, twins, triplets, quadruplets, septuplets.

Mutated: Malformed.

Neonatal: The first 30 days of life after birth.

Nocturnal emission: Ejaculation of semen during sleep.

Nonverbal language: The language of the motions, postures, and gestures of the body that is learned as part of communication.

Norms: Averages; can be used as guidelines for comparison concerning the age that specific abilities or skills are achieved or disappear.

Nurse practice acts: Defines the scope of practice for each level of professional practice in nursing.

Nursing caries: Tooth decay that occurs when the infant is put to bed while sucking on a bottle of milk or juice. The milk or juice pools in the mouth, allowing organisms to grow.

Object permanence: Knowing an object is there even though it is not within sight.

Occupational Health and Safety Act (OSHA): Standards of safety that must be maintained by employers to protect the health and safety of employees; mandates reporting of injuries sustained by workers.

Oedipus complex: Arises during the phallic stage of development. Freud suggested that little boys compete with their father for the mother's love and attention.

Operant conditioning: Involves behavioral consequences such as reward or punishment.

Ordinal position: Birth order; whether the infant is an only child, older child, youngest child, or middle child may influence the age and rapidity of mastering developmental tasks.

Oropharynx: The part of the anatomy that includes the mouth and throat.

Osteoporosis: The loss of bone mass.

Ovulation: Release of a matured egg from the ovary into the fallopian tube, which leads to the uterus.

Palliative care: Total care of patients whose disease is not responsive to curative therapy.

Parallel play: When a young child plays next to a friend but does not interact with the friend during play.

Personality: A unique combination of characteristics that results in the individual's recurrent pattern of behavior.

Pincer grasp: The ability to pick up small objects with the thumb and forefinger.

Plaque: A sticky, transparent mass of bacteria that grows on the surface and spreads to the roots of teeth.

Political action committees: A group that influences legislation by offering monetary contributions to legislators who support their needs and provides lobbying efforts to create an awareness of needed legislation.

Polypharmacy: The ingestion of multiple medications in 1 day.

Postformal operational thought: The process of integrating various points of view to develop knowledge and understanding.

Posttraumatic stress disorder (PTSD): The development of characteristic symptoms following an extreme traumatic stressor.

Preferred provider organization (PPO): An organization that contracts with professionals to provide care to a specific group of patients at an agreed-upon fee-for-service rate.

Preschool phase: Between 2 and 6 years of age.

Preverbal: Body language before the ability to speak.

Proximodistal: From the midline of the body to the periphery.

Puberty: The age at which sexual maturity occurs; having the functional ability to reproduce. Puberty involves physical and psychological changes.

Receptive language: Ability to understand words.

Relatedness: A sense of belonging.

Reproductive health: A term used to describe the health of the reproductive organs in all persons.

Sandwich generation: A period in middle adulthood when persons must deal with increased financial and emotional responsibilities related to their children and increased demands placed on them by their older and possibly dependent parents.

Scope of practice: "The identification of and legal limitations to the usual and customary skill practices of a professional. The usual and customary practices are determined by the educational preparation for that profession" (from *Nurse Practice Act, Business and Professional Code*).

Secondary sex characteristics: The development of pubic, facial, and body hair; also, in boys the enlargement and darkening of the scrotum and an increase in penis size; in girls the enlargement of breasts and darkening around the areola.

Senescence: A period in an adult's life in which the body begins to age and weaken.

Separation anxiety: When an infant cries or protests the parent leaving the room or a stranger approaching. Emerges after age 6 months.

Sexuality: Beliefs and behaviors that surround physiological responses, emotions, and sociocultural values. Involves communication, a sense of closeness, and mutual comfort.

Sexually transmitted disease: Disease that is transmitted through sexual intercourse and in some cases through oral copulation (oral sex).

Sibling rivalry: The competition between brothers and sisters, usually for parental attention and love.

SIDS: Sudden infant death syndrome.

Social cognition: Children begin to understand how their actions may affect other people. This enables children to get along better with peers and can enhance their self-concept.

Social learning theory: Involves exposure to and imitation of a behavior.

Somatic: Pertaining to the body.

Spermatogenesis: The production of sperm.

Stagnation: The failure to achieve generativity.

Standards of practice: Guidelines used to determine type and quality of care provided to patients.

Syndrome: A group of symptoms or signs of an abnormal condition.

Theory: A group of concepts that forms the basis for understanding observations. An accepted theory is logical, consistent, and integrates past and current research.

Therapeutic communication: A form of communication that involves accepting the patient's emotional outbursts and expressions and encouraging venting and verbalization.

Therapeutic presence: Remaining near the patient and family, or simply holding a hand, provides strength while facilitating expressions of emotions.

Toddler phase: Between the ages of 1 to 2 years.

Viable: Able to survive outside the uterus.

Virus vector: A virus that has the ability to enter specific cells in the body and act as a vehicle to carry substances to that cell.

Young adult: The ages between 20 and 39 years.

Bibliography and Internet Resources

CHAPTER 1 ■ *Healthy People 2010*

Berlinguer, G. (1999). Globalization and global health. *Int J Health*, 29(3), 579-595.

Brosco, J. (1999). The early history of the infant mortality rate in America: a refection upon the past and a prophecy of the future. *Pediatrics*, 103(2), 478-485.

Brundtland, G. *Fifth Global Conference on Health Promotion*. Mexico City, June 5, 2000, at www.who.int/director-general/speeches/200/20000605_mexico.html.

Centers for Disease Control and Prevention (CDC), National Center for Health Statistics. (2000). *Healthy People 2000 renew—review 1998–99*. Atlanta: CDC.

Davis, L., Okuboye, S., & Ferguson, S. (2000). Healthy People 2010: examining a decade of maternal-infant health. *Lifelines*, 4(3), 26-33.

U.S. Department of Health and Human Services (USDHHS). (1990). *Health: United States, 1989, and prevention profile,* Pub No (PHS) 90–1232. Hyattsville, MD: DHHS.

U.S. Department of Health and Human Services (USDHHS). (1990). *Healthy People 2010: national health promotion and disease prevention objectives*, Pub No 91–50213. Washington, DC: U.S. Government Printing Office.

Department of Health, Education and Welfare (DHEW). (1979). *Healthy People: the Surgeon General's report on health promotion and disease prevention*, PHS Pub No 79–55071. Washington, DC: DHEW.

U.S. Department of Health and Human Services (USDHHS). (1990). *Healthy People 2000: National health promotion and disease prevention objectives*, PHS Pub No 91–50213. Washington, DC: U.S. Government Printing Office.

Messias, D.H. Globalization, nursing and health for all. *Journal of Nursing Scholarship: An Official Publication of Sigma Theta Tau International Honor Society of Nursing*, 33(1), 9.

National Center for Health Statistics. (1999). *Health, United States 1999*. With health and aging chart book. Hyattsville, MD: DHHS.

National Center for Health Statistics. (1999). *Healthy People renew 1998–1999*. Hyattsville, MD, Washington, DC: U.S. Government Printing Office.

U.S. Department of Health and Human Services (USDHHS) Centers for Disease Control and Prevention. (1999). *Healthy People 2010: National Vital Statistics System*. McClean, VA: International Medical Publisher.

Singhn, G., & Yu, S. (1995). Infant mortality in US: trends, differentials, and projections 1950–2010. *American Journal of Public Health*, 85(17), 957-964.

U.S. Department of Health and Human Services (USDHHS). (2000). *Healthy People 2010* (2nd ed.). Washington, DC: U.S. Government Printing Office.

Velsor-Friedrich, B. (2000). Healthy People 2000/2010: healthy appraisal of the nation and future objectives. *Journal of Pediatric Nursing*, 15(1), 47-49.

WHO First Interenational Conference on Health Promotion, Ottowa Canada, Nov 21, 1986. www.who.int/hpr/archive/docs/ottowa.html.

Internet Resources

www.health.gov/healthypeople
www.cdc.gov/nchs/hphome.htm
www.who.int/director-general/speeches/200/20000605/mexico.html

CHAPTER 2 ■ *Government Influences on Health Care*

Advisory Commission On Consumer Protection and Quality in Health Care Industry. (1999). *Quality first: better health care for all Americans.* Washington, DC: U.S. Government Printing Office.

Burcham, M. (1999). Credentialing alternative medicine: a challenge for managed care organizations. *Manag Care Q, 7*(2), 39.

Glazer, G. (1999). Legislative policy issues related to interstate practice. *On-Line J Issues Nurs* May 4, 1999. www.nursingworld.org/ojin/tpclg/leg_2.htm

Harrington, C., & Estes, C. (1994). *Health policy and nursing,* Boston: Jones and Bartlett.

Kanen R., Ouslander, J., & Abrass, I. (1999). *Essentials of geriatrics.* New York: McGraw-Hill.

Knight, W. (1998) *Managed care: what it is and how it works.* Gaithersburg, MD: Aspen Publishers.

Lasseter, F. (1999). Legislative activities on interstate compact for mutual recognition on nursing regulations. *JAORN,*, 69, 647.

Levy, D. (Ed.). (1999). *State by state guide to managed care law.* Gaithersburg, MD: Aspen Publishers.

Mason, D., & Leavitt, J. (1998). *Policy and politics in nursing and health care.* Philadelphia: WB Saunders.

Milstead, J. (Ed.). (1999). *Health policy and politics: a nurses guide.* Gaithersburg, MD: Aspen Publishers.

Nies, M., & McEwen, M. (2001). *Community health nursing.* Philadelphia: WB Saunders.

U.S. Department of Health and Human Services (USDHHS). (2000). *Healthy People 2010* (2nd ed.). Washington, DC: U.S. Government Printing Office.

Internet Resources

www.dranonymous.com/dranon.html
www.healthcarelawnet.com/
www.bt.cdc.gov
www.NCSL.org
www.hpts.org

CHAPTER 3 ■ *The Influence of Family on Developing a Lifestyle*

American Psychiatric Association. (2000). *Diagnostic and statistical manual of mental disorders* (4th ed.), text rev. Washington, DC: American Psychiatric Association.

Andreason, M. (1994). Patterns of family life and TV consumption from 1945 to 1990s. In D. Zillman, J. Bryant, & A. Huston (Eds.), *Media, children and the family,* Hillsdale, NJ: Erlbaum.

Baronowski, T., & Nader, P. (1985). Family health behavior. In D. Turk & R. Kerns (Eds.), *Health, illness and family.* New York: Wiley [classic].

Bernhill, C., & Longo, D. (1978). Fixation and regression in the family life cycle. *Family Practice,* 17(4), 469.

Blackwell, D., & Blackwell, J. (2000). Building alternative families. *Lifelines AWHONN,* 3(5), 45–48.

Bowlby, J. (1951). *Maternal care and mental health.* New York: Columbia University Press [classic].

Bucher, L., Klemm, P., & Adepoju, J. (1996). Fostering cultural competence: a multicultural care plan. *The Journal of Nursing Education,* 35(7), 334.

Capizzano, J., Adams, G., & Sonenstein, F. (2000). *Childcare arrangements for children under five: variation across states.* Washington, DC: Urban Institute.

Dunn, J., et al. (2001). Family lives and friendships: the perspectives of children in step-single parent and non-step families. *Journal of Family Psychology,* 15(2), 272.

Duvall, E. & Miller, B. (1985). *Marriage and family development* (6th ed.). New York: Harper and Row [classic].

Emes, C. (1997). Is Mr. Pac-Man eating our children?: a review of the effect of videogames on children. *Canadian Journal of Psychiatry,* 42, 409.

Eth, S., & Pynoos, R. (Eds.). (1985). *PTSD in children*. Washington, DC: American Psychiatric Press [classic].

Feldman, R., Masalla, S., & Nadam, R. (2001). Cultural perspective on work and family: dual earner Israeli-Jewish and Arab families at the transition to parenthood. *Journal of Family Psychology*, 15(13), 492.

Fortunati, L., & Floerchinger-Franks, G. (2001). Men and family planning: what is their future role? *J Am Acad Nurse Pract*, 13(10), 473.

Friedman, M. (1992). *Family nursing, nursing theory and assessment*. New York: Appleton-Century-Croft.

Funk, K., & Buchman, D. (1996). Video and computer games in the 90s: children's time commitment and game preference. *Children Today*, 24(1), 12.

Funk, J. (1997). Re-evaluating importance of videogames. *Clinical Pediatrics*, 2, 86.

Furger, R. (1997). Your children are talking to strangers. *PC World*, 15(6), 35.

Hae-Jung Song, E., & Anderson, J. (2001). How violent videogames may violate children's health. *Contemp Pediatr*, 18(5), 102.

Havighurst, R. (1974). *Developmental tasks and education*. New York: David McKay [classic].

Jensen, P., & Shaw, J. (1993). Children as victims of war: current knowledge and future research needs. *Journal of the American Academy of Child and Adolescent Psychiatry*, 32, 697.

Klein, D., & White, D. (1996). *Family theories: an introduction*. Thousand Oaks, CA: Sage Publications.

Koepp, M., Gunn, R.N., Lawrence, A.D., et al. (1998). Evidence for striatal dopamine release during a video game. *Nature*, 393, 266.

Levine, M., Carey, W., & Crocker, A. (1999). *Developmental-behavioral pediatrics* (3rd ed.). Philadelphia: WB Saunders.

Meijer, A. (1985). Child psychiatric sequelae of maternal war stress. *ACTA Psychiatr Scand*, 75, 205.

Monahon, C. (1997). *Children and trauma: a guide for parents and professionals*. San Francisco: Jossey Bass.

Murray, R., & Zentner, J. (2000). *Nursing assessment and health promotion through the lifespan* (7th ed.). New York: Prentice Hall.

National Center for Family Centered Care. (1990). *What is family centered care?* Bethesda, MD: Association for Care of Children's Health.

Newton, M. (2000). Family centered care: current realities in parent participation, *Journal of Pediatric Nursing*, 26(2), 164.

Pfefferbaum, B., Seale, T.W., McDonald, N.B., et al. (2000). Post-traumatic stress 2 years after the Oklahoma City bombing in youths geographically distant from the explosion. *Psychiatry*, 63, 358.

Popenoe, D. (1989). The family transformed, *Fam Affairs*, 2, 1 [classic].

Schoffe, S., Mangelsdorf, S., & Frosch, C. (2001). Co-parenting, family process and family structure: implications for preschoolers externalizing behavior problems. *Journal of Family Psychology*, 15(13), 526.

Shaefer, R. (2002). *Sociology: a brief introduction* (4th ed.). Boston: McGraw-Hill.

Shelov, S., Bar-on, M., & Beard, L., (Eds.). (1995). Media violence: a statement of the American Academy of Pediatrics Committee on Communications. *Pediatrics*, 95, 949.

Smilkstein, G., Ashworth, C., & Montano, D. (1982). The validity and reliability of the family Apgar as a test of family function. *Journal of Family Practice*, 15, 303.

Smilkstein, G. (1984). The physician and family function. *Fam Systems Med*, 263-279. [classic].

Smilkstein, G. (1978). The family Apgar: a proposal for a family function test and it's use by physicians. *The Journal of Family Practice*, 6(6), 1231 [classic].

Sugar, M. (1992). Toddlers' traumatic memories, *J Ment Health*, 13, 245.

Sutterly, D. (1999). *Perspectives in human development*. Philadelphia: JB Lippincott.

Swerdlow, J. (1999). Global cultures. *National Geographic*, 196(2), 10-127.

U.S. Department of Health and Human Services (USDHHS). (1995). *Psychosocial issues for children and families in disasters*. Washington, DC: U.S. Government Printing Office.

White, J. (1991). *Dynamics of family development: a theoretical perspective*. New York: Guilford Press.

Internet Resources

www.NMHA.org

www.act.hhs.gov/prams/cb/dis/table/entryexit.htm

www.urban.org

CHAPTER 4 ■ *Theories of Development*

Arlin, P. (1975). Cognitive development in adulthood. A 5th stage? *Dev Psychol*, 11, 602 [classic].

Bandura, A. (1977). *Social learning theory*. Englewood Cliffs, NJ: Prentice-Hall [classic].

Brofenbrenner, U. (1979). *The ecology of human development*. Cambridge, Mass: Harvard University Press [classic].

DuVall, E. (1977). *Marriage and family development*. Philadelphia: JB Lippincott [classic].

Funder, D. (1993). *Studying lives through time: personality and development*. Washington, DC: American Psychology Association.

Gormly, A., & Brodzinsky, D. (1989). *Lifespan human development*. Philadelphia: Harcourt Brace [classic].

Havighurst, R. (1974). *Developmental tasks and education*. New York: D. McKay [classic].

Kohlberg, L. (1964). Development of moral character and moral ideology. In H. Hoffman, & L. Hoffman (Eds.), *Review of child development research*. New York: Russell Sage [classic].

Kegan, R. (1982). *The evolving of self: a theory of human development*. Cambridge, Mass: Howard Press [classic].

Levinson, D.J., Darrow, C.N., & Klein, E.B. (1978). *The seasons of a man's life*. New York: Knopf [classic].

Loevinger, J. (1979). *Scientific ways in the study of ego development*. Worchester, Mass: Clark University Press [classic].

Piaget, J. (1926). *The language of the child*. Philadelphia: Harcourt Brace [classic].

Skinner, B. (1987). *Verbal behavior*. New York: Appleton-Century-Croft [classic].

Vygotsky, L. (1962). *Thoughts and language*. Cambridge, Mass: MIT Press [classic].

CHAPTER 5 ■ *Prenatal Influences on Healthy Development*

Barker, D. (1998). *Mothers, babies and health in later life*. Philadelphia: Churchill-Livingstone.

Barker, D., et al. (1993). Relationship of small head circumference and thinness at birth to death from cardiovascular disease in adult life. *Br Med J*, 306, 422.

Brazelton, T. (1973). The *neonatal behavioral assessment scale*. Philadelphia: JB Lippincott [classic]

Bronfenbrenner, U., & Ceci, S. (1993). Heredity and environment and the question of "how?" In R. Plomin, & G. McLearn (Eds.), *Nature, nurture and psychology*. Washington, DC: American Psychological Association.

Burroughs, A. & Leifer, G. (2001). *Maternity nursing: an introductory text* (8th ed.). Philadelphia: WB Saunders.

Curhan, G., Willet, W.C., Rimm, E.B., et al. (1996). Birth weight and adult hypertension and obesity in women. *Circulation*, 94, 1310.

Flynn, J. (1987). Massive IQ gains in 14 Nations: what IQ tests really measure. *Psychological Bulletin*, 101, 171 [classic].

Gopnik, A., Meltzoff, A., & Kuhl, P. (1999). *The Scientist in the crib*. Harper Collins.

Goldberg, G., & Prentice, A. (1994). Maternal and fetal determinants of adult diseases. *Nutrit Rev*, 52, 191.

Leifer, G. (2003). *Introduction to maternity and pediatric nursing* (4th ed.). Philadelphia: WB Saunders.

Levine, M., Carey, W., & Crocker, A. (1999). *Developmental-behavioral pediatrics* (3rd ed.). Philadelphia: WB Saunders.

Plomin, R., McClearn, G.E., Smith, D.L., et al. (1994). DNA markers associated with high versus low IQ: The IQ Quantitive Trait Loci Project (QTL). *Behavior Genetics*, 24, 107.

Rich-Edwards, J. et al. (1997). Birth weight and the risk of cardiovascular disease in a cohort of women followed up since 1976. *Br Med J*, 315, 396.

Rubin, R. (1963). Maternal touch at first contact with the newborn infant. *Nursing Outlook*, 11, 828 [classic].

Sayer, A., Cooper, C., & Barker, D. (1997). Is lifespan determined in utero? *Archives of Disease in Children*, 77, 161.

Shaheen, S., et al. (1994). Relationship between pneumonia in early childhood and impaired lung function in late adult life. *Am J Resp Crit Care Med*, 149, 616.

Spahis, J. (2002). Human genetics: constructing a family pedigree. *The American Journal of Nursing*, 102(7), 44-50.

Stein, C., Kiemaran, K., & Shaheen, S. (1997). Relationship of fetal growth to adult lung function in South India. *Thorax*, 52, 895.

Tinkle, M., & Cheek, D. (2002). Human genomics: challenges and opportunities. *Journal of Obstetric, Gynecologic, and Neonatal Nursing*, 31(2), 188.

Williams, J. (2000). Impact of genome research on children and their families. *Journal of Pediatric Nursing*, 15(4), 207-211.

Internet Resources

www.jjpi.com/portal/jnj/jjpi
www.NHGRI.nih.gov/
www.ORNL.GOV/TechResources/human_genome/resource/elsi.hml
www.genesage.com

CHAPTER 6 ■ *The Infant*

American Heart Association (AHA). (2001). Dietary guidelines revised for the new millennium. *Clinician Rev*, 11(8), 58.

Atkinson, W., et al. (2002). General recommendations immunizations: recommendations of the advisory committee on immunization practices. *Morbidity and Mortality Weekly Report*, 51(RR2), 1–34.

Behrman, R., Kleigman, R., & Jensen, H. (2004). *Nelson's textbook of pediatrics* (17th ed.). Philadelphia: WB Saunders.

Betz, C. (2002). *Healthy Children 2010*: implications for pediatric nursing practice. *Journal of Pediatric Nursing*, 17(3), 153.

Biagroll, F. (2002). Proper use of child safety seats. *American Family Physician*, 65(10), 2085.

Cahill, J., & Wagner, C. (2002). Challenges in breastfeeding. *Contemp Pediatr*, 19(5), 94.

Erikson, E. (1994). *The life cycle completed: a review*. New York: WW Norton.

Evers, D. (2001). Teaching mothers about childhood immunizations. *MCN: The American Journal of Maternal Child Nursing*, 25(5), 253.

Fowles, E. (1999). Brazelton Neonatal Behavior Scale. *MCN: The American Journal of Maternal Child Nursing*, 24(6), 287.

Gaensbauer, T. (1995). Trauma in the preverbal period: symptoms, memories, and developmental impact. *The Psychoanalytic Study of the Child*, 50, 122.

Leifer, G. (2003). *Introduction to maternity and pediatric nursing* (4th ed.). Philadelphia: WB Saunders.

Levine, M., Carey, W., & Crocker, A. (1999). *Developmental behavioral pediatrics*, (3rd ed.). Philadelphia: WB Saunders.

Lund, C., Kuller, J., et al. (2001). Neonatal skin care. *Journal of Obstetric, Gynecologic, and Neonatal Nursing*, 30(1), 30.

Medoff-Cooper, B., et al. (2000). Nutritive sucking and neurobehavioral development in preterm infants. *MCN: The American Journal of Maternal Child Nursing*, 25(2), 64.

Monastersky, R. (2001). Look who's listening: new research shows babies employ many tricks to pick up language. *Chronicles of Higher Education*, July 6, 2001, p 14.

Moon, R: (2001). Are you talking to your parents about SIDS? *Contemp Pediatr*, 18(3), 94.

Olsen, R., & Barbaresi, W. (1998). Development in the first year of life. *Contemp Pediatr*, 15(7), 49.

Page-Geortz, S., McCammon, S., & Westdahl, C. (2001). Breastfeeding promotion. *Lifelines*, 5(1), 41.

Roberts, S., Dallal, G. (2001). New childhood growth charts. *Nutrition Reviews*, 59(2), 31.

Velsor-Fredrich, B. (2000). *Healthy People 2010*: health appraisal of the nation and future objectives. *Journal of Pediatric Nursing*, 15(1), 47.

Wallerstedt, C., & Fletcher, B. (2000). Teaching with toys. *Lifelines*, 4(4), 45.

Internet Resources

www.brightfutures.org/mentalhealth/index.HTML

www.jppi.com/portal/jnj/jjp

CHAPTER 7 ■ *Early Childhood*

American Academy of Pediatrics. (1998). Communication on psychological aspects of child and family health. Guidance for effective discipline. *Pediatrics*, 101, 723.

Banks, J.B. (2002). Childhood discipline: challenges for clinicians and parents, *American Family Physician*, 66(8), 1447-1452.

Behrman, R., Kliegman, R., & Jenson, H. (2004). *Nelson's textbook on pediatrics* (17th ed.). Philadelphia: WB Saunders.

Behrman, R., & Kliegman, R. (2002). *Nelson's essentials of pediatrics* (4th ed.). Philadelphia: WB Saunders.

Calkins, S. (2002). Does adverse behavior during toddlerhood matter? The results of difficult temperament on maternal perception of behavior. *Infant Ment Health J*, 23(4), 381.

Cech, D., & Marten, S. (2002). *Functional movement development across the lifespan* (2nd ed.). Philadelphia: WB Saunders.

Chabner, D. (2004). *The language of medicine* (7th ed.). Philadelphia: WB Saunders.

Fournier, R. (2002) Early clinical assessment for harsh childhood discipline strategies. *MCN: The American Journal of Maternal Child Nursing*, 27(1), 34.

Gottfried, A., & Bathurst, L. (1983). Hand preference across time related to intelligence to young girls, not boys. *Science*, 221, 1074 [classic].

Greenspan, S. (1996). Assessing the emotional and social functioning of infants and young children. In S. Meisels & E. Fenichel (Eds.). *New visions for the developmental assessment of infants and young children*. Zero to Three: Washington, DC.

Kinsey, A., Pomeroy, W., & Martin, C. (1948). *Sexual behavior in the human male*, Philadelphia: WB Saunders [classic].

Leifer, G. (2003). *Introduction to maternity and pediatric nursing* (4th ed.). Philadelphia: WB Saunders.

Levine, M., Carey, W., & Crocker, A. (1999). *Developmental-behavioral pediatrics* (3rd ed.). Philadelphia: WB Saunders.

Littleboy, L., Reed, M., & Thompson, J. (2000). *Special educational needs in early years. Care and education*. London: Bailliere-Tindall/Elsevier Science.

Monastersky, R. (2001). Look who's listening: new research shows babies employ many tricks to pick up language, *Chron Higher Ed*, July 6, 2001, p 14-16.

Olson, S., Bates, J., Sindy, J., & Shilling, E. (2002). Early developmental precursors of impulsive and inattentive behavior in infancy through middle childhood. *Journal of Child Psychology and Psychiatry*, 3(4), 435-448.

Zimmerman, M. (1994). *Diagnosing DSM-IV psychiatric disorder in primary care*. East Greenwood, RI: Psychiatric Press.

Internet Resources

www.aap.org

www.allergicchild.com

www.nfer.ac.uk/pubs/special.htm

CHAPTER 8 ■ *Middle Childhood*

American Academy of Pediatrics Committee on Psychosocial Aspects of Child and Family Health (1998). Guidance for effective discipline. *Pediatrics*, 101, 723.

Banks, J.B. (2002) Childhood discipline: challenges for clinicians and parents. *American Family Physician*, 66(8), 1447.

Betz, C., Hunsberger, M., & Wright, S. (1994). *Family-centered nursing care of children* (2nd ed.). Philadelphia: WB Saunders.

Behrman, R., Kleigman, R., & Jenson, H. (2004). *Nelson's textbook of pediatrics* (17th ed.). Philadelphia: WB Saunders.

Brazelton, T. (1992). *Touchpoints: your child's emotional and behavioral development*. Boston: Addison-Wesley.

Doswell, W. (2002). An overview of female childhood in societal context: implications for nurses and practice. *Journal of Pediatric Nursing*, 17(6), 391-394.

Elkind, D. (2001). *The hurried child: growing up too fast, too soon*. Cambridge, MD: Perseus Publishers.

Gale. (2001). *Encyclopedia of psychology* (2nd ed.). Gale Group

Guttmacher, A. (1999). *Teen pregnancy: overall trends and state by state information*. New York: Allen Guttmacher Institute.

Herrenkohl, R., & Russo, M. (2001). Abusive early child rearing and early childhood aggression, *Child Maltreatment*, 6, 3.

Leifer, G. (2003). *Introduction to maternity and pediatric nursing* (4th ed.). Philadelphia: WB Saunders.

Levine, M., Carey, W., & Crocker, A. (Eds.). (1999). *Developmental-behavioral pediatrics* (3rd ed.). Philadelphia: WB Saunders.

Monsen, R. (2002). The child in the community: nursing makes a difference. *Journal of Pediatric Nursing*, 17(6), 439-441.

Pinderhughes, E. (1998). Discipline responses: influence of parents, socioeconomic status, ethnicity, beliefs about parenting, stress and cognitive emotional processes. *Journal of Family Psychology*, 14, 380-400.

Valfre, M. (2001). *Foundations of mental health* (2nd ed.). St. Louis: Mosby.

Internet Resources

www.SIECUS.org

CHAPTER 9 ■ *Adolescence*

American Psychiatric Association (APA) (2000). *Diagnostic and statistical manual of mental disorders* (4th ed.), text rev. (DSM-IVTR) Washington, DC: APA.

Arner, H., Burgess, A., & Asher, J. (2001). Caring for pregnant teens: medico-legal issues for nurses,. *JOGNN*, 30(2), 230.

Association of State and Territorial Health Officials (ASTHO). (1999). Healthy People initiate to launch nation's health goals for the new century. *ASTHO Report*, 7(2), 1–10.

Behrman, R., Kleigman, R., & Jenson, H. (2004). *Nelson's textbook of pediatrics* (17th ed.). Philadelphia: WB Saunders.

Centers for Disease Control and Prevention (CDC) (1999). Youth risk behavior surveillance: National Alternative High School Risk Behavior Survey. *Morbidity and Mortality WeeklyReport*, 48(SS07): 1.

Guttmacher, A. (1999). *Teen pregnancy: overall trends and state by state information.* New York: Allen Guttmacher Institute.

Jackson, S., Jacob, M,. Landman-Peters, K., & Lonting, A. (2001). Cognitive strategies employed in trying to arrange a first date. *Journal of Adolescence*, 24(3), 267-279.

Juang, L., & Silbereisen, R. (2002). The relationship between adolescence academic capabilities, beliefs and parenting and school grades. *Journal of Adolescence*, 25(1), 3-18.

Leifer, G. (2003). *Introduction to maternity and pediatric nursing* (4th ed.). Philadelphia: WB Saunders.

Levine, M., Carey, W., & Crocker, A. (1999). *Developmental-behavioral pediatrics* (3rd ed.). Philadelphia: WB Saunders.

Kracke, B. (2002). Role of personality and peers in adolescents career exploration. *Journal of Adolescence*, 25(1), 19-30.

Meeks, W., Oosterwegel, A., & Volleberg, H. (2002). Parental and peer attachment and identity development in adolescence. *Journal of Adolescence*, 25(1), 93-106.

National Center for Health Statistics (NCHS), Division of Data Services. (2002). Teenage births in the U.S.; state trends 1991–2000. An update. *National Vital Statistics Report*, 50(9). 4pp(PHS):1120. Hyattsville, MD.

Nieder, T., & Sieffge-Krenke, I. (2001). Coping with stress in different phases of a romantic relationship *Journal of Adolescence*, 24(3), 297-310.

Reamy, B., & Slakey, J. (2001). Adolescent idiopathic scoliosis. *American Family Physician*, 64(1), 111.

Roth, M., & Parker J. (2001). Affective behavioral responses to friends who neglect their friends for a date partner. *Journal of Adolscence*, 24(3), 281.

Shulman, S., & Kipnis, O. (2001). Adolescents' romantic relationships. *Journal of Adolescence*, 24(3), 336.

Tarrant, M. North, A.C., Edridge, M.D., et al. (2001). Social identity in adolescence. *Journal of Adolescence*, 24(5), 596.

Tilton-Weaver, L., Bitunski, E., & Galambos, N. (2001). Five images of maturity in adolescence: what does "grown-up mean?" *Journal of Adolescence*, 24(2), 143-158.

U.S. Department of Health and Human Services (USDHHS). (2000). *Healthy People 2010.* Washington, DC: International Medical Publishing, McLean VA.

Zimmer-Gembeck, M., Siebenbruner, C., & Collins, W. (2001). Diverse aspects of dating, *Journal of adolescence*, 24(3), 313-333.

Internet Resources

www.itsyoursexife.com
www.aap.org/policy/0103.html
www.plannedparenthood.org
www.seventeen.com/sexsmarts

CHAPTER 10 ■ *Young Adulthood*

Benson, V., & Marano, M. (1994). *Current estimates from the National Health Interview Survey.* Atlanta: Centers for Disease Control and Prevention.

Centers for Disease Control and Prevention (CDC). (1999). *Achievements in public health 1900–1999.* Atlanta: CDC.

Centers for Disease Control and Prevention (CDC). (2000). Healthy mothers and babies. *Morbidity and Mortality Weekly Report,* 48(38), 849.

Commons, M., Richards, F., & Armon, C. (1982). *Beyond formal operations: Late adolescent and adult cognitive development.* New York: Praeger [classic].

Centers for Disease Control and Prevention (CDC). (2000). *Fact sheet on dating violence.* Atlanta: National Center for Injury Prevention and Control.

Gotchman, D. (Ed.). (1997). *Handbook of health behaviors research.* New York: Plenum Press.

Hatcher, R., et al. (1998). *Contraceptive technology* (17th ed.). New York: Ardent Media.

Kulasingam, S., Hughes, J.P., Kiviat, N.B., et al. (2002). Evaluation of HPV testing in primary screening for cervical abnormalities. *Journal of the American Medical Association,* 288, 1749-1757.

Leifer, G. (2003). *Introduction to maternity and pediatric nursing* (4th ed.). Philadelphia: WB Saunders

Levinson, D. Darrow, C., & Klein, E.B. (1978). *The seasons of a mans life.* New York: Knopf [classic].

Murstein, B. (1982). Marital choices. In B. Wolman (Ed.), *Handbook of developmental psychology.* Englewood Cliffs, NJ: Prentice Hall [classic].

Ravnikar, V., & Chen, E. (1994). Hysterectomies. Where are the indications? *Obstetrics and Gynecology Clinics of North America,* 21(2), 405.

Rawlins, P., Williams, S., & Beck,C. (1993). *Mental health psychiatric nursing.* St. Louis: Mosby.

Roberts, A. (1983). Overtraining affects male reproductive status. *Fertility and Sterility,* 60, 686 [classic].

Internet Resources

www.cdc.gov/ncipc/dvp/youpt/datviol.htm

www.oclc.org

CHAPTER 11 ■ *Middle Adulthood*

Calandra, J., & Petterson, R. (2001). Midlife sexuality. *Nurseweek,* 14(20), 17-20.

Carr, D. (2000). The older adult driver. *American Family Physician,* 61(1), 141-146.

Centers for Disease Control and Prevention (CDC). (2002). *2002–2003 recommended adult immunization schedule 2002–2003.* Atlanta: CDC. IMM 746.

Erikson, E. (1994). *The life cycle completed: a review.* New York: WW Norton.

George, S. (2002). The menopause experience: a woman's perspective. *Journal of Obstetric, Gynecologic, and Neonatal Nursing,* 31(1), 77-85.

Goldman, L., & Bennett, J. (2000). *Cecil's textbook of medicine* (21st ed.). Philadelphia: Saunders.

Harrington, D. (2002). Latest data on HRT and cardiovascular health. *Contemp Obstet Gynecol Suppl,* (10), 1-10.

Katz, A. (2002). Sexuality after hysterectomy. *Journal of Obstetric, Gynecologic, and Neonatal Nursing,* 31(3), 236.

Leifer, R. (1997). *The happiness project.* New York: Snow Lion Publications.

Masters, W., Johnson, V., & Kolodny, R. (1986). *Masters and Johnson on sex and human loving.* Boston: Little Brown [classic].

Mayo Clinic Health Oasis. (1999). *Screening tests: interactive guide for men.* Rochester, MN: Mayo Clinic.

Schwartz, M., Klein, A., & McLucas, B. (2001). Uterine artery embolization in treatment of fibroids. *Contemp Obstet Gynecol,* 46(8), 14.

Scheick, D. (2002). Mastering group leadership. *Psychosocial Nursing and Mental Health Services,* 40(9): 35-36.

Skolnick, A. (1991). *Embattled paradise: the American family in an age of uncertainty.* New York: Basic Books.

Waldron, I. (1997). Changing gender roles and gender differences in health behavior. In D Gochman (Ed.), *Handbook of health behavior research.* New York: Plenum Press.

Willis, S., & Reed, J. (1997) *Life in the middle.* San Diego: Academic Press.

Internet Resources

www.mayohealth.org/mayo/9906/htm/screenings_men.htm

www.cdc.gov/nccdphp/hrt.htm

www.nlm.nih.gov/medlineplus/hormonereplacementtherapy.html

CHAPTER 12 ■ *Late Adulthood*

American Association for Geriatric Psychiatry (AAGP). (2002). *Position statement: psychotherapeutic medications in nursing homes.* Bethesda, MD: AAGP.

American Association of Geriatric Psychiatry (AAGP). (2003). Geriatrics and mental health: the facts association of geriatric psychiatry, Bethesda, MD: AAGP.

Baumeister, R., & Leary, M. (1995). The need to belong: desire for interpersonal attachments as a fundamental human motivation. *Psychological Bulletin*, 117: 497.

Berliner, H. (1999). Abuse of older adults. *Clin Ref Syst*, p 5, Aug 1, 1999.

Brennan, F. (2000). Exercise prescriptions for older adults. *Sports Medicine*, 30(2), 19.

Carr, D. (2002). The older adult driver. *American Family Physician*, 61(1), 141.

Carstensen, L., Charles, S., et al. (1998). Emotions in the second half of life: current directions in psychological science. *Psychological Science*, 7, 144–149.

Centers for Disease Control and Prevention, National Center of Health Statistics (CDC). (1999). Characteristics of elderly home health care users. National home and hospice survey, USDHHS Pub No 2000. Rockville, MD: CDC.

Chambliss, D. (1998). Empirically validated treatments. *Appl Prevent Psychol*, 8, 281.

Cohen, C. (2001). Guiding seniors. *RN*, 64(2), 50.

Doughty, S. (2001). The postmenopausal woman. *Adv Nurse Pract*, 9(7), 35.

Ewing, J. (1984). Detecting alcoholism: the CAGE questionnaire. *Journal of the American Medical Association*, 252, 1905-1907 [classic].

Havighurst, R. (1974). Developmental tasks and education. New York: David McKay [Classic].

Koenig, H., Pappas, P., Holsinger, T., & Bocher, J. (1995). Assessing diagnostic approaches to depression in medically ill older adults. *Journal of the American Geriatrics Society*, 43, 472.

Kumar, S. (1999). WHO sets agenda for care of elderly. *Lancet*, 353, (91): 161, 353-361.

Kurtzweil, P., Scogen, F., & Rosen, G. (1996). A test of the fail-safe N for self help programs. *Profess Psychol Res Pract*, 27, 629-630.

Leifer, G. (2003). *Introduction to maternity and pediatric nursing* (4th ed.). Philadelphia: WB Saunders.

Leuchter, A.(1994). Brain structure and functional correlates of late life depression. In C Schneider, et al. (Eds.), *Diagnosis and treatment of depression in later life*. Washington, DC: American Psychological Press.

Lobo, R. (2000). Menopause. In L. Goldman & J Bennett (Eds.), *Textbook of medicine*. Philadelphia: WB Saunders.

Morrow, D., Leirer, B., Altieri, P., & Fitzsimmons, C. (1994). When expertise reduces age differences in performance. *Psychology and Aging*, 9, 134.

Norcross, J., Santrock, J.W., Smith, T.P., et al. (2000). *Authoritative guide to self help resources in mental health*. New York: Guilford Press.

Ojta, C., Fraga, P., & Forciea, M. (2001). Antiaging therapy. *Hospital Practices*, 36(6), 43.

Porter, S., & Hanley, E. (2001). The musculoskeletal effects of smoking. *J Am Acad Orthoped Surg*, 9, 9-17.

Qualls, S., & Beles, A. (Eds.). (2000). *Psychology and the aging revolution*. Washington, DC: American Psychological Association.

Salthouse, T., & Coon, V. (1999). Interpretation of differential deficits: the case of aging and mental arithmetic. *Journal of Experimental Psychology. Learning, Memory, and Cognition*, 20(5), 1172-1182.

Terri, L., Curtis, J., Gallagher-Thompson, D., & Thompson, C. (1996). Cognitive-behavioral therapy with depressed older adults. In C Schneider, et al, *Diagnosis and treatment of depression in later life*. Washington, DC: American Psychiatric Press.

U.S. Department of Health and Human Services (USDHHS). (2000). *Healthy people 2010* (2nd ed.). Washington, DC: U.S. Government Printing Office.

World Health Organization (WHO). (1997). The Heidelberg guidelines for promoting physical activity among older persons. *J Aging Phys Act*, 5(1), 8.

Wilcox, S., King, A., & Brassington, G. (1999). Physical activity preferences of middle age and older adults. *J Aging Phys Act*, 7, 386.

Zelinski, E., & Burnight, K. (1997). 16-year longitudinal and time lag changes in memory and cognition in older adults. *Psychology and Aging*, 12, 503.

Internet Resources

www.aoa.gov/aoa/stats/profile/6.html

www.agingstats.gov

www.DHHS.gov/aging

www.infoaging.org

www.census.gov/prod/pubs

www.aagponline.org/proffacts_mh.asp

CHAPTER 13 ■ *Geriatrics: Advanced Old Age*

Baldwin, K., & Shaul, M. (2001). When your patient can no longer live independently. *J Gerontol Nurs*, 27(11),10.

Berlinger, J. (2001). Domestic violence. *Nursing*, 31(8), 58.

Brennan, F. (2002). Exercise prescriptions for older adults, *Sports Medicine*, 30(2), 19.

Butler, R. (1990) A disease called ageism. *Journal of the American Geriatrics Society*, 38(2), 178-180 [editorial].

Butler, R. (1969). Age-ism: another form of bigotry. *Gerontologist*, 9(4), 243-246, [classic].

Buttaro, T.M., Trybulski, J.A., Bailey, P.P., & Sandberg-Cook, J. (2003). *Primary care: a collaborative practice.* (2nd ed.). St. Louis: Mosby.

Catania, J.A. (1989). Older Americans and AIDS: transmission risks and primary prevention research needs. *Gerontologist*, 29, 373.

Christiansen, H., & Grzybowksi, J. (1993). *Biology of aging*. Toronto: Mosby.

Cohen, C. (2001). Guiding seniors. *RN*, 64(2), 50.

Cummings, E., & Henry, W. (1961). *Growing old*. New York: Basic Books [classic].

Domrose, C. (2002). Seasons of change. *Nurseweek*, 15(12), 15.

Ebersole, P., & Hess, P. (1998). *Toward healthy aging*. St. Louis: Mosby.

Felton, B. (2001). Conceptualizing resilience in women older than 85. *J Gerontol Nurs*, 27(1), 46.

Finch, C., & Schneider, E. (2000). Biology of aging. In L. Goldman & J. Bennett (Eds.), *Cecil's textbook of medicine* (21st ed.). Philadelphia: WB Saunders.

Friedman, H. (2002). *Health psychology*. New York: Prentice-Hall.

Fuller, G. (2000). Falls in the elder. *American Family Physician*, 61(7), 2159-2168.

Gallo, J., Reichel, W., & Andersen, L. (1995). *Handbook of geriatric assessment* (2nd ed.). Frederick, MD: Aspen Publishers.

Goldman, L., & Bennett, J.C. (2000). *Cecil textbook of medicine* (21st ed., vol. 1). Philadelphia: WB Saunders.

Gurvich, T., & Cunningham, J. (2000). Appropriate use of psychotropic drugs in nursing homes, *American Family Physician*, 61(5), 1437-1446.

Guyton, A.C., & Hall, J. E. (2001). *Textbook of medical physiology* (10th ed.). Philadelphia: WB Saunders.

Hamilton, S. (2001). Detecting dehydration and malnutrition in the elderly. *Nursing*, 31(12), 56-57.

Ivey, J. (2001) Somebody's grandma and grandpa: children's responses to contact with elders, *MCN: The American Journal of Maternal Child Nursing*, 26(1), 23.

Kane, R., Ouslander, J., & Abrass, J. (1999). *Essentials of clinical geriatrics* (4th ed.). New York: McGraw-Hill.

Masters, W., & Johnson, V. (1976). *The pleasure bond*. New York: Bantam [classic].

Miller, K., Zylstra, R., & Standridge, J. (2000). The geriatric patient: a systematic approach to maintaining health. *American Family Physician*, 61(4), 1089-1104.

Paice, J. (2003). Sexuality and chronic pain. *The American Journal of Nursing*, 103(1), 87.

Pickering, S., & Thompson, J.S. (1998). *Promoting positive practice in nursing older people: perspectives on quality of life*. London: Baillieré-Tindall.

Resnick, B. (2001). Motivating older adults to engage in self-care. *Patient Care for Nurse Pract*, 4(9), 13-15.

Speroff, L. (2001). Postmenopausal estrogen therapy. *Contemp Obstet Gynecol*, 46(5).30.

Sulmassy, D., & McIlvane, J. (2002). Dying dissatisfied. *Arch Int Med*, 162(18), 2098-2114.

U.S. Department of Health and Human Services (USDHHS) (2000). Healthy people 2010 (2nd ed.). Washington, DC: U.S. Government Printing Office.

U.S. Preventative Services Task Force (USPSTF). (2002). *Screening for osteoporosis in postmenopausal women: guide to clinical preventative services* (3rd ed.). Washington, DC: Office of Disease Prevention and Health Promotion, U.S. Government Printing Office.

Waillant, G. (2002). *Aging well*. New York: Little Brown.

World Health Organization (WHO). (1986). *Concepts for sexual health*, Copenhagen: WHO.

Internet Resources

www.nimh.nih.gov/publicat/elderlydepsuicide.cfm

www.suicidology.org/older_men_and_women.htm

www.lastacts.org/files/files/misc/meansfull.pdf

www.preventiveservices.ahrq.gov

CHAPTER 14 ■ *Planning for the End of a Generation*

American Academy of Pediatrics Committee on Bioethics and Committee on Hospital Care. (2000). Palliative care for children. *Pediatrics*, 106, 351.

American Nurses Association (ANA). (2001). *A new code of ethics for nurses. ANA's code of ethics project task force with interpretive statements*. Washington, DC: ANA.

Baldwin, K., & Shaul, M. (2001). When your patient can no longer live independently. *Gerontol Nurs*, 27(11), 10.

Bednash, G., & Ferrel, B. (2002). *Nursing care at the end of life*. Sacramento: CEU for Nurses CME Resource American Nurses Credentialing Center.

Bluebond-Langner, M. (1996). *In the shadow of illness. Parents of siblings of the chronically ill child*. Princeton, NJ: Princeton University Press.

Bowden, V. (2002). End of life care: a priority issue for pediatric nurses. *J Ped Nurs*, 17(6), 456.

Enright, B., & Marwit, S. (2002). The diagnosis of complicated grief: a closer look, *Journal of Clinical Psychology*, 58(7), 747-758.

Feifel, F. (1977). *The meaning of death to children: new meanings of death*. New York: McGraw-Hill [classic].

Ferrel, B., & Coyle, N. (Eds.). (2001). *Textbook of palliative nursing*. New York: Oxford Press.

Field, M., & Cassel, C. (1997). *Approaching death: improving care at the end of life. Report of the Institute of Medicine Task Force*. Washington, DC: National Academy Press.

Forbes, S. (2001). This is heaven's waiting room: end of life in one nursing home. *Gerontol Nurs*, 27(11), 37.

Friedman, H. (2002). *Health psychology* (2nd ed.). New York: Prentice Hall.

Fry, V. (1995). *Part of me died too: stories of creative survival among bereaved children*. New York: Penguin Putnam.

Geiter, H. (2002). The spiritual side of nursing. *RN*, 65(5), 46.

Grubb, L. (2002) Hearing is the last to go. *RN*, 65(1), 51.

Kübler-Ross, E. (1969). *On death and dying: what the dying have to teach doctors, nurses, clergy and their families*. New York: Macmillan [Classic].

LaDuke, S. (2001). Terminal dyspnea and palliative care. *The American Journal of Nursing*, 101(11), 26-30.

Lewis, L., Brecker, M., Reaman, G., & Sahler, O. (2002). How you can help meet the needs of the dying child. *Contemp Pediatr*, 19(4), 147-159.

Meisel, A. (2000). *The right to die*, (Vol.s 1–2). New York: Aspen Law and Business.

National Hospice and Palliative Care Organization (NHPCO). (1996). *New findings address escalating end of life debate*. Alexandria, VA: NHPCO.

Nelson, L. (1995). When a child dies: practical and sensitive advice for helping parents through their worst nightmare. *The American Journal of Nursing*, 95(3), 61-64.

Paice, J.A. (2002). Managing psychological conditions in palliative care. *The American Journal of Nursing*, 102(11), 36-43.

Periyakoil, V., & Hallenbeck, J. (2002). Identifying and managing preparatory grief and depression at end of life. *American Family Physician*, 65(5), 883-890.

Post, S., Puchalski, C., & Larson, D. (2000). Physicians and patient spirituality: professional boundaries, competency and ethics. *Ann Int Med*, 132, 578.

Ramer-Chrastek, J. (2000). Hospice care for a terminally ill child in the school setting. *J School Nurs*, 16(2), 52-56.

Rivlin, D. (2001). Books for children when a child's friend dies. *Contemp Pediatr*, 18(10), 134.

Scanlon, C. (2003). Ethical concerns in end-of-life care. *The American Journal of Nursing*, 103(1), 48-55.

Silverman, P. (2000). *Never too young to know: death in children's lives*. Oxford, UK: Oxford University Press.

Stanley, K. (2002). The healing power of presence: respite from the fear of abandonment. *Oncology Nursing Forum*, 29(6), 935-940.

Stephenson, J. (2000). Palliative and hospital care needed for children with life threatening conditions. *Journal of the American Medical Association*, 284(19), 2437-2438.

World Health Organization (WHO). (1990). *Cancer pain relief and palliative care*. Technical Report Series 804, Geneva, Switzerland: WHO.

Internet Resources

www.lastacts.org

www.prc.coh.org

www.AmericanHospice.org

www.NPR.org/programs/death

www.soros.org/death/about_us.htm

www.aacn.nche.edu/ELNEC/index.htm

CHAPTER 15 ■ *Bereavement*

Alexander, K. (2001). The one thing you can never take away; perinatal bereavement photographs. *MCN: The American Journal of Maternal Child Nursing*, 26(3), 123.

American Psychiatric Association (APA). (2000). *Diagnostic and statistical manual of mental disorders* (4th ed.), text rev. (DSM-IV: TR) Washington DC: APA.

Bowlby, J. (1980). *Attachment and loss* (vol. 3). New York: Basic Books [classic].

Bowlby, J. (1960). Grief and mourning in infancy and childhood. *The Psychoanalytic Study of the Child*, 15:9:52 [classic].

Cote-Arsenault, D., Bidlack, D., & Humm, A. (2001). Women's emotions and concerns during pregnancy, following pregnancy loss. *MCN: The American Journal of Maternal Child Nursing*, 26(3), 128.

Erikson, E. (1994). *The life cycle completed: a review*. New York: WW Norton.

Felton, B., & Hall, J. (2001). Overcoming adversity from illness and loss. *Gerontol Nurs*, 27(11), 46.

King, A. (1994). *Suddenly alone*. Wilsonville, OR: Book Partners.

Kübler-Ross, E. (1969). *On death and dying: what the dying have to teach doctors, nurses, clergy and their families*. New York: Macmillan [classic].

Leifer, G. (2003). *Introduction to maternity and pediatric nursing* (4th ed.). Philadelphia: WB Saunders.

Lewis, L., Breckher, M., Reaman, G., & Sahler, O. (2002). How you can help meet the needs of dying children. *Contemp Pediatr*, 19(4), 147.

Lindeman, E. (1944). The symptomatology and management of acute grief. *The American Journal of Psychiatry*, 101, 144 [classic].

Lipson, J.G., Dibble, S.L., & Minarik, P.A. (1996). *Culture & nursing care: a pocket guide*. San Francisco: UCSF Nursing Press.

Schulz, R. (1978). *The psychology of death, dying and bereavement*. Boston: Addison-Wesley [classic].

Smith, S.F., Duell, D.J., & Martin, B.C. (2000). *Clinical nursing skills: basic to advanced skills*. New York: Prentice Hall.

Viorst, J. (1986). *Necessary losses*. New York: Simon & Schuster [classic].

Vyieyanthi, P., & Hollenbeck, J. (2002). Identifying and managing prepatory grief and depression at end of life. *American Family Physician*, 65(5), 883.

Wheeler, S., & Austen, J. (2001). Impact of early pregnancy loss on adolescents. *American Journal of Maternal Child Nursing*, 26(3), 154.

Zonnebelt-Smenge, S., & Vries, R. (2001). *The empty chair: handling grief on holidays and special occasions*. Grand Rapids, MI: Baker Books.

Zunin, L., & Zunin, H. (1991). *The art of condolence*. New York: HarperCollins.

Internet Resources

www.aarp.org/griefprograms/home.html

www.adec.org

www.aplacetoremember.com

www.compassionbooks.com

www.finalthoughts.com/rc_html

www.modimes.com

www.nmha.org/reassurance/childcoping.cfm

APPENDIX A

www.phppo.cdc.Gov/PHTN/webcast/ADUL:T_imm03

Index

Page numbers followed by a *t* indicate tables, page numbers followed by an *f* indicate figures, and page numbers followed by a *b* indicate boxes.